Neurobiology of Obesity

Obesity is one of the prime contributors to ill health in modern society, affecting around 20–25% of the population. It can cause or exacerbate a variety of health problems and is often associated with several other diseases including type 2 diabetes, coronary heart disease and certain types of cancer. Significant progress has been made in understanding the role of the nervous system and, in particular, the complex interplay between a range of orexigenic and anorectic agents within specific hypothalamic nuclei in the regulation of energy balance, appetite and adiposity. Several different neuronal pathways, neurotransmitters and hormones have been identified as major players in the regulation of feeding behavior and body weight and these are now being targeted as having therapeutic potential. Written for academic researchers and graduate students, *Neurobiology of Obesity* is a concise overview of recent developments in this field, written by leading international experts.

JENNI HARVEY is currently a Wellcome Research Career Development Fellow in the Department of Pharmacology and Neuroscience at the University of Dundee. The main focus of her research is to investigate the role of the endocrine peptides, leptin and insulin, in both normal and pathological function in extrahypothalamic regions of the brain, including the hippocampus and cerebellum.

DOMINIC J. WITHERS is Professor of Diabetes and Endocrinology at the Centre for Diabetes and Endocrinology at University College London. His research interests include the role of hormone and nutrient-sensing signaling pathways in the regulation of energy homeostasis by the central nervous system and in pancreatic beta cell function.

Neurobiology of Obesity

JENNI HARVEY
Department of Pharmacology and
Neuroscience, University of Dundee

DOMINIC J. WITHERS
Centre for Diabetes
and Endocrinology,
University College London

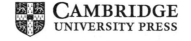

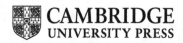

CAMBRIDGE
UNIVERSITY PRESS

Shaftesbury Road, Cambridge CB2 8EA, United Kingdom

One Liberty Plaza, 20th Floor, New York, NY 10006, USA

477 Williamstown Road, Port Melbourne, VIC 3207, Australia

314–321, 3rd Floor, Plot 3, Splendor Forum, Jasola District Centre, New Delhi – 110025, India

103 Penang Road, #05–06/07, Visioncrest Commercial, Singapore 238467

Cambridge University Press is part of Cambridge University Press & Assessment, a department of the University of Cambridge.

We share the University's mission to contribute to society through the pursuit of education, learning and research at the highest international levels of excellence.

www.cambridge.org
Information on this title: www.cambridge.org/9780521860338

© Cambridge University Press & Assessment 2008

First published 2008

A catalogue record for this publication is available from the British Library

ISBN   978-0-521-86033-8   Hardback

Contents

Preface

In the twenty-first century, obesity affects around 20–25% of the population and it is now one of the prime contributors to ill health in modern society. Obesity can cause or exacerbate a variety of health problems and it is often associated with a number of other diseases including type II diabetes mellitus, coronary heart disease and certain types of cancer. The incidence of obesity and related diseases is steadily increasing such that obesity is now regarded as a global epidemic. In recent years, major advances have been made in determining the role of the central nervous system, in particular specific hypothalamic nuclei, in regulating energy balance. From such studies it is apparent that a highly intricate neural system involving a complex interplay between a range of orexigenic and anorectic agents controls food intake and body weight. Thus, a greater understanding of the key neurotransmitter molecules, their related signal transduction pathways and molecular targets, as well as the neuronal pathways that control release of these neurotransmitters is vital if novel therapeutic targets for the treatment of obesity and related diseases are to be uncovered. This book provides a concise overview of recent developments in this field. As an introduction, Professor Bloom gives an outline of the factors that are known to play a key role in regulating energy balance and the development of obesity in humans. Professor Clement considers the genetics of human and rodent body weight regulation as the use of genetic technologies has markedly increased our understanding of dysfunctions in body weight regulation. The hypothalamus is a key region of the brain that adjusts both the drive to eat and energy expenditure in response to a range of signals. Professor Ahima reviews the role of particular medial hypothalamic structures in this regulatory process, and introduces the concept that a range of distinct, but molecular signals interact to control food intake. In the following chapter, Dr Niswender reviews the evidence implicating leptin and insulin as key hormones that provide afferent information to the brain as well as the recent advances made in determining the sites and mechanisms of action of these adipostats. This aspect is expanded on by Dr Sutherland and Professor Ashford, who provide an overview of the signaling capability of leptin and insulin receptors and discuss how specific signaling pathways may impact on feeding behavior. The potential development of specific therapeutic agents directed against signaling pathways regulated by leptin and insulin for the treatment of obesity is also discussed. This is followed by a detailed review by Dr Strack and Professor Levin of various animal models of diet-induced obesity and how these compare with human obesity. In addition to leptin and insulin, findings from both genetic and pharmacological studies have implicated melanocortins, opiates and the gut hormone ghrelin in hypothalamic regulation of energy homeostasis. The role of these agents is dealt with in depth in reviews by Professors Low, Levine and Horvath, respectively. Drs Della-Fera and Baile discuss the role of the CNS in regulating the levels of adipose tissue, whereas in the final review, Dr Halford provides a detailed overview of the therapeutic strategies to treat obesity.

Contributors

Rexford S. Ahima
University of Pennsylvania School of Medicine
Department of Medicine
Division of Endocrinology, Diabetes and Metabolism
Philadelphia
Pennsylvania 19104
USA

Mike Ashford
Division of Pathology and Neurosciences
University of Dundee
Ninewells Hospital and Medical School
Dundee DD1 9SY
UK

Clifton A. Baile
University of Georgia
444 Animal Science Complex
Athens
GA 30602–2771
USA

Stephen R. Bloom
Department of Metabolic Medicine
Division of Investigative Science
Imperial College London
Hammersmith Campus
Du Cane Road
London W12 0NN
UK

Richard J. Bodnar
Department of Psychology and
Neuropsychology Doctoral Sub-Program
Queens College
City University of New York
USA

Karine Clément
Hôtel-Dieu Service de Nutrition
Place du Parvis Notre-Dame
75004 Paris
France

Mary Anne Della-Fera
University of Georgia
444 Animal Science Complex
Athens
GA 30602–2771
USA

Benjamin C. T. Field
Department of Metabolic Medicine
Division of Investigative Science
Imperial College London
Hammersmith Campus
Du Cane Road
London W12 0NN
UK

Jason C. G. Halford
School of Psychology
Eleanor Rathbone Building
Bedford Street South
University of Liverpool
Liverpool, L69 7ZA
UK

Mark W. Hamrick
Medical College of Georgia
Augusta
GA 30912–2000
USA

Tamas Horvath
Department of Obstetrics, Gynecology and Reproductive Sciences
Yale University School of Medicine
New Haven
Connecticut 06520
USA

Barry E. Levin
Neurology Service (127C)
Veterans Affairs Medical Center
385 Tremont Avenue
East Orange
New Jersey 07018–1095
USA

Allen S. Levine
Minnesota Obesity Center
Department of Food Sciences and Nutrition
University of Minnesota
St. Paul
MN 55108
USA

Malcolm J. Low
Center for the Study of Weight Regulation
Mail code L481
Oregon Health & Science University
3181 SW Sam Jackson Park Road
Portland
OR 97239–3098
USA

Kevin D. Niswender
Diabetes, Endocrinology and Metabolism
715 Preston Research Building
Vanderbilt University Medical Center
2220 Pierce Avenue
Nashville
TN 37232–6303
USA

Neel S. Singhal
University of Pennsylvania School of Medicine
Department of Medicine
Division of Endocrinology, Diabetes and Metabolism
Philadelphia
Pennsylvania 19104
USA

Caroline J. Small
Department of Metabolic Medicine
Division of Investigative Science
Imperial College London
Hammersmith Campus
Du Cane Road
London W12 0NN
UK

Alison M. Strack
Neurology Service (127C)
Veterans Affairs Medical Center
385 Tremont Avenue
East Orange
New Jersey 07018–1095
USA

Calum Sutherland
Division of Pathology and Neurosciences
University of Dundee
Ninewells Hospital and Medical School
Dundee DD1 9SY
UK

Virginie Tolle
UMR. 549 INSERM-Université Paris V
IFR Broca Ste-Anne
Paris
France

1

Introductory chapter

BENJAMIN C. T. FIELD, CAROLINE J. SMALL
AND STEPHEN R. BLOOM

Obesity is a global phenomenon, a disease which is spread by increasing urbanization and which causes major morbidity and mortality. Over the last two decades it has reached unprecedented and dramatic levels in industrially developed countries but the rise in prevalence affects almost every part of the world. It is already placing huge burdens on the health systems of many countries. Its potential to cause disability amongst working-age populations worldwide, particularly as a result of complications of diabetes, makes it imperative to work towards both preventative and curative solutions.

Yet, despite the fact that obesity has become such a widespread disease, there remains within the medical community a tradition of stigmatizing individual sufferers. Doctors and other health professionals have tended to provide what is seen as self-evident advice, namely, to consume less food and to expend more energy through physical activity. The subsequent failure of patients to lose weight, despite good advice, and in the face of complications of their condition, is then viewed as evidence of an inability to control lifestyles and to resist urges. At the root of this view lies an historical absence of knowledge of the hugely complex and fascinating innate homeostatic mechanism which controls satiety and energy balance: a mechanism that has evolved over millions of years, has seen humankind through feast and famine, and has run into trouble only since the advent of mechanization. This absence of knowledge, and the resulting lack of effective remedies, has made it convenient for doctors to blame their patients for perceived failings of self-control.

Neurobiology and Obesity, ed. Jenni Harvey and Dominic J. Withers. Published by Cambridge University Press. © Cambridge University Press 2008

Nonetheless, the last decade has seen a number of important advances in understanding of the anatomical and molecular basis of the satiety circuits. This knowledge has been translated rapidly into a wide range of drug development programs, offering the prospect that a range of safe and effective antiobesity treatments will become available within the next 10 years. The current chapter aims to set the scene for discussion of these advances by describing the scale, medical consequences and causes of the global obesity crisis, and by reviewing how the development of novel antiobesity compounds may be informed by knowledge of the relative merits of currently available treatments.

1.   Definition of obesity

Adipose tissue functions as an energy store, the principal role of which is to improve the chance of survival during prolonged food deprivation. This fact underlies the celebration of obesity as an indicator of health in some rural African cultures and may explain in part the ambivalence of many in Western cultures towards the categorization of obesity as a disease. Nevertheless, an excess of body fat is causally associated with an increased risk of developing diabetes, hypertension, cardiovascular disease, respiratory disease, osteoarthritis and cancer and it is this association which is crucial to the medical definition of obesity.

The World Health Organization (WHO) currently recommends that body mass index (BMI) is used as the standard tool for both clinical and epidemiological assessment of adiposity. This is a pragmatic choice which is acceptable to patients and proven to be robust when performed by trained personnel (WHO, 1995). The association between BMI and total adiposity, body fat distribution and risk of complications is strong but nonetheless varies between populations. In particular, in comparison to Europeans, individuals in some Asian populations tend, at any given BMI, to have greater amounts of total body fat, greater ratios of visceral to subcutaneous fat and, hence, a greater risk of developing complications (WHO Expert Consultation, 2004). In recognition of this, a modification to the previous international classification of obesity has been agreed (see Table 1.1) (WHO Expert Consultation, 2004; WHO Global InfoBase Team, 2005) and work on the utility of waist circumference measurement in addition to BMI is in progress. Recently published epidemiological surveys, such as the INTERHEART study (Yusuf et al., 2005), may hasten the process of incorporating a measure of abdominal obesity into an international classification.

The rapid rise in prevalence of obesity in the developed world is well-documented. In the UK the prevalence in adults almost tripled between 1980 and 1998 (National Audit Office, 2001) and similar increases have been observed in the USA (Flegal et al., 1998, 2002), Canada (Katzmarzyk, 2002;

Table 1.1 *World Health Organization classification of body weight including additional subdivisions of BMI introduced in 2004, intended to provide additional 'public health action points', particularly for Asian populations (WHO Expert Consultation, 2004).*

Principal categories	Sub-categories		BMI (kg/m^2)	Additional BMI subdivisions for epidemiological reporting
Underweight			< 18.50	
		Severe thinness	< 16.00	
		Moderate thinness	16.00–16.99	
		Mild thinness	17.00–18.49	
Normal range			18.50–24.99	18.50–22.99
				23.00–24.99
Overweight			≥ 25.00	
	Pre-obese		25.00–29.99	25.00–27.49
				27.50–29.99
	Obese		≥ 30.00	
		Obese class I	30.00–34.99	30.00–32.49
				32.50–34.99
		Obese class II	35.00–39.99	35.00–37.49
				37.50–39.99
		Obese class III	≥ 40.00	

Tremblay *et al.*, 2002; Katzmarzyk & Ardern, 2004) and Australia (de Looper & Bhatia, 2001). It was estimated recently that obesity is responsible for 30 000 deaths per annum in the UK (National Audit Office, 2001). This figure is likely to rise as a result of the increasing prevalence of obesity in children and, hence, of the development of complications at ever younger ages (Bundred *et al.*, 2001; McCarthy *et al.*, 2003; Lobstein *et al.*, 2004).

Whilst the prevalence of obesity in developed countries has been systematically studied for several decades, it is only since the introduction of the WHO classification that global comparisons have been possible. The first truly global survey of body weight (WHO Global InfoBase Team, 2005) showed that 75.6% of males aged 15 years and over living in the USA are overweight (BMI ≥ 25) and 36.5% of the same population are frankly obese (BMI ≥ 30). The corresponding figures for the UK are 65.7% and 21.6% respectively. These results come as no surprise but an unwelcome finding of the report is that obesity is not confined to the developed world but is also becoming prevalent in middle and low income countries (see Figure 1.1).

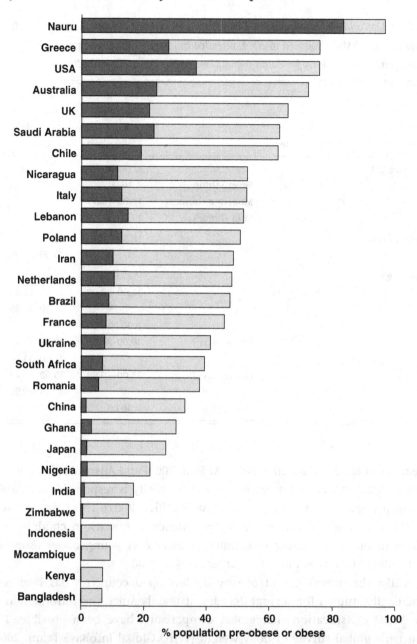

Figure 1.1 Prevalence of obesity (BMI ≥ 30.00; dark grey bars) and pre-obesity (BMI 25.00 to 29.99; light grey bars) in males aged 15 years and above in selected countries. The combined length of the dark and light grey bars is representative of the proportion of each population classified as overweight i.e. BMI ≥ 25.00. Data from World Health Organization SuRF Report 2 (WHO Global InfoBase Team, 2005).

In particular, heavily populated countries such as China and India have experienced rapid changes in recent years. The absolute increase between 2002 and 2005 in numbers of overweight adult males in the two countries combined was almost ten times greater than the increase seen in the USA (WHO Global Infobase Team, 2005). The implication of these findings and of predicted increases in prevalence is that, whilst obesity has until recently been viewed as predominantly affecting developed countries, it is rapidly becoming widespread throughout the world. The inevitable consequence is that huge, global health problems are being stored up for the near future.

2.   Complications of obesity

The most devastating human and economic consequences of the rise in prevalence of obesity are likely to arise from an increased incidence of type 2 diabetes mellitus. Obesity is well established as a prime risk factor for the development of insulin resistance and diabetes (Sims et al., 1973; Wannamethee & Shaper, 1999; Stevens et al., 2001). The strength of the association is particularly well illustrated by a prospective cohort study of 114 281 women (Colditz et al., 1995) in which subjects with a BMI between 22.0 and 22.9 had a threefold increase in risk of developing type 2 diabetes compared with those with a BMI less than 22. For individuals with BMIs from 25.0 to 26.9, from 29.0 to 30.9 and in a range above 35.0, the risks were 8 times, 27 times and 93 times greater respectively. Type 2 diabetes mellitus, already a common illness in developed countries, is becoming increasingly common worldwide (Amos et al., 1997; King et al., 1998; Wild et al., 2004). The inevitable consequence of this is that diabetic complications, including retinopathy, nephropathy, neuropathy, peripheral vascular disease, stroke and ischaemic heart disease, will become increasingly common.

Of even greater concern is the fact that obesity and, hence, diabetes are occurring at ever younger ages. Complications of diabetes, which have hitherto been confined mainly to the elderly population, are thus beginning to appear earlier in life. Type 2 diabetes mellitus is increasingly being reported in children (Fagot-Campagna et al., 2000; Ramachandran et al., 2003; Lobstein & Jackson-Leach, 2006) and a recent study of Canadian adults aged 18 to 33 who had developed type 2 diabetes in childhood revealed the devastating damage which may be caused. In a group of 58 patients, seven had died, two of whom had been on dialysis, another three were still alive on dialysis, one had become blind and one had had a toe amputated. The rate of pregnancy loss amongst the women was 38% (Dean & Flett, 2002).

In addition to its role in causing diabetes mellitus, obesity is an important independent risk factor for hypertension and dyslipidemia (Brown et al., 2000; Wilson et al., 2002) and for pro-inflammatory states (Ford, 1999), which together are components of the metabolic syndrome and are implicated in atherogenesis (Ridker et al., 1997; Pickup & Mattock, 2003). It is thus unsurprising that obesity is strongly associated with the risk of developing cardiovascular disease (Fang et al., 2003), acute thrombotic events (Wolk et al., 2003), atrial fibrillation (Wang et al., 2004) and heart failure (Kenchaiah et al., 2002). Indeed, in a 20-year epidemiological study of the inhabitants of two Scottish towns, obesity was associated with 9 additional cardiovascular deaths and 36 additional cardiovascular hospital admissions for every 100 affected subjects (Murphy et al., 2006).

Obesity results in impaired respiratory function both through mechanical forces, including inhibition of diaphragmatic movement by intra-abdominal fat, and by reducing the capacity of individuals to undertake physical activity. Epidemiological studies have demonstrated a clear association between obesity and asthma (Ford, 2005), obstructive sleep apnea (Resta et al., 2001) and obesity hypoventilation syndrome (Olson & Zwillich, 2005). Both obstructive sleep apnea and obesity hypoventilation syndrome are risk factors for the development of cor pulmonale, diabetes and hypertension. Prospective studies have shown that weight loss results in improvement of symptoms (Avenell et al., 2004; Ford, 2005; Kalra et al., 2005).

Obesity is a major cause of reproduction-related morbidity in women. It reduces the safety of some commonly used forms of contraception, increases the risk of anovulatory infertility (Linné, 2004) and reduces the likelihood of successful in vitro fertilization treatment (Fedorcsák et al., 2004; Lintsen et al., 2005). Fortunately, weight loss improves outcomes in women undergoing treatment for anovulatory infertility (Crosignani et al., 2003). In women who become pregnant, obesity increases the risk of gestational diabetes, hypertension, pre-eclampsia, foetal macrosomia, intrauterine death, emergency caesarean section, wound infection, genital tract infection, postpartum hemorrhage and birth trauma (Sebire et al., 2001; Nohr et al., 2005).

There is also an extensive literature, derived from large cohort studies, describing the increased risk that obese individuals run of developing various cancers, in particular, carcinomas of the esophagus, stomach, colon, rectum, liver, gallbladder, pancreas and kidney and hematopoietic malignancies including leukemia, myeloma and non-Hodgkin's lymphoma. In addition, obese men are at increased risk of developing prostate carcinoma and obese women are at increased risk of cancers of the breast, endometrium, cervix and ovary (Calle et al., 2003; Batty et al., 2005; Hampel et al., 2005). There are several potential mechanisms by which obesity may result in malignancy. The risk of esophageal cancer is likely to be derived mainly from gastro-esophageal reflux but other alimentary tract cancers have been postulated to occur more commonly as a result of hyperinsulinaemia causing increased mitogenic signalling at the insulin-like growth factor-1 (IGF-1) receptor (Giovannucci, 1995). Post-menopausal breast and endometrial carcinoma, as well as prostate carcinoma, may occur more commonly because excess adipose tissue is a major source of circulating sex hormones (Bianchini et al., 2002; Calle & Kaaks, 2004).

The mechanical stress exerted by obese individuals on their lower limbs is responsible for a large increase in risk of developing osteoarthritis of the knees (Hart & Spector, 1993; Stürmer et al., 2000). Furthermore, weight loss reduces the risk of osteoarthritis (Felson et al., 1992) and, especially in combination with exercise, has been shown to ameliorate symptoms and improve the functional capacity of sufferers (Messier et al., 2004).

Lastly, obese individuals in most societies are disadvantaged socio-economically and psychologically. They are more likely to take long-term sick leave (Vingard et al., 2005), more likely to be depressed (Heo et al., 2005; Sjöberg et al., 2005; Herva et al., 2006) and have reduced earning potential compared with the non-obese (Baum & Ford, 2004). Whether the latter observation reflects a causal relationship is unclear but further study of trends in the USA may provide useful information since, although it continues to affect lower income groups disproportionately, the prevalence of obesity has increased more quickly over the last 30 years in higher than lower income social groups (Chang & Lauderdale, 2005).

3.   Causes of obesity

A recent review of genetic studies of obesity concluded that over 600 separate genes, markers and chromosomal regions are linked to obesity phenotypes (Pérusse et al., 2005). A small number of these constitute recently described monogenic obesity syndromes, including leptin and leptin receptor mutations, which are characterized principally by severe early onset obesity. Another small group is known to be responsible for the classical pleiotropic obesity syndromes, such as Bardet–Biedl and Prader–Willi syndromes, in which obesity is just one of several diagnostic characteristics (Farooqi & O'Rahilly, 2005). Although the study of such syndromes sheds considerable light on the pathophysiology of obesity, they are nonetheless exceptional: BMI is a continuous variable within populations and, although obesity tends to run in families, it is not, with few exceptions, inherited in classical Mendelian fashion.

It follows that the vast majority of genes identified by linkage studies may have only small individual effects on body weight. Nonetheless their additive effects, as judged from twin, family and adoption studies, are likely to account for between 40% and 70% of variation in BMI within populations (Maes et al., 1997). This view is reinforced by a prospective study of chronic overfeeding in monozygotic twins which found that the variance in weight gained was three times greater between unrelated subjects than within twin pairs (Bouchard et al., 1990).

If inheritance is such an important factor though, why should there have been an unprecedented increase in the prevalence of obesity over the last 30 years? The most likely explanation is that evolutionary pressure exerted over many millennia of uncertain food supply has favored the survival of individuals possessing 'thrifty' genotypes, a term originally coined by J. V Neel in relation to the risk of developing diabetes mellitus (Neel, 1962). According to the thrifty genotype hypothesis, individuals who were adept at storing excess energy as adipose tissue in times of plenty would have been protected from the worst ravages of famine.

It is only in recent decades that the mechanization of food production and transport, along with a prolonged period of relative peace, has rendered food shortages virtually non-existent for the populations of developed countries. At the same time, marketing pressures have tended to favor the production of highly palatable, energy-dense, cheap, processed foods which are widely available and intensively advertised, especially to children. Fast food has become an increasingly prominent component of modern diets (Nielsen et al., 2002) and seems to play a role in promoting excessive energy intake (Ebbeling et al., 2004). These environmental changes have revealed a widespread predisposition to obesity which has been propagated by the erstwhile evolutionary advantage of the thrifty genotype. Furthermore, there is preliminary evidence that increases in energy intake in pre- and postnatal life may have long-term programming effects on hypothalamic satiety centers, thus enhancing the effect of a pre-existing genetic predisposition to obesity (Prentice, 2005). Within the space of just one or two generations, the thrifty genotype has been rendered not simply irrelevant but positively harmful.

It would be wrong, however, to view technology and prosperity, or, indeed, our genetic inheritance, as the villains of the piece. We are stuck with our thrifty genotypes and would not wish to compensate by returning to a more precarious food supply system. On many levels the situation might be ameliorated by education and re-education: of national and local policy-makers, of schoolteachers, of parents and of children. In particular, progress on prevention may be made by reducing exposure to snacks, confectionery, fast food and vending machines (Vereecken *et al.*, 2005; Rolls *et al.*, 2006). Such measures are far less expensive than dealing with the medical consequences of obesity. For a rapidly increasing number of people, however, preventative measures will have come too late: the need for effective obesity treatments has never been greater.

4.   Treatments for obesity

The current range of choices for treating obesity is limited, the central problem being that appetite must continue to be controlled after initial loss of weight. A combination of dieting and increased physical activity is effective only when pursued vigorously and consistently. There has been a renewal of medical interest recently in the optimum constituents of weight-reducing diets, in part at least because of the commercial success of highly restrictive diets such as that proposed by Atkins (1972). It is likely that diets rich in protein have a greater satiating effect than other forms of weight-reducing diet (Rolls *et al.*, 1988; Barkeling *et al.*, 1990) but this does not necessarily translate into greater weight-reducing efficacy. Furthermore, even patients enrolled in randomized controlled trials have difficulty adhering to weight-reducing diets and typically achieve very modest weight loss (Dansinger *et al.*, 2005).

Unexpected adverse effects have led to the withdrawal of several antiobesity drugs in recent years, including phentermine, fenfluramine and dexfen-fluramine, and regulatory scrutiny has thus become particularly stringent on potential newcomers to the market. This approach is entirely justifiable, particularly since patients may need to continue treatment for several decades. Of the treatments currently available, orlistat (Xenical, Roche Products Ltd), a pancreatic lipase inhibitor which works by reducing intestinal absorption of dietary fats, has been shown to cause an additional 3–4% weight loss over and above that achieved by diet alone in a 2-year period but at the expense of adverse effects which include anal leakage of oily faeces. Rebound weight gain occurs after cessation of treatment (Foxcroft & Milne, 2000). Sibutramine (Reductil, Abbott Laboratories Ltd), an inhibitor of serotonin and noradrenaline reuptake in the central nervous system (CNS), which reduces appetite and increases energy expenditure (Hansen *et al.*, 1998), has been shown to result in a similar amount of weight loss (Finer, 2002). Its use is limited by side effects including tachycardia and hypertension and it is licensed for a maximum of one year's treatment in the UK. Again, rebound weight gain occurs after cessation of treatment (Wirth & Krause, 2001).

Apart from the licensed antiobesity medications, a number of currently available drugs, including fluoxetine, sertraline, buproprion, zonisamide and topiramate, are used on an unlicensed basis. A recent meta-analysis of published trials (Li *et al.*, 2005) found that there was little evidence to support the use of either fluoxetine or sertraline but that buproprion and topiramate have weight-reducing effects broadly similar to both sibutramine and orlistat. The same may also be true for zonisamide but the supporting data comprise only a single randomized controlled trial at present (Gadde *et al.*, 2003).

Bariatric surgery is the only treatment currently available which routinely results in substantial, permanent weight loss. Procedures may be purely restrictive, for instance gastric banding or gastroplasty, or use a more complicated reconstructive technique incorporating gastric bypass, for instance Roux-en-Y gastric bypass or biliopancreatic diversion. The latter operations are more efficacious in terms of initial weight loss, sustainability of weight loss and resolution of pre-existing metabolic conditions such as type 2 diabetes mellitus and hyperlipidemia (Biertho *et al.*, 2003; Sjöström *et al.*, 2004; Scopinaro *et al.*, 2005). The perioperative mortality rate in experienced centers for Roux-en-Y gastric bypass is typically about 0.5% (Buchwald *et al.*, 2004). A recent study has raised concern about hospital readmission rates after Roux-en-Y gastric bypass (Zingmond *et al.*, 2005) but the procedure is nonetheless considered by many to offer the most appropriate compromise between efficacy and operative safety (Sjöström *et al.*, 2004; Haslam & James, 2005; le Roux & Bloom, 2005).

The mechanism by which Roux-en-Y gastric bypass cause sustained weight loss are intriguing. The reduction in gastric volume required for a successful result is less than that required for purely restrictive procedures. Furthermore, post-operative malabsorption is usually transient because of gut adaptation. Nonetheless, not only does Roux-en-Y gastric bypass result in a dramatic reduction in appetite, as assessed by meal frequency and preference for calorie-dense substances (Halmi *et al.*, 1981; Kenler *et al.*, 1990; Brolin *et al.*, 1994), it also causes rapid resolution of hyperglycemia and hyperinsulinemia, typically within a few days of the operation and well in advance of significant weight loss (Kellum *et al.*, 1990; Schauer *et al.*, 2003). It is likely that these advantageous metabolic changes are caused by profound alterations in gut hormone secretion which occur as a direct result of the procedure (Cummings *et al.*, 2004; le Roux *et al.*, 2006). A greater understanding of these changes will be vital to the ongoing search for novel treatments.

The development of novel antiobesity medications has become a very active research area over the last decade, propelled by a recognition of the growing scale of the clinical problem, by the current lack of safe and effective treatments, and by the discovery of leptin, which invigorated the whole field and led to an understanding of the molecular basis of the hypothalamic satiety circuits. The targets of compounds currently under development include intestinal nutrient absorption, stimulation of metabolic rate and modulation of either CNS neurotransmitter systems or peripheral signals of satiety and energy balance (Jandacek & Woods, 2004; Wasan & Looije, 2005; Powell, 2006). While these approaches all offer some promise, they may not all bear the same risk of adverse effects.

With regard to compounds targeting intestinal nutrient absorption, it is likely that gastrointestinal effects will be prominent, either as a result of utilization of nutrients by colonic bacterial flora or, as with orlistat, because of anal leakage. In contrast, adverse effects of drugs which stimulate metabolic rate are unlikely to be confined to the gut. Thyroxine has long been misused as a weight loss drug, despite the attendant risks of cardiac arrhythmia and loss of lean body mass, while amphetamine and related compounds were withdrawn because of concerns over their addictive potential (Colman, 2005). Several other approaches to stimulating metabolic rate are under consideration, including 3-adrenoceptor stimulation, modulation of uncoupling protein activity, and tissue-specific alteration of type 2 iodothyronine deiodinase activity. The challenge will be to develop compounds which avoid cardiovascular effects in particular.

The identification of many of the neurotransmitter systems associated with hypothalamic and extrahypothalamic satiety circuits has led to the development of a plethora of compounds, with the neuropeptide Y and serotonin receptors being particularly closely studied (Jandacek & Woods, 2004). The principal drawback of targeting CNS neurotransmitters is that each neurotransmitter typically possesses multiple functions in many different centers within the CNS. Apparently specific compounds may thus have diverse effects, some of which may be undesirable. An example of this is rimonabant, a cannabinoid-1 receptor antagonist manufactured by Sanofi-Aventis which has been the subject of prolonged scrutiny by European and American drug licensing agencies: in two phase III trials, the most common reason for discontinuation of treatment was depression (Després et al., 2005; Van Gaal et al., 2005).

Perhaps the most promising approach is to reduce appetite by modulating satiety signals emanating from the gut, the principal advantage being that, unlike neurotransmitters, circulating gut hormones do not typically have a wide range of unrelated effects. Furthermore, adverse effects are likely to be limited to the gastrointestinal tract and will mainly consist of amplification of the sensations associated with eating a large meal, such as nausea. Gut hormone-based therapies may thus provide novel antiobesity medications which combine the efficacy and durability of bariatric surgery but avoid the associated risks. Small-scale randomized controlled trials examining the use of peptide YY_{3-36} (Batterham et al., 2003) and oxyntomodulin (Wynne et al., 2005) in obese humans show promising results. Exenatide, a peptide with glucagon-like peptide-1 (GLP-1) receptor agonist properties which is resistant to breakdown by dipeptidyl peptidase IV (DPPIV), was recently approved for use as a treatment for type 2 diabetes mellitus in the USA. It has been shown in phase III studies to combine an insulinotropic effect on glycaemic control with the capacity to cause weight loss (DeFronzo et al., 2005; Kendall et al., 2005). A further small-scale trial in lean volunteers suggests that the use of combinations of gut hormones may, by mimicking normal physiology more closely, be even more effective than using single hormones (Neary et al., 2005).

Lastly, in addition to peripheral hormonal signals, attempts are also being made to modulate neural signals from the gut, either directly, using vagus nerve electrodes, or indirectly, by using electrical stimulation to slow gastric emptying. Whilst work on direct vagal stimulation remains at a preclinical stage, trials of a gastric stimulation system, the rights to which were purchased by Medtronic in 2005, are in progress.

5.   Conclusions

The history of drug treatment for obesity is littered with stories of dashed hopes and medical disasters. To reflect on this is no bad thing, since it reminds us of the scale of scientific endeavor still required and also of the paramount importance of patient safety. Nonetheless, anxieties over potential adverse effects, along with a desire to adhere closely to an evidence-based ethic, have led to a number of perverse licensing decisions in recent years. No treatment, past or present, provides durable weight loss beyond the end of the course, except for bariatric surgery. The very reason for the success of bariatric surgery is likely to be that the hormonal, as well as anatomical, changes persist. There should therefore be an expectation that novel medications will be licensed for indefinite use in patients shown to respond during an appropriate trial period. Furthermore, whilst for some patients it will be advantageous for their physicians to insist on substantial weight loss prior to commencing treatment, for others the same approach may be perceived as alienating and counterproductive.

Whatever the eventual identities of successful treatments, there can be no doubt that research into the neurobiology of obesity has become vigorous and hugely productive. The imperative to develop successful preventative strategies and effective treatments is absolutely clear and yet, in many ways, the insights provided by research in this area are more interesting still: the study of the control of appetite and of its interactions with other behavioral and metabolic systems offers a fascinating glimpse into the inner workings of the brain.

References

Amos, A. F., McCarty, D. J. & Zimmet, P. (1997). The rising global burden of diabetes and its complications: estimates and projections to the year 2010. *Diabetic Med.* **14**, S1–85.

Atkins, R. (1972). *Dr. Atkins' Diet Revolution: The High Calorie Way to Stay Thin Forever.* New York: D. McKay Co.

Avenell, A., Broom, J., Brown, T. J. *et al.* (2004). Systematic review of the long-term effects and economic consequences of treatments for obesity and implications for health improvement. *Health Technol. Assess.* **8**, 138.

Barkeling, B., Rossner, S. & Bjorvell, H. (1990). Effects of a high-protein meal (meat) and a high-carbohydrate meal (vegetarian) on satiety measured by automated computerized monitoring of subsequent food intake, motivation to eat and food preferences. *Int. J. Obes.* **14**, 743–51.

Batterham, R. L., Cohen, M. A., Ellis, S. M. *et al.* (2003). Inhibition of food intake in obese subjects by peptide YY3-36. *N. Engl. J. Med.* **349**, 941–8.

Batty, G. D., Shipley, M. J., Jarrett, R. J., Breeze, E., Marmot, M. G. & Davey Smith, G. (2005). Obesity and overweight in relation to organ-specific cancer mortality in London (UK): findings from the original Whitehall study. *Int. J. Obes.* **29**, 1267–74.

Baum, C. L. & Ford, W. F. (2004). The wage effects of obesity: a longitudinal study. *Health Econ.* **13**, 885–99.

Bianchini, F., Kaaks, R. & Vainio, H. (2002). Overweight, obesity, and cancer risk. *Lancet Oncol.* **3**, 565–74.

Biertho, L., Steffen, R., Ricklin, T. *et al.* (2003). Laparoscopic gastric bypass versus laparoscopic adjustable gastric banding: a comparative study of 1200 cases. *J. Am. Coll. Surg.* **197**, 536–47.

Bouchard, C., Tremblay, A., Despres, J. P. *et al.* (1990). The response to long-term overfeeding in identical twins. *N. Engl. J. Med.* **322**, 1477–82.

Brolin, R. L., Robertson, L. B., Kenler, H. A. & Cody, R. P. (1994). Weight loss and dietary intake after vertical banded gastroplasty and Roux-en-Y gastric bypass. *Ann. Surg.* **220**, 782–90.

Brown, C. D., Higgins, M., Donato, K. A. *et al.* (2000). Body mass index and the prevalence of hypertension and dyslipidaemia. *Obes. Res.* **8**, 605–19.

Buchwald, H., Avidor, Y., Braunwald, E. *et al.* (2004). Bariatric surgery: a systematic review and meta-analysis. *J. Am. Med. Assoc.* **292**, 1724–37.

Bundred, P., Kitchiner, D. & Buchan, I. (2001). Prevalence of overweight and obese children between 1989 and 1998: population based series of cross sectional studies. *Br. Med. J.* **322**, 326–8.

Calle, E. E. & Kaaks, R. (2004). Overweight, obesity and cancer: epidemiological evidence and proposed mechanisms. *Nat. Rev. Cancer* **4**, 579–91.

Calle, E. E., Rodriguez, C., Walker-Thurmond, K. & Thun, M. J. (2003). Overweight, obesity, and mortality from cancer in a prospectively studied cohort of U.S. adults. *N. Engl. J. Med.* **348**, 1625–38.

Chang, V. W. & Lauderdale, D. S. (2005). Income disparities in body mass index and obesity in the United States, 1971–2002. *Arch. Intern. Med.* **165**, 2122–8.

Colditz, G. A., Willett, W. C., Rotnitzky, A. & Manson, J. E. (1995). Weight gain as a risk factor for clinical diabetes mellitus in women. *Ann. Intern. Med.* **122**, 481–6.

Colman, E. (2005). Anorectics on trial: a half century of federal regulation of prescription appetite suppressants. *Ann. Intern. Med.* **143**, 380–5.

Crosignani, P., Colombo, M., Vegetti, W., Somigliana, E., Gessati, A. & Ragni, G. (2003). Overweight and obese anovulatory patients with polycystic ovaries: parallel improvements in anthropometric indices, ovarian physiology and fertility rate induced by diet. *Hum. Reprod.* **18**, 1928–32.

Cummings, D. E., Overduin, J. & Foster-Schubert, K. E. (2004). Gastric bypass for obesity: mechanisms of weight loss and diabetes resolution. *J. Clin. Endocrinol. Metab.* **89**, 2608–15.

Dansinger, M. L., Gleason, J. A., Griffith, J. L., Selker, H. P. & Schaefer, E. J. (2005). Comparison of the Atkins, Ornish, Weight Watchers, and Zone diets for weight loss and heart disease risk reduction. *J. Am. Med. Assoc.* **293**, 43–53.

de Looper, M. & Bhatia, K. (2001). *Australian Health Trends 2001. AIHW Cat. No. PHE 24.* Canberra: Australian Institute of Health and Welfare.

Dean, H. & Flett, B. (2002). Natural history of type 2 diabetes diagnosed in childhood: long term follow-up in young adult years (abstract 99-OR). *Diabetes*, **51 (Suppl. 2)**, A24.

DeFronzo, R. A., Ratner, R. E., Han, J., Kim, D. D., Fineman, M. S. & Baron, A. D. (2005). Effects of exenatide (exendin-4) on glycemic control and weight over 30 weeks in metformin-treated patients with type 2 diabetes. *Diabetes Care*, **28**, 1092–100.

Després, J.-P., Golay, A. & Sjöström, L. (2005). Effects of rimonabant on metabolic risk factors in overweight patients with dyslipidaemia. *N. Engl. J. Med.* **353**, 2121–34.

Ebbeling, C. B., Sinclair, K. B., Pereira, M. A., Garcia-Lago, E., Feldman, H. A. & Ludwig, D. S. (2004). Compensation for energy intake from fast food among overweight and lean adolescents. *J. Am. Med. Assoc.* **291**, 2828–33.

Fagot-Campagna, A., Pettitt, D. J., Engelgau, M. M. *et al.* (2000). Type 2 diabetes among North American children and adolescents: an epidemiologic review and a public health perspective. *J. Pediatr.* **136**, 664–72.

Fang, J., Wylie-Rosett, J., Cohen, H. W., Kaplan, R. C. & Alderman, M. H. (2003). Exercise, body mass index, caloric intake, and cardiovascular mortality. *Am. J. Prev. Med.* **25**, 283–9.

Farooqi, I. S. & O'Rahilly, S. (2005). Monogenic obesity in humans. *Annu. Rev. Med.* **56**, 443–58.

Fedorcsák, P., Dale, P. O., Storeng, R. *et al.* (2004). Impact of overweight and underweight on assisted reproduction treatment. *Hum. Reprod.* **19**, 2523–8.

Felson, D. T., Zhang, Y., Anthony, J. M., Naimark, A. & Anderson, J. J. (1992). Weight loss reduces the risk for symptomatic knee osteoarthritis in women: the Framingham study. *Ann. Intern. Med.* **116**, 535–9.

Finer, N. (2002). Sibutramine: its mode of action and efficacy. *Int. J. Obes.* **26 (Suppl. 4)**, S29–33.

Flegal, K. M., Carroll, M. D., Kuczmarski, R. J. & Johnson, C. L. (1998). Overweight and obesity in the United States: prevalence and trends, 1960-1994. *Int. J. Obes.* **22**, 39-47.

Flegal, K. M., Carroll, M. D., Ogden, C. L. & Johnson, C. L. (2002). Prevalence and trends in obesity among US adults, 1999-2000. *J. Am. Med. Assoc.* **288**, 1723-7.

Ford, E. S. (1999). Body mass index, diabetes, and c-reactive protein among U.S. adults. *Diabetes Care* **22**, 1971-7.

Ford, E. S. (2005). The epidemiology of obesity and asthma. *J. Allergy Clin. Immunol.* **115**, 897-909.

Foxcroft, D. R. & Milne, R. (2000). Orlistat for the treatment of obesity: rapid review and cost-effectiveness model. *Obes. Rev.* **1**, 121-6.

Gadde, K. M., Franciscy, D. M., Wagner, H. R. II & Krishnan, K. R. R. (2003). Zonisamide for weight loss in obese adults: a randomized controlled trial. *J. Am. Med. Assoc.* **289**, 1820-5.

Giovannucci, E. (1995). Insulin and colon cancer. *Cancer Causes Control* **6**, 164-79.

Halmi, K. A., Mason, E., Falk, J. R. & Stunkard, A. (1981). Appetitive behavior after gastric bypass for obesity. *Int. J. Obes.* **5**, 457-64.

Hampel, H., Abraham, N. S. & El-Serag, H. B. (2005). Meta-analysis: obesity and the risk for gastroesophageal reflux disease and its complications. *Ann. Intern. Med.* **143**, 199-211.

Hansen, D. L., Toubro, S., Stock, M. J., Macdonald, I. A. & Astrup, A. (1998). Thermogenic effects of sibutramine in humans. *Am. J. Clin. Nutr.* **68**, 1180-6.

Hart, D. J. & Spector, T. D. (1993). The relationship of obesity, fat distribution and osteoarthritis in women in the general population: the Chingford study. *J. Rheumatol.* **20**, 331-5.

Haslam, D. W. & James, W. P. T. (2005). Obesity. *Lancet* **366**, 1197-209.

Heo, M., Pietrobelli, A., Fontaine, K. R., Sirey, J. A. & Faith, M. S. (2006). Depressive mood and obesity in U.S. adults: comparison and moderation by sex, age, and race. *Int. J. Obes.* **30**, 513-19.

Herva, A., Laitinen, J., Miettunen, J., Veijola, J., Karvonen, J. T., Läksy, K. & Joukamaa, M. (2006). Obesity and depression: results from the longitudinal northern Finland 1966 birth cohort study. *Int. J. Obes.* **30**, 520-7.

Jandacek, R. J. & Woods, S. C. (2004). Pharmaceutical approaches to the treatment of obesity. *Drug Discov. Today* **9**, 874-80.

Kalra, M., Inge, T., Garcia, V. *et al.* (2005). Obstructive sleep apnea in extremely overweight adolescents undergoing bariatric surgery. *Obes. Res.* **13**, 1175-9.

Katzmarzyk, P. T. (2002). The Canadian obesity epidemic: an historical perspective. *Obes. Res.* **10**, 666-74.

Katzmarzyk, P. T. & Ardern, C. I. (2004). Overweight and obesity mortality trends in Canada, 1985-2000. *Can. J. Public Health* **95**, 16-20.

Kellum, J. M., Kuemmerle, J. F., O'Dorisio, T. M. *et al.* (1990). Gastrointestinal hormone responses to meals before and after gastric bypass and vertical banded gastroplasty. *Ann. Surg.* **211**, 763-70.

Kenchaiah, S., Evans, J. C., Levy, D. *et al.* (2002). Obesity and the risk of heart failure. *N. Engl. J. Med.* **347**, 305–13.

Kendall, D. M., Riddle, M. C., Rosenstock, J. *et al.* (2005). Effects of exenatide (exendin-4) on glycemic control over 30 weeks in patients with type 2 diabetes treated with metformin and a sulphonylurea. *Diabetes Care* **28**, 1083–91.

Kenler, H. A., Brolin, R. E. & Cody, R. P. (1990). Changes in eating behavior after horizontal gastroplasty and Roux-en-Y gastric bypass. *Am. J. Clin. Nutr.* **52**, 87–92.

King, H., Aubert, R. E. & Herman, W. H. (1998). Global burden of diabetes, 1995–2025. *Diabetes Care* **21**, 1414–31.

le Roux, C. W. & Bloom, S. R. (2005). Why do patients lose weight after Roux-en-Y gastric bypass? *J. Clin. Endocrinol. Metab.* **90**, 591–2.

le Roux, C. W., Aylwin, S. J. B., Batterham, R. L. *et al.* (2006). Gut hormone profiles following bariatric surgery favor an anorectic state, facilitate weight loss, and improve metabolic parameters. *Ann. Surg.* **243**, 108–14.

Li, Z., Maglione, M., Tu, W. *et al.* (2005). Meta-analysis: pharmacologic treatment of obesity. *Ann. Intern. Med.* **142**, 532–46.

Linné, Y. (2004). Effects of obesity on women's reproduction and complications during pregnancy. *Obes. Rev.* **5**, 137–43.

Lintsen, A. M. E., Pasker-de, Jong P. C. M., de Boer, E. J. *et al.* (2005). Effects of subfertility cause, smoking and body weight on the success rate of IVF. *Hum. Reprod.* **20**, 1867–75.

Lobstein, T. & Jackson-Leach, R. (2006). Estimated burden of paediatric obesity and co-morbidities in Europe. Part 2. Numbers of children with indicators of obesity-related disease. *Int. J. Pediatr. Obes.* **1**, 33–41.

Lobstein, T., Baur, L. & Uauy, R. (2004). Obesity in children and young people: a crisis in public health. *Obes. Rev.* **5 (Suppl. 1)**, 4–85.

McCarthy, H. D., Ellis, S. M. & Cole, T. J. (2003). Central overweight and obesity in British youth aged 11–16 years: cross sectional surveys of waist circumference. *Br. Med. J.* **326**, 624–6.

Maes, H. H. M., Neale, M. C. & Eaves, L. J. (1997). Genetic and environmental factors in relative body weight and human adiposity. *Behav. Genet.* **27**, 325–51.

Messier, S. P., Loeser, R. F., Miller, G. D. *et al.* (2004). Exercise and dietary weight loss in overweight and obese older adults with knee osteoarthritis: the arthritis, diet, and activity promotion trial. *Arthritis Rheum.* **50**, 1501–10.

Murphy, N. F., MacIntyre, K., Stewart, S., Hart, C. L., Hole, D. & McMurray, J. J. V. (2006). Long-term cardiovascular consequences of obesity: 20-year follow-up of more than 15000 middle-aged men and women (the Renfrew-Paisley study). *Eur. Heart J.* **27**, 96–106.

National Audit Office (2001). *Tackling Obesity in England. Report by the Comptroller and Auditor General.* London: The Stationery Office.

Neary, N. M., Small, C. J., Druce, M. R. *et al.* (2005). Peptide YY_{3-36} and glucagon-like peptide-1_{7-36} inhibit food intake additively. *Endocrinology* **146**, 5120–7.

Neel, J. V. (1962). Diabetes mellitus: a "thrifty" genotype rendered detrimental by "progress"? *Am. J. Hum. Genet.* **14**, 353–62.

Nielsen, S. J., Siega-Riz, A. M. & Popkin, B. M. (2002). Trends in food locations and sources among adolescents and young adults. *Prev.Med.* **35**, 107–13.

Nohr, E. A., Bech, B. H., Davies, M. J., Frydenberg, M., Henriksen, T. B. & Olsen, J. (2005). Prepregnancy obesity and fetal death: a study within the Danish national birth cohort. *Obstet. Gynecol.* **106**, 250–9.

Olson, A. L. & Zwillich, C. (2005). The obesity hypoventilation syndrome. *Am. J. Med.* **118**, 948–56.

Pérusse, L., Rankinen, T., Zuberi, A. *et al.* (2005). The human obesity gene map: the 2004 update. *Obes. Res.* **13**, 381–90.

Pickup, J. C. & Mattock, M. B. (2003). Activation of the innate immune system as a predictor of cardiovascular mortality in type 2 diabetes mellitus. *Diabet. Med.* **20**, 723–6.

Powell, D. R. (2006). Obesity drugs and their targets: correlation of mouse knockout phenotypes with drug effects in vivo. *Obes. Rev.* **7**, 89–108.

Prentice, A. M. (2005). Early influences on human energy regulation: thrifty genotypes and thrifty phenotypes. *Physiol. Behav.* **86**, 640–5.

Ramachandran, A., Snehalatha, C., Satyavani, K., Sivasankari, S. & Vijay, V. (2003). Type 2 diabetes in Asian-Indian urban children. *Diabetes Care* **26**, 1022–5.

Resta, O., Foschino-Barbaro, M. P., Legari, G. *et al.* (2001). Sleep-related breathing disorders, loud snoring and excessive daytime sleepiness in obese subjects. *Int. J. Obes.* **25**, 669–75.

Ridker, P. M., Cushman, M., Stampfer, M. J., Tracy, R. P. & Hennekens, C. H. (1997). Inflammation, aspirin, and the risk of cardiovascular disease in apparently healthy men. *N. Engl. J. Med.* **336**, 973–9.

Rolls, B. J., Hetherington, M. & Burley, V. J. (1988). The specificity of satiety: the influence of foods of different macronutrient content on the development of satiety. *Physiol. Behav.* **43**, 145–53.

Rolls, B. J., Roe, L. S. & Meengs, J. S. (2006). Reductions in portion size and energy density of foods are additive and lead to sustained decreases in energy intake. *Am. J. Clin. Nutr.* **83**, 11–17.

Schauer, P. R., Burguera, B., Ikramuddin, S. *et al.* (2003). Effect of laparoscopic Roux-en-Y gastric bypass on type 2 diabetes mellitus. *Ann. Surg.* **238**, 467–85.

Scopinaro, N., Marinari, G. M., Camerini, G. B., Papadia, F. S. & Adami, G. F. (2005). Specific effects of biliopancreatic diversion on the major components of metabolic syndrome. *Diabetes Care*, **28**, 2406–11.

Sebire, N. J., Jolly, M., Harris, J. P. *et al.* (2001). Maternal obesity and pregnancy outcome: a study of 287213 pregnancies in London. *Int. J. Obes.* **25**, 1175–82.

Sims, E. A., Danforth, E. Jr., Horton, E. S., Bray, G. A., Glennon, J. A. & Salans, L. B. (1973). Endocrine and metabolic effects of experimental obesity in man. *Recent Prog. Horm. Res.* **29**, 457–96.

Sjöberg, R. L., Nilsson, K. W. & Leppert, J. (2005). Obesity, shame, and depression in school-aged children: a population-based study. *Pediatrics* **116**, 389–92.

Sjöström, L., Lindroos, A., Peltonen, M. *et al.* (2004). Lifestyle, diabetes and cardiovascular risk factors 10 years after bariatric surgery. *N. Engl. J. Med.* **351**, 2683–93.

Stevens, J., Couper, D., Pankow, J. et al. (2001). Sensitivity and specificity of anthropometrics for the prediction of diabetes in a biracial cohort. *Obes. Res.* **9**, 696–705.

Stürmer, T., Günther, K. P. & Brenner, H. (2000). Obesity, overweight and patterns of osteoarthritis: the Ulm osteoarthritis study. *J. Clin. Epidemiol.* **53**, 307–13.

Tremblay, M. S., Katzmarzyk, P. T. & Willms, J. D. (2002). Temporal trends in overweight and obesity in Canada, 1981–1996. *Int. J. Obes.* **26**, 538–43.

Van Gaal, L. F., Rissanen, A. M., Scheen, A. J., Ziegler, O. & Rössner, S. (2005). Effects of the cannabinoid-1 receptor blocker rimonabant on weight reduction and cardiovascular risk factors in overweight patients: 1-year experience from the RIO-Europe study. *Lancet* **365**, 1389–97.

Vereecken, C. A., Bobelijn, K. & Maes, L. (2005). School food policy at primary and secondary schools in Belgium-Flanders: does it influence young people's food habits? *Eur. J. Clin. Nutr.* **59**, 271–7.

Vingard, E., Lindberg, P., Josephson, M. et al. (2005). Long-term sick-listing among women in the public sector and its associations with age, social situation, lifestyle, and work factors: a three-year follow-up study. *Scand. J. Public Health* **33**, 370–5.

Wang, T. J., Parise, H., Levy, D. et al. (2004). Obesity and the risk of new-onset atrial fibrillation. *J. Am. Med. Assoc.* **292**, 2471–7.

Wannamethee, S. G. & Shaper, A. G. (1999). Weight change and duration of overweight and obesity in the incidence of type 2 diabetes. *Diabetes Care* **22**, 1266–72.

Wasan, K. M. & Looije, N. A. (2005). Emerging pharmacological approaches to the treatment of obesity. *J. Pharm. Pharmaceut. Sci.* **8**, 259–71.

World Health Organization (1995). *Physical Status: The Use and Interpretation of Anthropometry. Report of a WHO Expert Consultation. WHO Technical Report Series Number 854.* Geneva: World Health Organization.

WHO Expert Consultation (2004). Appropriate body-mass index for Asian populations and its implications for policy and intervention strategies. *Lancet* **363**, 157–63.

WHO Global InfoBase Team (2005). *The SuRF Report 2. Surveillance of Chronic Disease Risk Factors: Country-level Data and Comparable Estimates.* Geneva: World Health Organization.

Wild, S., Roglic, G., Green, A., Sicree, R. & King, H. (2004). Global prevalence of diabetes: estimates for the year 2000 and projections for 2030. *Diabetes Care* **27**, 1047–53.

Wilson, P. W. F., D'Agostino, R. B., Sullivan, L., Parise, H. & Kannel, W. B. (2002). Overweight and obesity as determinants of cardiovascular risk: the Framingham experience. *Arch. Intern. Med.* **162**, 1867–72.

Wirth, A. & Krause, J. (2001). Long-term weight loss with sibutramine. A randomized controlled trial. *J. Am. Med. Assoc.* **286**, 1331–9.

Wolk, R., Berger, P., Lennon, R. J., Brilakis, E. S. & Somers, V. K. (2003). Body mass index: a risk factor for unstable angina and myocardial infarction in patients with angiographically confirmed coronary artery disease. *Circulation* **108**, 2206–11.

Wynne, K., Park, A. J., Small, C. J. *et al.* (2005). Subcutaneous oxyntomodulin reduces body weight in overweight and obese subjects: a double-blind, randomized, controlled trial. *Diabetes* **54**, 2390–5.

Yusuf, S., Hawken, S., Ôunpuu, S. *et al.*, INTERHEART Study Investigators (2005). Obesity and the risk of myocardial infarction in 27 000 participants from 52 countries: a case-control study. *Lancet* **366**, 1640–9.

Zingmond, D. S., McGory, M. L. & Ko, C. Y. (2005). Hospitalization before and after gastric bypass surgery. *J. Am. Med. Assoc.* **294**, 1918–24.

2

Genetics of human and rodent body weight regulation

KARINE CLÉMENT

1.   Introduction

Obesity has become a major public health problem owing to its prevalence, which stands at more than 25% in certain countries, and its alarming increase in children. Classically, obesity results from the interaction between environmental factors such as overeating and/or reduction in physical activity and hereditary factors. The role of environmental, behavioral and socioeconomic factors in individuals with different biological susceptibilities has been recognized. Although the complexity of obesity was noted early in the last century (Mayer, 1953), the contribution of genetic factors in determining obesity has been emphasized by numerous epidemiological studies carried out in large and different populations (twins brought up together or separately, adopted children, nuclear families, etc.). These studies have been extensively reviewed elsewhere (Sorensen, 1995). According to such studies, 30–80% of weight variation might be attributed to genetic factors.

Obesity is also characterized by a high phenotype heterogeneity linked to the different stages in weight evolution. Each stage in the development towards obesity (weight gain, weight maintenance and chronicization, variable response to treatment, comorbidities occurrence) could presumably be associated with different molecular mechanisms (Figure 2.1). At present we do not know any of the molecular mechanisms regulating the passage from one stage to another. Molecular approaches in obesity have been predominantly aimed at discovering whether there are naturally occurring mutations that influence

Neurobiology and Obesity, ed. Jenni Harvey and Dominic J. Withers. Published by Cambridge University Press. © Cambridge University Press 2008

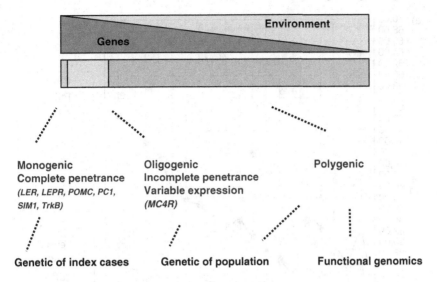

Figure 2.1 Role of genetics in human obesity and common approaches.

the rapidity and severity of fat mass accumulation, as well as genetic variations in candidate genes or genomic regions that are generally associated with some obesity phenotypes, and not to a specific phase in the evolution toward obesity.

The contribution of genetic factors in obesity can be summarized as below (Figure 2.2):

- Single mutations contribute to the development of obesity in humans and rodents. These forms of monogenic obesity are rare, very severe and generally commence in childhood (Farooqi & O'Rahilly, 2004). Research concerning single mutations was conducted within individuals characterized by specific biochemical or hormonal abnormalities (Farooqi & O'Rahilly, 2004).

- Several genetic variants interact with an "at risk" environment in common obesities (i.e. polygenic obesity). Here each susceptibility gene, taken in isolation, would only have a slight effect on weight, however the cumulative contribution of these genes would become significant when interacting with environmental factors predisposing their phenotypic expression (e.g. overeating, reduction in physical activity, hormonal changes, socioeconomical factors etc.). Thus, the common disease/common variant hypothesis has been proposed (Lander, 1996) and suggests that the genetic risk for obesity is due to disease-promoting common alleles. As a consequence, the percentage of obesity attributed to them (attributable risk) could be high. This hypothesis is a popular one in multifactorial diseases. Alternatively,

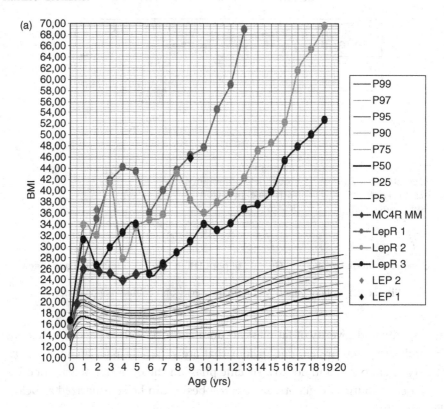

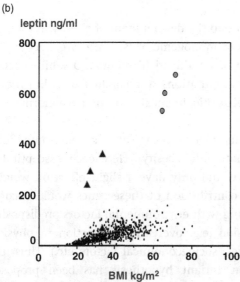

Figure 2.2 Evolution of body mass index in LEPR deficient patients and leptin
levels. (a). Curves in orange, brown and green are body mass index (BMI) curves
of patients carrying the LEPR mutation. For comparison, the pink and the black
diamonds are the BMI measured in the two leptin deficient cousins at 2 years and 9 years

the risk for common obesity could also be due to the cumulative effect of several loci, each with multiple disease-predisposing alleles but of low frequency (oligogenic obesity) (Pritchard, 2001).

Herein an up-to-date survey of genes that have been studied in human obesity is presented, with more emphasis placed on studies where the role of genes in the central nervous system, notably in the leptin/melanocortin axis, is discussed. Focus will be given on naturally occurring mutations in mice and humans. We do not discuss here the different genetic syndromes associated with obesity, as reviewed in Chung & Leibel (2005). We will conclude the chapter on the role of genetic variations in common forms of obesity.

2.   Rare monogenic obesity

Linkage studies, mouse models (knock-out, transgenesis) and spontaneous mutations as well as pharmacological studies, have discovered the primary role of the leptin/melanocortin pathway in regulating energy homeostasis (Coll et al., 2004). The physiological importance of these pathways is thoroughly discussed in the other book chapters. The role of these pathways in humans has been unraveled by the discovery that naturally occurring mutations in mice have their human counterparts (Figure 2.3).

2.1   Leptin and leptin receptor deficiencies

Several mouse and rat models of obesity stem from single gene mutations that affect the production or signaling of the leptin hormone. The discovery

Caption for Figure 2.2 (cont.)

(Montague et al., 1997) and the curve in blue is the BMI evolution of a patient carrying a homozygous MC4R mutation. Black line is BMI reference curve for the French populations (50th percentile). Grey lines are reference BMI curves. Upper grey/brown lines are 99, 97, 95, 90, 75th percentiles. Lower grey/brown lines are 25 and 5th percentiles.

(b). Leptin levels in a French family carrying the leptin receptor mutation. Orange circles are the level of leptin in the three homozygous carriers of the leptin receptor mutation and triangles depict leptin levels in heterozygous carriers of the family. The leptin levels are compared with that of 800 subjects with a wide BMI range (black crosses). One subject of the family (triangle in the black cloud of dots) with the leptin receptor wild type allele has leptin levels related with corpulence. The high leptin levels in the family is related to this particular homozygous mutation in the human leptin receptor gene that results in a truncated leptin receptor lacking both the transmembrane and the intracellular domains. The truncated receptor is secreted into blood and binds the majority of serum leptin, markedly increasing bound and total leptin as demonstrated in Lahlou et al. (2000).

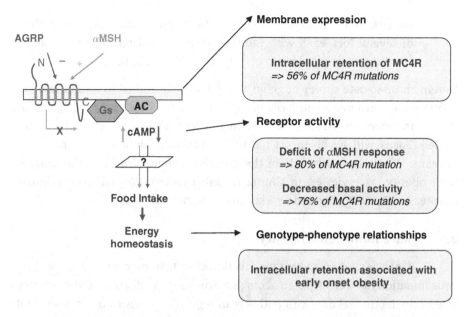

Figure 2.3 Summary of functional anomalies found in MC4R mutations. Five melanocortin receptors, termed MC1R through MC5R, have been characterized thus far. As illustrated by MC4R, they belong to the G protein-coupled receptor (GPCR) superfamily and signal through adenylyl cyclase-proteine kinase A (AC) activation by coupling to Gs. After stimulation, cAMP is produced. This figure summarizes the principal functional consequences associated with the mutations in humans. The percentages shown here refer to Lubrano-Berthelier *et al.* (2003a). AGRP: agouti-related peptide.

of the leptin (LEP) and leptin receptor (LEPR) gene mutations in *ob/ob* and *db/db* mice was a result of 40 intense years of research where the animal phenotypes were first described and then after careful and elegant investigations into the dysfunctional biology underlying these animals, the hypothesis was raised regarding their perturbed regulation of body weight. Then exploiting the progress made with modern molecular tools in genome sequencing and genome wide scanning, positional cloning led to the discovery that the LEP and LEPR genes were mutated. All mutations lead to nonfunctional LEP or LEPR in these mice or rats as summarized in Table 2.1. The resulting consequence of these mutations is an early massive increase in fat mass related to an abnormal control of energy balance and endocrine abnormalities, as illustrated in Table 2.2. Depending on the genetic background, some mice develop glucose intolerance, dyslipidemia and diabetes. Major perturbations in the CNS pathways regulating food intake and energy expenditure have been largely described in obese rodents (Table 2.1).

Table 2.1 *Major steps leading to the discovery of leptin and leptin receptor mutations*

Study	Description	Main hypothesis or findings
(Kennedy, 1953)	Experiments in rats	Signals produced by adipose tissue could influence food intake
(Coleman, 1973)	Parabiosis of *ob* and *db* mice with normal mice	Mouse phenotype results in loss of function of a circulating molecule or of its receptor
(Bahary et al., 1990), (Friedman et al., 1991)	Genetic crossing in *db* and *ob* mice	Molecular maps of *db* and *ob* regions. Human homologous regions are on chromosome 1 (LEPR) and 7 (LEP)
(Zhang et al., 1994)	Positional cloning in the leptin gene region Leptin gene sequencing in *ob/ob* mice	LEP gene and leptin hormone are discovered. LEP$^{ob/ob}$ mice carries a C105T mutation converting an Arg to stop codon in the LEP gene.
(Tartaglia et al., 1995)	Positional cloning of leptin receptor gene	LEPR is discovered. LEPR$^{db/db}$ mice carries a G106T mutation leading to nucleotide insertion and stop codon.
(Montague et al., 1997) (Strobel et al., 1998)	Sequencing human subjects with morbid obesity and low leptin	Consanguineous families with children carrying homozygous mutations in LEP gene
(Clement et al., 1998)	Sequencing human subjects with morbid obesity and high leptin	Consanguineous families with sisters carrying homozygous mutation in the LEPR gene

A few years after the discovery of leptin, families carrying LEP gene mutations were recognized (Montague *et al.*, 1997; Strobel *et al.*, 1998; Farooqi *et al.*,
2001) in addition to families with a mutation in the LEPR gene (Clement *et al.*,
1998). Similar to animal models, carriers of these mutations have severe early
onset obesity, within the first few months of life, and several endocrinal dysfunctions. Additionally, afflicted individuals had impulsive patterns of eating
behavior and food-seeking disorder similar to those observed in patients with
Prader–Willi syndrome. Evaluating body composition in LEPR mutation carriers showed a large amount of total body fat mass ($> 50\%$). Resting energy
expenditure was related to the level of corpulence in humans, which is in
contrast with animal models typically characterized with a decrease in energy
expenditure and hypothermia. In patients with a mutation in LEP or LEPR
genes, the complete failure to enter puberty was related to hypogonadotrophic

Table 2.2 *Human and rodent mutations affecting the leptin and the melanocortin pathways*

Gene	Transmission	Rodent model	Human obesity	Associated phenotypes
Leptin	Recessive	Mice (Lep$^{ob/ob}$)	Severe, from the first days of life. Hyperphagia	Gonadotrophic and thyrotrophic insufficiency
Leptin receptor	Recessive	Rat (Lepr^{fa}, lepr^{fak}) Lepr^{db} Db^{3j}, db^{Pas})	Severe, from the first days of life	Gonadotrophic, thyrotrophic and somatotrophic insufficiency
Proopiomelanocortin (POMC)	Recessive	Agouti mutations	Severe, from the first month of life	ACTH insufficiency. Mild hypothyroidism. Ginger hairs
Proconvertase 1 (PC1)	Recessive	Fat mouse	Considerable, from the first month of life	Gonadotrophic and corticotrophic insufficiency Hyperproinsulinaemia. Other dysfunction of gut peptides
Melanocortin 4 receptor (MC4R)	Dominant		Early onset, variable severity, large size	No other phenotype

hypogonadism. Thyrotrophic insufficiency of central origin was also observed. Insufficient somatotrophic secretion was described in females with a leptin receptor mutation. Such findings are in agreement with data produced in mice with a nonfunctional LEP and LEPR where a stunted growth curve was observed. A high rate of infection associated with a deficiency in T cell number and function was identified, suggesting a role of leptin in immunity (Farooqi & O'Rahilly, 2005).

The prospective follow up of some patients carrying LEP (Ozata et al., 1999) or LEPR mutations revealed that spontaneous pubertal development might occur as well as the normalization of thyroid mild dysfunction in adulthood (K. Clément, unpublished observation). In contrast to ob/ob and db/db mice with hypercorticosteronemia, humans with leptin and leptin receptor deficiency scored normal in tests for hypothalamic-pituitary-adrenal function although some mild alteration could not be excluded, as described below.

Leptin-deficient children and adults, similar to that seen in rodents (Halaas et al., 1997) greatly benefited from subcutaneous injections of leptin which resulted in a loss of fat mass with a major effect on reducing food intake and improving other dysfunctions such as immune functions (Farooqi et al., 2002). In humans, an interesting detailed microanalysis of eating behavior of three leptin-deficient adults prior to and following 3 months of leptin treatment, revealed a reduction in overall food consumption, a slower rate of eating and a decreased duration of eating at every meal (Ozata et al., 1999; Williamson et al., 2005). These findings supported a role for leptin in influencing an individual motivation to eat before each meal (Williamson et al., 2005). In a separate study, hormonal and metabolic changes were evaluated before and after leptin treatment (Licinio et al., 2004). Leptin treatment was able to induce aspects of puberty even in adults, as illustrated by the effect of leptin treatment in one 27-year-old adult male with hypogonadism. In two women aged between 35–40 years, leptin treatment led to regular menstrual periods and hormonal peaks of progesterone evoking a pattern of ovulation. Although cortisol deficiency was not initially found in leptin-deficient patients, 8 months of leptin treatment modified the pulsatility of cortisol with a greater morning rise of cortisol. Leptin could have a previously unsuspected impact on human hypothalamic-pituitary-adrenal function in humans. Metabolic parameters of leptin-deficient patients improved in parallel with weight loss.

Because of a nonfunctional LEPR, leptin treatment is useless in LEPR deficient females. Since 1998, the clinical situation of the two sisters in the family under study (Clement et al., 1998) deteriorated with an exacerbation of weight that reached more than 220 kg at 20 years of age. The oldest sister rapidly developed renal insufficiency leading to dialysis one year later. Further investigation including kidney biopsy under polarized light and immunohistochemistry led to the diagnosis of kidney amyloidosis AA. Exhaustive clinical, biological and radiological investigations did not detect any common cause of secondary amyloidosis. However, serum amyloid A (SAA) depositions were found in the adipose tissue of both sisters. The coincidence of SAA overexpression in the adipose tissue and renal amyloidosis in extreme adiposity related to LEPR mutation prompted a series of investigations which showed that SAA is produced by adipocyte cells and suggested that it might contribute to the systemic complications associated with human obesity. The presence of SAA in adipose tissue was also found in morbidly obese subjects with a normal LEPR sequence (Poitou *et al.*, 2005b).

Factors that could possibly bypass normal leptin delivery systems are being developed but are not yet currently available for the treatment of these patients. The ciliary neurotrophic factor (CNTF) is nevertheless one of these candidate molecules; it activates downstream signaling molecules such as STAT-3 in the hypothalamus area that regulates food intake, even when administered systemically. Treatment with CNTF in humans and animals, including *db/db* mice induced substantial loss of fat mass (Sleeman *et al.*, 2000). The neurotrophic factor, Axokine, an agonist for CNTF receptor, is under development by the Regeneron Company, for the potential treatment of obesity and its metabolic associated complications (Preti, 2003).

Recent studies suggest that the phenotype in mice, and perhaps humans deficient in LEP and LEPR, is due primarily to a default in leptin signaling in the CNS rather than in the periphery. Short isoforms of LEPR are found in peripheral organs while the physiologically active long isoform of LEPR (Ob-Rb) is considered to be mainly expressed in the CNS. In addition to its central action on food intake and energy expenditure, leptin may also have direct peripheral effects on non-adipose tissues (i.e. muscle, liver, hematopoetic, bone cells) to exert a role in different functional pathways such as angiogenesis, inflammation and immunity, fat oxidation and bone remodeling. In an elegant recent study, the targeted deletion of the LEPR gene in peripheral tissues (thus expression was maintained in the brain) did not lead to obesity, suggesting that the peripheral effect of leptin could be predominantly mediated via the CNS (de Luca *et al.*, 2005).

2.2   *Proopiomelanocortin-derived peptides deficiency*

The proopiomelanocortin (POMC) protein participates in transmitting the leptin signal from the periphery to the hypothalamus during a central homeostatic response. The production of POMC in the CNS is stimulated by leptin and the post-translational process of the protein gives rise to the production of different peptides harboring many functional properties (Seeley et al., 2004). The nature of the POMC-derived peptides depends on the type of endoproteolytic enzymes which are specific to certain areas of the brain. In the anterior pituitary, the presence of proconvertase 1 (PC1) enzyme allows the production of ACTH and β- lipotropin peptides, while the presence of both PC1 and PC2 in the hypothalamus regulates the production of α-, β-, γ-MSH and β-endorphins. The peptides derived from POMC exert their action via different melanocortin receptors located throughout the organism such as melano-cortin 4 receptor, MC4R and MC3R (brain), MC2R (adrenal gland) and MC1R (skin). Antagonizing these receptors with either naturally occurring molecules or simply through removal of the ligand leads to a highly recognizable phenotype. The lethal yellow agouti, the first mouse model of monogenic obesity, recapitulated aspects of this phenotype with severe obesity and yellow coat color (Bultman et al., 1992). The mutation results in a widespread ectopic expression of the agouti protein. The molecular defined mechanism for the expression of the agouti protein is due to a chromosome deletion at the agouti locus that results in the fusion of agouti coding sequence with the promoter elements of the Raly gene which encodes a ubiquitous protein. The yellow coat color is due to the antagonism by agouti of MC1R in the skin and obesity related to MC4R blockade in the brain (Michaud et al., 1994). The character-ization of the agouti protein also led to the discovery of agouti-related protein (AGRP) which can competitively antagonize POMC-derived peptides at the MC4R in the hypothalamus (Ollmann et al., 1997; Stutz et al., 2005). Genetic manipulation of POMC produced a phenotype resembling that of lethal yellow agouti mice. POMC-knockout mice become obese through a loss of anorexi-genic action of α-MSH on MC4R expressing neurons. They have no adrenal functions due to the lack of ACTH production and they present variable alterations in coat pigmentation as a consequence of the absence of α-MSH in the skin where it acts through MC1R (Slominski et al., 2005). Thus, blocking MC1R function with either the agouti protein or through the absence of α-MSH, results in a lack of production of a dark pigment, eumelanin and the production of the red pigment pheomelanin.

The phenotype of children with mutations that completely prevent POMC-derived peptides production is similar to that of POMC-deficient mice. Six families carrying a POMC mutation (Krude et al., 1998, 2003) have been described (Farooqi et al., 2006) Obese children with a POMC deficiency have an adreno-corticotrophic hormone deficiency that can lead to acute adrenal insufficiency from birth. The patients coming from Germany, Slovenia, the Netherlands and Switzerland are homozygous or compound heterozygous for POMC gene mutations. Similar to leptin signal-deficient patients, POMC-deficient children have a normal resting metabolism. They display mild central hypothyroidism that necessitates hormonal replacement (Krude *et al.*, 2003). The reason for this mild anomaly in the thyrotrophic axis is unknown despite the proposed influence of the melanocortin peptides on the hypothalamic pituitary axis (reviewed in Martin *et al.*, 2005). Most, but not all, POMC-deficient children have red hair and hypopigmentation. In some POMC-deficient mice, a normal pigmentation and hair color phenotype suggests that either the mouse MC1R has sufficient basal activity to trigger and sustain in vivo eumelanogenesis or that redundant non-melanocortin pathways compensate for this deficiency (Slominski *et al.*, 2005). Pigmentation varies greatly between individuals and particularly among ethnic groups, because of several differences in melanin (size, shape, density and type) and multiple polymorphisms in MC1R that influence its basal activity (Carroll *et al.*, 2005). Several observations, including an unpublished one from our group, suggest that the skin and hair phenotype might vary according to the ethnic origin of POMC mutation carriers (Challis *et al.*, 2002; Farooqi *et al.*, 2006) however further clarification on the skin phenotype is required prior to drawing conclusions. In the POMC-deficient children, a 3-month trial using a MC4R agonist had little effect on either weight or food intake (Krude *et al.*, 2003; Faroogi *et al.*, 2006) possibly due to the low affinity of the agonist. Nevertheless, POMC-deficient individuals might benefit from the new MC4R agonists currently under development.

2.3   *Proconvertase deficiency*

Mutations in enzymes involved in the processing of prohormones have also been described. Proconvertases such as carboxypeptidase E (Cpe) are essential for many prohormones processing including POMC, proinsulin and other gut hormones. The recessive fat mouse (Cpe^{fat}), characterized with hyperinsulinemia and the late onset of obesity, carries a Ser202Pro missence mutation in the Cpe gene (Naggert *et al.*, 1995). This Cpe^{fat} phenotype is reminiscent of the phenotype of an obese English patient in whom a mutation of Prohormone Convertase 1 (PC1) was found (Jackson *et al.*, 1997).

This woman displayed postprandial hypoglycemic malaises and fertility disorders. The delayed postprandial malaise was explained by the accumulation of proinsulin stemming from the lack of PC1 which is involved in insulin maturation. The absence of POMC maturation due to the PC1 mutation causes a dysfunctional melanocortin pathway and explains the obese phenotype (Jackson *et al.*, 1997). The discovery of a second case of PC1 deficiency has revealed default of processing of other hormones (Jackson *et al.*, 2003). A congenital PC1 deficiency leading to severe diarrhea due to severe small intestinal dysfunction was found in a very young obese girl, suggesting a possible role for PC1 in human intestinal absorptive function. To reinforce this hypothesis, the first PC1-deficient patient was re-examined and a milder intestinal phenotype was discovered. The processing of several intestinal prohormones – progastrin and proglucagon – was found to be altered, explaining, at least in part, the intestinal phenotype.

2.4   Other rare monogenetic forms

Naturally occurring mutations in mice have their human counterpart except the tubby mouse that displays late onset obesity, hyperinsulinemia and neuro-sensory defects (Carroll et al., 2004). Nevertheless the tubby gene (TUB) is a plausible candidate gene notably because of its expression in CNS areas playing a role in energy metabolism, its proposed role in insulin signaling and the contribution of TUB gene in the accumulation of fat in experimental models of *Caenorhabditis elegans* (Mukhopadhyay et al., 2005). The precise function of the TUB protein remains to be identified and the discovery of obese individuals lacking a functional TUB gene would help in validating its role in human body weight regulation.

In this regard, the role of new candidate genes was illustrated by the recent discovery of rare cases of monogenic obesity.

A severely obese young female who has a de novo balanced translocation between chromosomes 1p22.1 and 6q16.2 was identified. At 6 months the baby had a rate of early weight gain comparable to that of LEP or LEPR-deficient subjects and a voracious appetite but an increased linear growth. This translocation underlying her phenotype was due to the disruption of the single-minded homologue 1 (SIM1) gene located on chromosome 6 (Figure 2.3). This gene codes for a transcription factor that has a demonstrated role in murine development of the supraoptic and paraventricular nuclei of the hypothalamus (Holder et al., 2000).

The neurotrophic tyrosine receptor (TRKB) for the brain-derived neurotrophic factor (BDNF) is involved in the central regulation of food intake (Xu et al., 2003). The genetic manipulation of BDNF revealed that haploinsufficiency leads to obesity, hyperphagia and aggressiveness in mice (Lyons et al., 1999). A de novo heterozygous mutation in the NTRK2 gene, that encodes TRKB, was also described in an 8-year-old boy with early onset obesity, a mental retardation, developmental delay and anomalies in higher neurological functions such as early memory, learning and nociception (Yeo et al., 2004). This mutation leads to impairment in receptor autophosphorylation and alters the signaling to MAP kinase.

These studies emphasize the specific interest in exploring subgroups of obese phenotype in order to discover the role of novel candidate genes and gene products in the etiopathogenicity of obesity. In future genetic screening, the role of gene-encoding transcription factors and their target genes with a role in hypothalamus nuclei formation may be considered candidates in patients with obesity and hypothalamic hormonal dysfunctions. Whether or not these genes, including SIM1, might modulate the function of leptin and melanocortin in the control of food intake and energy expenditure is currently being investigated by specialists in the field. This line of research seems especially promising following the findings in which BDNF signaling via its receptor TRKB was found to be part of the MC4R mediated pathway (Xu *et al.*, 2003).

3.   Obesity with monogenic influence

3.1   *Mutations in the melanocortin 4 receptor*

Considering the pivotal role of the melanocortin pathway in the control of food intake and the discovery of syndromic obesity associated with melanocortin dysfunction, the MC4R gene became a candidate of choice for genetic studies in human obesity. The hypothesis that a dysfunction of MC4R could lead to obesity was reinforced by the study of MC4R knockout mice. These mice develop a morbid obesity and increased linear growth. Heterozygous mice display signs of intermediate obesity with variable degrees of severity with males being less affected than females. The use of MC4R pharmacological agonists in rodents reduces food intake, while antagonists of this receptor increase it (Huszar *et al.*, 1997; Butler, 2006).

These findings were followed by the discovery of mutations in the human MC4R gene. In 1998, together with the group of Steve O'Rahilly in Cambridge, we reported one of the first two frameshift mutations in MC4R that resulted in a truncated form of this protein in severely obese families (Vaisse *et al.*, 1998; Yeo *et al.*, 1998). Since then, more than 90 different mutations affecting the amino-acid composition in the protein have been described in different populations of German, French, English, Danish and American children and adults (Vaisse *et al.*, 1998; Hinney *et al.*, 1999; Farooqi *et al.*, 2000; Vaisse *et al.*, 2000; Dubern *et al.*, 2001a; Jacobson *et al.*, 2002; Miraglia Del Giudice *et al.*, 2002; Larsen *et al.*, 2004). They include frameshift, inframe deletion, nonsense and missense mutations, located throughout the coding sequence of the MC4R gene. To date, no mutation with a functional consequence has been described in the promoter region. The frequency of these mutations has been assessed as being between 0.5–3% of obesity cases (Carroll *et al.*, 2005).

Functional studies of MC4R mutations provided arguments for the patho-
genicity of such genetic alterations that are not common polymorphisms. The
response to a melanocortin agonist of mutant MC4R was commonly assayed.
After ligand binding, MC4R activation stimulates Gs protein with a subsequent
increase in cAMP levels. The production of intracellular cAMP in response to
αMSH demonstrated a broad heterogeneity in the activation of the different
MC4R mutants, ranging from normal or partial activation to a total absence of
activation (Vaisse et al., 2000; Yeo et al., 2003). More thorough functional
investigations were also performed for many, but unfortunately not all,
mutations. An intracellular transport defect of the mutated receptor, by
intracellular retention, was identified for the majority of MC4R mutations
found in childhood obesity (Lubrano-Berthelier et al., 2003a, 2003b), which
proffers a possible explanation for the impaired response to the agonist. MC4R
is constitutively active, meaning that it is basally active in the absence of a
ligand. Agouti-related peptide (AGRP) acts as an inverse agonist (Nijenhuis
et al., 2001). Therefore MC4R could have an inhibitory action on food intake, in
the absence of the ligand. The systematic study of basal activity of several
MC4R mutations has shown that an alteration in this activity may be the
only functional anomaly found, in particular for mutations located in the
N-terminal extra-cytoplasmic domain of this receptor (Srinivasan et al., 2004).
Thus, a tonic satiety signal, provided by the constitutive activity of MC4R could
be required for the long-term regulation of energy balance. It is generally
accepted that MC4R mutations cause obesity by a haploinsufficiency mechanism rather than a dominant negative activity. Since the role of homo- and
hetero-dimerization in G protein synthesis and maturation is proposed, some
dominant negative effect of MC4R mutations cannot be fully excluded. A
previous study has suggested a dominant negative effect for the D90N mutant
of MC4R (Biebermann et al., 2003). Efforts are now being made towards a
classification of MC4R mutations based on their functional consequences and
association with the subphenotypes of obesity (Lubrano-Berthelier et al., 2006).

Subjects homozygous for MC4R mutations develop severe forms of obesity
with very early development (Farooqi et al., 2000; Lubrano-Berthelier et al.,
2004). In contrast to the alterations in leptin and melanocortin pathways
described above, no endocrine abnormalities have been described in carriers of
MC4R gene alteration. The obese phenotype of MC4R mutations in heterozygotic carriers remains a matter of debate. Obesity usually has an autosomal
codominant mode of transmission in most of the families studied. Penetrance
of the disease is incomplete and the clinical expression associated to MC4R
mutations vary. Nevertheless a role for MC4R mutations in the facilitation of
early-onset obesity is widely accepted. An association between disorders of

feeding behavior such as "binge eating" and MC4R gene sequence changes have been described (Branson *et al.*, 2003), however, this finding currently remains very controversial (Farooqi *et al.*, 2003b; Gotoda, 2003; Herpertz *et al.*, 2003; Hebebrand *et al.*, 2004). Noteworthy to this study, patients with both MC4R mutations and common MC4R with and without functional consequences were grouped together to analyze genotype–phenotype correlations. The study of resting metabolic rate in some children or adults carrying MC4R mutations revealed that the basal energy expenditure was always related to the level of corpulence. This finding is in close agreement with a recent study in animal models (Cre/lox MC4R mice) showing that MC4R-expressing neurons in the paraventricular hypothalamus control food intake but not energy expenditure (Balthasar *et al.*, 2005). In children, bone mineral density increases in carriers of MC4R mutants were observed (Farooqi *et al.*, 2003b). The increased bone density observed in MC4R-deficient patients may be caused, at least in part, by a decrease in bone resorption. A decrease in bone resorption markers was indeed identified in patients with MC4R homozygous mutations (Elefteriou *et al.*, 2005). As a general rule, clinical analysis, even if carefully performed, does not allow for the easy detection of obesity stemming from MC4R mutation from the phenotype of common forms of early-onset obesity. After examining more than 769 obese adults and lean subjects, we recently showed that obese adults carrying functionally relevant MC4R mutations are not significantly characterized with either binge-eating disorder or a history of early-onset obesity. Rather, the onset and severity of the obesity in the carriers is related to the functional severity of the MC4R mutations (Lubrano-Berthelier *et al.*, 2006). The absence of a distinguishable phenotype in adults does not exclude that children carrying a MC4R mutation might express a phenotype (accelerated growth, hyperinsulinemia, anomalies of food intake behavior) that attenuates during adulthood (Farooqi *et al.*, 2003a). Overall MC4R mutations might be strong predictors for the development of obesity but the role of the environment as well as other genetic variants might be not negligible in the phenotypic expression of obesity. As shown by Irani and colleagues, the obese phenotype of MC4R KO mice can be overcome if regular exercise is started at an early stage (Irani *et al.*, 2005). Hyperphagia is particularly observed when fed with a high fat diet. Potentially modulating genetic factors located either in MC4R gene or other candidate genes might also modulate the phenotype (Dempfle *et al.*, 2004). A common V103I variant studied in more than 7500 subjects was negatively associated with obesity but no functional consequence of this variant on MC4R function was described (Heid *et al.*, 2005). The search for MC4R mutations in large general populations is also necessary to estimate their global frequency in populations not especially recruited for obesity gene studies (Govaerts *et al.*, 2005) and to explore possible gene–gene, gene–environment interaction. It is also essential to pursue the precise functional characterization of naturally occurring MC4R mutations carried by obese subjects. This will be useful in therapeutic intervention aiming at improving melanocortin action in the control of body weight homeostasis.

3.2   *Other suspected genes*

The MC3R gene has been the source of genetic investigation in obese and diabetic subjects because of its recognizable role in the control of body weight homeostasis (Tao, 2005). However, different functions in controlling body weight homeostasis were attributed to MC3R and MC4R. MC3R appears to be involved in increasing feeding efficiency while having only minor effects on the control of food intake itself. MC3R KO mice have increased fat and reduced lean body mass. In contrast with MC4R KO animals, MC3R KO mice are not hyperphagic (Huszar *et al.*, 1997; Marsh *et al.*, 1999; Chen *et al.*, 2000) and are prone to high fat diet-induced obesity.

Rare genetic data have been produced regarding naturally occurring mutations in the MC3R gene as reviewed by Tao (2005). One published study reported the occurrence of a MC3R mutation (Ile183Asn) in a nuclear family originating from India. This mutation was not found in the small number of lean subjects examined by the authors. The Ile183Asn mutation was observed in a severely obese 13-year-old girl and her obese father, but the other members of the family carrying the wild type allele were also obese or overweight. This case report is insufficient to reach a conclusion concerning the definitive role of MC3R I183N mutation in the pathogenesis of obesity within this family. Nevertheless the functional analysis of this mutation revealed a defect in the activation of MC3R in response to an agonist. Further genetic and functional studies are necessary to clarify the role of MC3R in the pathogenesis of obesity and abnormalities of fat partitioning, especially in humans.

Rare mutations in the POMC genes were also found in obese individuals with no other visible phenotype. In children from the UK, the frequency of an Arg236Gly mutation in POMC was mildly increased in obese subjects and a functional analysis revealed that the mutation prevented the normal processing of β-MSH and B-endorphin, resulting in an aberrant fusion protein (Challis *et al.*, 2002). Although able to bind MC4R, this aberrant peptide leads to a decrease in the activation of the receptor. In the same cohort, five unrelated probands were heterozygous for a rare missense variant in the region encoding beta-MSH, Tyr221Cys. The mutation was not found in lean controls suggesting association with obesity. The variant peptide was impaired in its ability to activate signaling through MC4R (Lee *et al.*, 2006). A loss-of-function missense mutation within the coding region for β-MSH (Y5C-β-MSH) was found in obese members of a family. It was suggested that the lack of functional β-MSH critically reduces the amount of MSH peptide in the POMC/MC4R signaling pathway, leading to mismanagement in weight (Biebermann *et al.*, 2006). Functional mutations in β-MSH might then be associated with obesity. The question remains whether POMC and MC3R may be considered as oligogenes such as MC4R.

4.   Polygenic obesity

4.1   *General and theoretical approach*

The genetic study of common forms of obesity is based on the analysis of variations in genomic DNA (genetic polymorphism or single nucleotide polymorphism, SNP) situated within or near candidate genes (Figure 2.2). Different strategies are utilized; linkage and association studies in family or in unrelated individuals. The aims are to determine whether an association exists between an allele of a gene and obesity traits (Hebebrand *et al.*, 2003; Perusse *et al.*, 2005). For this purpose, DNA and clinical data banks have been constituted in Europe and in the USA. A summary of these genetic studies, which concern a large number of genes and chromosomal regions, is reported each year in the international journal *Obesity* (Perusse *et al.*, 2005). It is impossible to provide details into all these studies; therefore we have focused on some genes encoding adiposity signals and specific brain factors.

4.2   *Genomic regions*

With the concept of genetic polymorphism and the development of powerful molecular tools, it is feasible to "rapidly" explore the genome of the families with common obesity. The objective is a systematic examination of all chromosomes in the families of obese subjects thanks to highly polymorphic markers and methods of analysis capable of detecting increased allelic sharing in obese sibpairs. This task is performed in the absence of knowledge regarding gene functions and aims at identifying known or novel genes predisposing an individual to obesity. The use of powerful molecular and statistical tools allows the genes to be positioned and eventually cloned; however it is not trivial to identify the specific gene when certain genomic linked regions are composed of thousands of nucleic acids. Nevertheless, these approaches have been applied to different cohorts throughout the world such as in families with extreme obesity occurring during adulthood or childhood (European and

American studies), families recruited from the general population (Quebec family study), and particular groups (Pima Indians, Mexican Americans, African Americans and Amish), among others (Perusse et al., 2005). This strategy has revealed several chromosomal locations linked with obesity. At least seven genes located on chromosomes 2, 5, 6, 10, 11, 19 and 20 have been significantly implicated in common obesity (all references in Perusse et al., 2005). Some loci might be more specific to morbid obesity or a childhood obesity (Saar et al., 2003; Meyre et al., 2005). A few regions have been confirmed in different populations; for example the 2p21 region seems to play a role in the variability of circulating leptin levels in French, Mexican American and African American people. The region on chromosome 10 is a region linked to obesity in French, German Caucasian and Amish cohorts. When considered together linking all chromosomal regions with obesity is far more complex than considering the results individually. All chromosomes, with the exception of Y, have been implicated and more than 200 chromosomal regions have been linked to different phenotypes such as fat mass, the distribution of adipose tissue, the occurrence of a metabolic syndrome, resting energy expenditure, energy and macronutrient intake, weight variation, the levels of circulating leptin and insulin; however it is important to note that most studies are based on the crude assessment of body mass index (BMI). Interactions between several chromosomal regions such as on chromosomes 10 and 20, and 2 and 13, have been found. These regions may interact to influence extreme obesity (Dong et al., 2004). This is a Sisyphean task to keep an updated view of all regions linked to obesity, particularly because a large number of non-significant and unreplicated results are produced. A further challenge is to identify the genes explaining the increase in polymorphism allele sharing in linked regions. When this has been completed and potential candidate genes hypothesized, the predisposing allelic variations must then be determined. The confirmation of the gene implication in the pathogenesis of the disease is another key issue.

4.3   Candidate genes

The choice of a candidate gene in obesity research is based on several criteria including the physiological role of its encoded protein in the mechanism of obesity, its chromosomal location in a region linked to obesity in human or animal models, the phenotypic consequences of its genetic manipulation (Knockout, transgenesis, floxed) in rodent models and eventually the in vitro functional characteristics of mutations or variations in this gene. The pattern of gene expression in critical tissues regulating weight management, or even its modification of expression in response to an environmental stress, can be used. However, it is rare that all these criteria are considered.

To briefly summarize 15 years of genetic analysis in obese populations in different countries, the "candidate gene" approach has not revealed the preponderant and unambiguous role of genes in the etiopathogenicity of common obesity and even recent studies are not definite, as illustrated with glutamate decarboxylase-2 GAD2 (discussed below). The reasons for this lack of reproducibility with most association and linkage studies tend to lie with a poor statistical power to detect modest effect, a lack of control over type 1 error rate, population stratification and an over-interpretation of marginal data. Other influencing factors may also affect reproducibility such as environmental factors which may vary within a population and are known to strongly influence the development of obesity. Similarly to the issues raised with linkage studies, it is rather difficult to isolate substantial results from sets of noisy data.

A very large number of genes and polymorphisms have been examined. These genes are implicated in controlling food intake, energy expenditure, lipid and glucose metabolism and more recently in inflammatory processes (Table 2.3). Table 2.3 shows examples of the most studied genes in independent populations. Of note, positive but also negative associations were found for all the gene variants. As with many other candidates, the genes implicated in the monogenic forms of obesity do not seem to play a more preponderant role in the development of common forms of obesity than others. Nevertheless they might not be excluded as potential targets for multi-factorial obesities and have been studied in different populations as previously reviewed (Poitou *et al.*, 2005a).

4.4   *Genes involved in the leptin/melanocortin axis*

Some associations and linkage between obesity phenotypes and the leptin or leptin receptor gene regions have been found (Table 2.3 and Poitou *et al.*, 2005a). POMC was also considered as a strong positional candidate. In Mexican Americans, variants located in the 3' and 5' untranslated region, with no functional impact on the protein, and haplotypes revealed association with leptin levels (Hixson *et al.*, 1999). How genetic variation in POMC (or another nearby gene) could contribute to leptin serum levels' variability remains to be discovered. In other populations, most of the polymorphisms located in the POMC gene were initially not associated with obese-related phenotypes and no functional influence could be predicted. In a larger recent study comprised of 1428 subjects from 248 non-obese families in the UK, not specifically recruited

Table 2.3 *Examples of candidate genes associated with obesity phenotypes in humans*

Genes (Code)	Locus	Animal model/phenotype	Human obesity locus (N)	Functional genetic variants
Food intake				
Leptin (LEP)	7q31	ob/ob mice/ severe obesity	Yes	No
Leptin receptor (LEPR)	1p31	db/db mice/ severe obesity	Yes	No
Agouti-related peptide (AGRP)	16q22	Transgenic/ obese KO/ non-obese	Yes	Yes (promoter activity)
Dopamine D2 receptor (DRD2)	11q23.2	KO/ non-obese	No	Decreased number of receptor
Energy metabolism				
Uncoupling protein 1 (UCP1)	4q28-q31	KO and transgenics/ reduced adiposity	No	No
Uncoupling protein (UCP2)	11q13	KO/ non-obese	Yes	Yes (change in UCP2 mRNA)
Uncoupling protein (UCP3)	11q13	KO/ non-obese	Yes	No
β3 adrenergic receptor (B3-AR)	9p12	KO/ increased adiposity	Yes	Decreased activity
G protein beta 3 subunit gene (GNB3)	12p13.3	no	Yes	Yes (modified G protein activation)
Adipose tissue metabolism				
Adiponectin (ACDC)	3q27	KO/ diet-induced insulin resistance	Yes	yes
Peroxisome proliferator activated receptor γ (PPARγ)	3p25	KO/ decreased brown adipose tissue	No	Decreased activity
Tumour necrosis factor α (TNFα)	6p21.3	KO/ increased adiposity under high fat diet	Yes	Yes (transcriptional activity)
β2 adrenergic receptor (β2-AR)	5q31-q32	KO/ increased adiposity under high fat diet	Yes	Decreased activity

Table 2.3 (*cont.*)

Genes (Code)	Locus	Animal model/phenotype	Human obesity locus (N)	Functional genetic variants
Interleukin 6 (IL6)	7p21	KO/ mature onset obesity	No	Yes
Lipasehormone sensitive (LIPE)	19q13.2	KO/ reduced abdominal fat mass/ resistance to diet-induced obesity	Yes	Yes in 1 study (decreased adipocyte lipolysis)
Glucocorticoid receptor (NCR3C1)	5q31	Floxed/ age-dependent modified adiposity	Yes	Differential response to glucocorticoids
Lipid and glucose metabolism				
Insulin (INS)	11p15.5	No	Yes	Yes
LDL receptor	19p13	No	Yes	No

Notes: This list of candidate gene is not exhaustive and the classification by function is arbitrary since these genes may participate in several functions. The genes selected are among the most studied ones in the genetics of human obesity. We selected genes showing positive association in more than 5 *independent* studies. The "animal model" column shows a spontaneous animal model or one created by genetic manipulations of invalidation (Knockout, KO), overexpression or floxed. Positive as well as negative associations have been found between single nucleotide polymorphisms (SNPs) located in all genes and obesity phenotypes. The "functional genetic variant" column shows the existence of genetic variants with functional consequences described in vitro.

for the genetic study of obesity, an association was found between variants spanning the POMC gene (variants located in the 3' and 5' region) and the waist/hip ratio (WHR) but not with BMI or leptin levels. However, the proportion of the variance in WHR attributed to the genetic variation was relatively small (1.1%) (Baker *et al.*, 2005). As described in Chapter 3, the potential contribution of POMC in the genetic predisposition to obesity mainly stems up to now from direct gene screening that revealed several rare mutations of low frequency associated with obesity (Carroll *et al.*, 2005). Studies in AGRP were also performed. Mutation screening of the AGRP gene coding region in obese children did not reveal significant mutations (Dubern *et al.*, 2001). A non-conservative amino acid substitution, Ala67Thr in the AGRP gene was moderately associated with abdominal adiposity in middle-age subjects (Argyropoulos *et al.*, 2002). This polymorphism was also associated with lower body weight in a small group of subjects belonging to the Quebec family study with the largest effect being observed on body fat mass; however no functional effect for this mutation was found in the various studies (Marks *et al.*, 2004; de Rijke *et al.*, 2005). In black populations, a functional −38C>T mutation (Bai *et al.*, 2004) in the AGRP gene promoter was also associated with leanness and type of macronutrient intake (Loos *et al.*, 2005).

Common polymorphisms of MC4R and MC3R were also found in both obese and lean populations. As noted above, a meta-analysis and a large screening of the Val103Ile variant of MC4R revealed that this variant is associated with a decreased BMI. Chromosome 20q13, where the MC3R gene is located, is a region that has been linked with obesity and type 2 diabetes in several studies (Perusse *et al.*, 2005). Attempts to associate common MC3R variants with obesity-related phenotypes, including body fat partitioning, were generally disappointing or irreproducible (Li *et al.*, 2000; Boucher *et al.*, 2002; Schalin-Jantti *et al.*, 2003) even if recent studies suggested the possible association between MC3R common variants and obesity (Yiannakouris *et al.*, 2004; Feng *et al.*, 2005). Regarding the TUB gene, in type 2 diabetic subjects it showed significant associations between several SNPs and the level of corpulence (Mak *et al.*, 2006; Shiri-Sverdlov *et al.*, 2006). In general, more systematic investigation of SNPs spanning genes in the melanocortin pathway in large obese and non-obese populations is still needed to decipher their role in the contribution to the polygenic nature of obesity.

4.5   *Genes identified by positional cloning*

The identification of new genes implicated in obesity may also be achieved by an alternate strategy: positional cloning. Three recent studies have revealed a significant difference in the SNP frequency between populations of obese subjects and controls. These SNPs are located in the gene encoding *SLC6A14* (solute carrier family 6 [neurotransmitter transporter], member 14) on chromosome X (Suviolahti *et al.*, 2003), *GAD2* on chromosome 10 (Boutin *et al.*, 2003) and ecto-nucleotide pyrophosphatase/phosphodiesterase 1 gene (*ENPP1/PC-1*) on chromosome 6 (Meyre *et al.*, 2005). The *SLC6A14* gene is of interest because it codes for an amino acid transporter able to regulate the availability of tryptophan during the synthesis of serotonin and thus may affect the regulation of appetite and mood. The genetic association with the *SLC6A14* gene was replicated in an independent French population (Durand *et al.*, 2004), but other screening in the large cohort collected in Europe and North America is necessary, as are functional studies aimed at unraveling the physiopathological role of variations in *SLC6A14* (Tiwari & Allison, 2003).

The gene *GAD2* encodes the 65kDa subunit of the glutamic acid decarboxylase enzyme (GAD65) which catalyzes the formation of GABA (γ-aminobutyric acid) that interacts with neuropeptide Y (NPY) in the hypothalamus to stimulate food intake. Three SNPs showed an association with morbid obesity in a French population. In the families, the SNPs segregate with obesity and an association was observed in a case-control study prompting a protective effect to be attributed to the wild-type allele. The role of one SNP located in the *GAD2* promoter was strengthened by a functional study revealing that the allele most frequently found in obese subjects exhibits greater transcriptional activity than the wild allele (Boutin *et al.*, 2003). This offers a possible explanation for the increase in hypothalamic GABA and the subsequent increase in food intake. This success story derived from a positional cloning strategy was dampened by the findings in a very large population of 2359 subjects comprised of more than 600 families of German origin, i.e. four times as many subjects as in the first report. In two independent case-control studies, the authors were unable to confirm the association of *GAD2* gene with severe obesity. No detectable effect for the *GAD2* promoter SNP was observed on transcription in cell lines using a reporter gene assay (Swarbrick *et al.*, 2005). This study illustrates once again the issues raised by genetic studies in humans affected by multifactorial diseases. If the reasons for the conflicting *GAD2* results may be attributed to usual caveats complicating the interpretation of genetic studies, the discrepancies in functional data are more problematic and will require clarification. Whether the linkage previously found on chromosome 10 is due to the impact of another candidate gene will also need to be investigated in the future.

4.6   *Gene–environment interaction*

Although the essential role of gene–gene and gene–environment interactions is fundamental to the progression of obesity, it is amazing to find that these interactions are little covered in genetic studies. This holds particularly true for genes involved in the leptin and melanocortin-signaling pathways. Most studies explored the effect of candidate gene variants on spontaneous weight gain or on the response to intervention promoting weight loss by either diet or gastric surgery in humans. Genetic variations of adrenoceptors, uncoupling proteins and PPARγ were the most investigated, yet the number of subjects studied remain limited (Perusse *et al.*, 2005) as reviewed by Verdich (Verdich *et al.*, 2004)

5.   Lessons learned from genetic studies

Combined genetic studies in rodents and rare human cases opened a new avenue of research in the field of obesity. Thanks to the characterization of some human mutations, it is clear that leptin and its target pathway have a fundamental role in energy balance and in the regulation of endocrine functions in humans. Monogenic obesity related to LEP and LEPR dysfunctions represent biological models of extreme obesity. Most of these cases associating severe obesity and endocrine abnormalities are very rare. In contrast, obesity associated with MC4R mutations is the most frequent situation of human obesity with identified genetic influence discovered to date. Classically a trait is considered to be oligogenic when two or more genes work together to produce a given phenotype. In the obesity context, this would imply that few genes might be determining the obese phenotype. Whether or not there are forms of obesity equivalent to MC4R-linked ones is yet to be discovered. Further investigation of genes implicated in the melanocortin pathway will probably provide this information in the future.

By looking at the complex picture of susceptibility genes in frequent cases of obesity, one might keep in mind that most genetic studies have mainly produced a large repertoire of predisposing alleles of diverse importance. Allelic gene variations are not necessarily sufficient for the expression of an obese phenotype. This might be true both for genes involved in the CNS and in the peripheral control of body weight regulation. Apart from the issues related to statistics as discussed above, one can note that the studies discussed here produced a list of common variants that may modify the risk of obesity occurring but only with a small degree of certainty. Even if confirmed or replicated in independent studies, these susceptibility alleles have to be incorporated in the overall picture of the many possible contributing environmental factors that may equally have strong effects (Ardlie *et al.*, 2002). The genetic background (characterized by the combination of multiple allelic variations), epigenetic or environmental factors that may include diet, exercise, stress, hormonal, socioeconomic factors and the developmental stage of epigenetic events may intervene in the occurrence, development and maintenance of obesity (Figure 2.1). Furthermore, it is conceivable individuals with a high genetic susceptibility to weight gain will have a potential to react to their environment only at certain points during their lifetime. This raises the issue of the appropriateness of future genetic testing for complex diseases such as obesity in which prevention is not a trivial task.

6.   Conclusion

With the establishment of DNA and clinical databanks of disparate cohorts of unrelated patients and of families, decisive progress in the understanding and management of obesity can be expected; however the best success has come from the study of extreme forms of obesity and syndromic obesity. The integrated study of hereditary characteristics within the genome and the function, regulation and interaction of genes is improving our approach to disease management with the ultimate goal of impacting on public health.

Acknowledgements

The program of genetic research on obesity in French families is supported by the Department of Clinical Research/Assistance Publique Hôpitaux de Paris (Hospital Clinical Research Programme) and a grant from the ANR (French National Research Agency, GIP-ANR). I warmly thank David Mutch and Michèle Guerre-Millo for their constructive comments when elaborating the manuscript.

References

Ardlie, K. G., Lunetta, K. L. & Seielstad, M. (2002). Testing for population subdivision and association in four case-control studies. *Am. J. Hum. Genet.* **71**, 304–11.

Argyropoulos, G., Rankinen, T., Neufeld, D. R. *et al.* (2002). A polymorphism in the human agouti-related protein is associated with late-onset obesity. *J. Clin. Endocrinol. Metab.* **87**, 4198–202.

Bahary, N., Leibel, R. L., Joseph, L. & Friedman, J. M. (1990). Molecular mapping of the mouse db mutation. *Proc. Natl. Acad. Sci. USA* **87**, 8642–6.

Bai, F., Rankinen, T., Charbonneau, C. *et al.* (2004). Functional dimorphism of two hAgRP promoter SNPs in linkage disequilibrium. *J. Med. Genet.* **41**, 350–3.

Baker, M., Gaukrodger, N., Mayosi, B. M. *et al.* (2005). Association between common polymorphisms of the proopiomelanocortin gene and body fat distribution: a family study. *Diabetes* **54**, 2492–6.

Balthasar, N., Dalgaard, L. T., Lee, C. E. *et al.* (2005). Divergence of melanocortin pathways in the control of food intake and energy expenditure. *Cell* **123**, 493–505.

Biebermann, H., Krude, H., Elsner, A. *et al.* (2003). Autosomal-dominant mode of inheritance of a melanocortin-4 receptor mutation in a patient with severe early-onset obesity is due to a dominant-negative effect caused by receptor dimerization. *Diabetes* **52**, 2984–8.

Biebermann, H., Castaneda, T. R., van Landeghem, F. *et al.* (2006). A role for beta-melanocyte-stimulating hormone in human body-weight regulation. *Cell Metab.* **3**, 141–6.

Boucher, N., Lanouette, C. M., Larose, M. *et al.* (2002). A +2138InsCAGACC polymorphism of the melanocortin receptor 3 gene is associated in human with fat level and partitioning in interaction with body corpulence. *Mol. Med.* **8**, 158–65.

Boutin, P., Dina, C., Vasseur, F. *et al.* (2003). GAD2 on Chromosome 10p12 is a candidate gene for human obesity. *PLoS Biol* **1**, E68.

Branson, R., Potoczna, N., Kral, J. G. *et al.* (2003). Binge eating as a major phenotype of melanocortin 4 receptor gene mutations. *N. Engl. J. Med.* **348**, 1096–103.

Bultman, S. J., Michaud, E. J. & Woychik, R. P. (1992). Molecular characterization of the mouse agouti locus. *Cell* **71**, 1195–204.

Butler, A. A. (2006). The melanocortin system and energy balance. *Peptides* **27**, 281–90.

Carroll, K., Gomez, C. & Shapiro, L. (2004). Tubby proteins: the plot thickens. *Nat. Rev. Mol. Cell Biol.* **5**, 55–63.

Carroll, L., Voisey, J. & van Daal, A. (2005). Gene polymorphisms and their effects in the melanocortin system. *Peptides* **26**, 1871–85.

Challis, B. G., Pritchard, L. E., Creemers, J. W. *et al.* (2002). A missense mutation disrupting a dibasic prohormone processing site in pro-opiomelanocortin (POMC) increases susceptibility to early-onset obesity through a novel molecular mechanism. *Hum. Mol. Genet.* **11**, 1997–2004.

Chen, A. S., Marsh, D. J., Trumbauer, M. E. *et al.* (2000). Inactivation of the mouse melanocortin-3 receptor results in increased fat mass and reduced lean body mass. *Nat. Genet.* **26**, 97–102.

Chung, W. K. & Leibel, R. L. (2005). Molecular physiology of syndromic obesities in humans. *Trends Endocrinol. Metab.* **16**, 267–72.

Clement, K., Vaisse, C., Lahlou, N. *et al.* (1998). A mutation in the human leptin receptor gene causes obesity and pituitary dysfunction. *Nature* **392**, 398–401.

Coleman, D. L. (1973). Effects of parabiosis of obese with diabetes and normal mice. *Diabetologia* **9**, 294–8.

Coll, A. P., Farooqi, I. S., Challis, B. G., Yeo, G. S. & O'Rahilly, S. (2004). Proopiomelanocortin and energy balance: insights from human and murine genetics. *J. Clin. Endocrinol. Metab.* **89**, 2557–62.

de Luca, C., Kowalski, T. J., Zhang, Y. *et al.* (2005). Complete rescue of obesity, diabetes, and infertility in db/db mice by neuron-specific LEPR-B transgenes. *J. Clin. Invest.* **115**, 3484–93.

de Rijke, C. E., Jackson, P. J., Garner, K. M. *et al.* (2005). Functional analysis of the Ala67Thr polymorphism in agouti related protein associated with anorexia nervosa and leanness. *Biochem. Pharmacol.* **70**, 308–16.

Dempfle, A., Hinney, A., Heinzel-Gutenbrunner, M. *et al.* (2004). Large quantitative effect of melanocortin-4 receptor gene mutations on body mass index. *J. Med. Genet.* **41**, 795–800.

Dong, C., Li, W. D., Li, D. & Price, R. A. (2004). Interaction between obesity-susceptibility loci in chromosome regions 2p25-p24 and 13q13-q21. *Eur. J. Hum. Genet.* **13**, 102–8.

Dubern, B., Clement, K., Pelloux, V. *et al.* (2001). Mutational analysis of melanocortin-4 receptor, agouti-related protein, and alpha-melanocyte-stimulating hormone genes in severely obese children. *J. Pediatr.* **139**, 204–9.

Durand, E., Boutin, P., Meyre, D. *et al.* (2004). Polymorphisms in the amino acid transporter solute carrier family 6 (neurotransmitter transporter) member 14 gene contribute to polygenic obesity in French Caucasians. *Diabetes* **53**, 2483–6.

Elefteriou, F., Ahn, J. D., Takeda, S. *et al.* (2005). Leptin regulation of bone resorption by the sympathetic nervous system and CART. *Nature* **434**, 514–20.

Farooqi, I. S. & O'Rahilly, S. (2004). Monogenic human obesity syndromes. *Recent Prog. Horm. Res.* **59**, 409–24.

Farooqi, I. S. & O'Rahilly, S. (2005). Monogenic obesity in humans. *Annu. Rev. Med.* **56**, 443–58.

Farooqi, I. S., Yeo, G. S., Keogh, J. M. *et al.* (2000). Dominant and recessive inheritance of morbid obesity associated with melanocortin 4 receptor deficiency. *J. Clin. Invest.* **106**, 271–9.

Farooqi, I. S., Keogh, J. M., Kamath, S. *et al.* (2001). Partial leptin deficiency and human adiposity. *Nature* **414**, 34–5.

Farooqi, I. S., Matarese, G., Lord, G. M. *et al.* (2002). Beneficial effects of leptin on obesity, T cell hyporesponsiveness, and neuroendocrine/metabolic dysfunction of human congenital leptin deficiency. *J. Clin. Invest.* **110**, 1093–103.

Farooqi, I. S., Keogh, J. M., Yeo, G. S. *et al.* (2003a). Clinical spectrum of obesity and mutations in the melanocortin 4 receptor gene. *N. Engl. J. Med.* **348**, 1085–95.

Farooqi, I. S., Yeo, G. S. & O'Rahilly, S. (2003b). Binge eating as a phenotype of melanocortin 4 receptor gene mutations. *N. Engl. J. Med.* **349**, 606–9.

Farooqi, I. S., Drop, S., Clements, A. *et al.* (2006). Heterozygosity for a POMC-null mutation and increased obesity risk in humans. *Diabetes.* **55**, 2549–53.

Feng, N., Young, S. F., Aguilera, G. et al. (2005). Co-occurrence of two partially inactivating polymorphisms of MC3R is associated with pediatric-onset obesity. *Diabetes* **54**, 2663–7.

Friedman, J. M., Leibel, R. L., Siegel, D. S., Walsh, J. & Bahary, N. (1991). Molecular mapping of the mouse ob mutation. *Genomics* **11**, 1054–62.

Gotoda, T. (2003). Binge eating as a phenotype of melanocortin 4 receptor gene mutations. *N. Engl. J. Med.* **349**, 606–609; author reply 606–609.

Govaerts, C., Srinivasan, S., Shapiro, A. et al. (2005). Obesity-associated mutations in the melanocortin 4 receptor provide novel insights into its function. *Peptides* **26**, 1909–19.

Halaas, J. L., Boozer, C., Blair-West, J., Fidahusein, N., Denton, D. A. & Friedman, J. M. (1997). Physiological response to long-term peripheral and central leptin infusion in lean and obese mice. *Proc. Natl. Acad. Sci. USA* **94**, 8878–83.

Hebebrand, J., Friedel, S., Schauble, N., Geller, F. & Hinney, A. (2003). Perspectives: molecular genetic research in human obesity. *Obes. Rev.* **4**, 139–46.

Hebebrand, J., Geller, F., Dempfle, A. et al. (2004). Binge-eating episodes are not characteristic of carriers of melanocortin-4 receptor gene mutations. *Mol. Psychiatry* **9**, 796–800.

Heid, I. M., Vollmert, C., Hinney, A. et al. (2005). Association of the 103I MC4R allele with decreased body mass in 7937 participants of two population based surveys. *J. Med. Genet.* **42**, e21.

Herpertz, S., Siffert, W. & Hebebrand, J. (2003). Binge eating as a phenotype of melanocortin 4 receptor gene mutations. *N. Engl. J. Med.* **349**, 606–9.

Hinney, A., Schmidt, A., Nottebom, K. et al. (1999). Several mutations in the melanocortin-4 receptor gene including a nonsense and a frameshift mutation associated with dominantly inherited obesity in humans. *J. Clin. Endocrinol. Metab.* **84**, 1483–6.

Hixson, J. E., Almasy, L., Cole, S. et al. (1999). Normal variation in leptin levels is associated with polymorphisms in the proopiomelanocortin gene, POMC. *J. Clin. Endocrinol. Metab.* **84**, 3187–91.

Holder, J. L., Jr., Butte, N. F. & Zinn, A. R. (2000). Profound obesity associated with a balanced translocation that disrupts the SIM1 gene. *Hum. Mol. Genet.* **9**, 101–8.

Huszar, D., Lynch, C. A., Fairchild-Huntress, V. et al. (1997). Targeted disruption of the melanocortin-4 receptor results in obesity in mice. *Cell* **88**, 131–41.

Irani, B. G., Xiang, Z., Moore, M. C., Mandel, R. J. & Haskell-Luevano, C. (2005). Voluntary exercise delays monogenetic obesity and overcomes reproductive dysfunction of the melanocortin-4 receptor knockout mouse. *Biochem. Biophys. Res. Commun.* **326**, 638–44.

Jackson, R. S., Creemers, J. W., Ohagi, S. et al. (1997). Obesity and impaired prohormone processing associated with mutations in the human prohormone convertase 1 gene. *Nat. Genet.* **16**, 303–6.

Jackson, R. S., Creemers, J. W., Farooqi, I. S. et al. (2003). Small-intestinal dysfunction accompanies the complex endocrinopathy of human proprotein convertase 1 deficiency. *J. Clin. Invest.* **112**, 1550–60.

Jacobson, P., Ukkola, O., Rankinen, T. *et al.* (2002). Melanocortin 4 receptor sequence variations are seldom a cause of human obesity: the Swedish Obese Subjects, the HERITAGE Family Study, and a Memphis cohort. *J. Clin. Endocrinol. Metab.* **87**, 4442–6.

Kennedy, G. C. (1953). The role of depot fat in the hypothalamic control of food intake in the rat. *Proc. R. Soc. Lond. B. Biol. Sci.* **140**, 578–96.

Krude, H., Biebermann, H., Luck, W., Horn, R., Brabant, G. & Gruters, A. (1998). Severe early-onset obesity, adrenal insufficiency and red hair pigmentation caused by POMC mutations in humans. *Nat. Genet.* **19**, 155–7.

Krude, H., Biebermann, H., Schnabel, D. *et al.* (2003). Obesity due to proopiomelanocortin deficiency: three new cases and treatment trials with thyroid hormone and ACTH 4-10. *J. Clin. Endocrinol. Metab.* **88**, 4633–40.

Lahlou, N., Clement, K., Carel, J. C. *et al.* (2000). Soluble leptin receptor in serum of subjects with complete resistance to leptin: relation to fat mass. *Diabetes* **49**, 1347–52.

Lander, E. S. (1996). The new genomics: global views of biology. *Science* **274**, 536–9.

Larsen, L. H., Echwald, S. M., Sorensen, T. I., Andersen, T., Wulff, B. S. & Pedersen, O. (2004). Prevalence of mutations and functional analyses of melanocortin 4 receptor variants identified among 750 men with juvenile-onset obesity. *J. Clin. Endocrinol. Metab.* **90**, 219–24.

Lee, Y. S., Challis, B. G., Thompson, D. A. *et al.* (2006). A POMC variant implicates beta-melanocyte-stimulating hormone in the control of human energy balance. *Cell Metab.* **3**, 135–40.

Li, W. D., Joo, E. J., Furlong, E. B. *et al.* (2000). Melanocortin 3 receptor (MC3R) gene variants in extremely obese women. *Int. J. Obes. Relat. Metab. Disord.* **24**, 206–10.

Licinio, J., Caglayan, S., Ozata, M. *et al.* (2004). Phenotypic effects of leptin replacement on morbid obesity, diabetes mellitus, hypogonadism, and behavior in leptin-deficient adults. *Proc. Natl. Acad. Sci. USA* **101**, 4531–6.

Loos, R. J., Rankinen, T., Rice, T. *et al.* (2005). Two ethnic-specific polymorphisms in the human Agouti-related protein gene are associated with macronutrient intake. *Am. J. Clin. Nutr.* **82**, 1097–101.

Lubrano-Berthelier, C., Cavazos, M., Dubern, B. *et al.* (2003a). Molecular genetics of human obesity-associated MC4R mutations. *Ann. N Y Acad. Sci.* **994**, 49–57.

Lubrano-Berthelier, C., Durand, E., Dubern, B. *et al.* (2003b). Intracellular retention is a common characteristic of childhood obesity-associated MC4R mutations. *Hum. Mol. Genet.* **12**, 145–53.

Lubrano-Berthelier, C., Le Stunff, C., Bougneres, P. & Vaisse, C. (2004). A homozygous null mutation delineates the role of the melanocortin-4 receptor in humans. *J. Clin. Endocrinol. Metab.* **89**, 2028–32.

Lubrano-Berthelier, C., Dubern, B., Lacorte, J. M. *et al.* (2006). Melanocortin 4 receptor mutations in a large cohort of severely obese adults: prevalence, functional classification, genotype-phenotype relationship and lack of association with binge eating. *J. Clin. Endocrinol. Metab.* **91**, 1811–18.

Lyons, W. E., Mamounas, L. A., Ricaurte, G. A. et al. (1999). Brain-derived neurotrophic factor-deficient mice develop aggressiveness and hyperphagia in conjunction with brain serotonergic abnormalities. Proc. Natl. Acad. Sci. USA 96, 15 239–44.

Mak, H. Y., Nelson, L. S., Basson, M., Johnson, C. D. & Ruvkun, G. (2006). Polygenic control of Caenorhabditis elegans fat storage. Nat. Genet. 38, 363–8.

Marks, D. L., Boucher, N., Lanouette, C. M. et al. (2004). Ala67Thr polymorphism in the Agouti-related peptide gene is associated with inherited leanness in humans. Am. J. Med. Genet. A. 126, 267–71.

Marsh, D. J., Hollopeter, G., Huszar, D. et al. (1999). Response of melanocortin-4 receptor-deficient mice to anorectic and orexigenic peptides. Nat. Genet. 21, 119–22.

Martin, N. M., Smith, K. L., Bloom, S. R. & Small, C. J. (2005). Interactions between the melanocortin system and the hypothalamo-pituitary-thyroid axis. Peptides 27, 333–9.

Mayer, J. (1953). Genetic, traumatic and environmental factors in the etiology of obesity. Physiol. Rev. 33, 472–508.

Meyre, D., Bouatia-Naji, N., Tounian, A. et al. (2005). Variants of ENPP1 are associated with childhood and adult obesity and increase the risk of glucose intolerance and type 2 diabetes. Nat. Genet. 37, 863–7.

Michaud, E. J., Bultman, S. J., Klebig, M. L. et al. (1994). A molecular model for the genetic and phenotypic characteristics of the mouse lethal yellow (Ay) mutation. Proc. Natl. Acad. Sci. USA 91, 2562–6.

Miraglia Del Giudice, E., Cirillo, G., Nigro, V. et al. (2002). Low frequency of melanocortin-4 receptor (MC4R) mutations in a Mediterranean population with early-onset obesity. Int. J. Obes. Relat. Metab. Disord. 26, 647–51.

Montague, C. T., Farooqi, I. S., Whitehead, J. P. et al. (1997). Congenital leptin deficiency is associated with severe early-onset obesity in humans. Nature 387, 903–8.

Mukhopadhyay, A., Deplancke, B., Walhout, A. J. & Tissenbaum, H. A. (2005). C. elegans tubby regulates life span and fat storage by two independent mechanisms. Cell Metab. 2, 35–42.

Naggert, J. K., Fricker, L. D., Varlamov, O. et al. (1995). Hyperproinsulinaemia in obese fat/fat mice associated with a carboxypeptidase E mutation which reduces enzyme activity. Nat. Genet. 10, 135–42.

Nijenhuis, W. A., Oosterom, J. & Adan, R. A. (2001). AgRP(83-132) acts as an inverse agonist on the human-melanocortin-4 receptor. Mol. Endocrinol. 15, 164–71.

Ollmann, M. M., Wilson, B. D., Yang, Y. K. et al. (1997). Antagonism of central melanocortin receptors in vitro and in vivo by agouti-related protein. Science 278, 135–8.

Ozata, M., Ozdemir, I. C. & Licinio, J. (1999). Human leptin deficiency caused by a missense mutation: multiple endocrine defects, decreased sympathetic tone, and immune system dysfunction indicate new targets for leptin action, greater central than peripheral resistance to the effects of leptin, and spontaneous correction of leptin-mediated defects. J. Clin. Endocrinol. Metab. 84, 3686–95.

Perusse, L., Rankinen, T., Zuberi, A. *et al.* (2005). The human obesity gene map: the 2004 update. *Obes. Res.* **13**, 381–490.

Poitou, C., Lacorte, J. M., Coupaye, M. *et al.* (2005a). Relationship between single nucleotide polymorphisms in leptin, IL6 and adiponectin genes and their circulating product in morbidly obese subjects before and after gastric banding surgery. *Obes. Surg.* **15**, 11–23.

Poitou, C., Viguerie, N., Cancello, R. *et al.* (2005b). Serum amyloid A: production by human white adipocyte and regulation by obesity and nutrition. *Diabetologia* **48**, 519–28.

Preti, A. (2003). Axokine (Regeneron). *IDrugs* **6**, 696–701.

Pritchard, J. K. (2001). Are rare variants responsible for susceptibility to complex diseases? *Am. J. Hum. Genet.* **69**, 124–37.

Saar, K., Geller, F., Ruschendorf, F. *et al.* (2003). Genome scan for childhood and adolescent obesity in German families. *Pediatrics* **111**, 321–7.

Schalin-Jantti, C., Valli-Jaakola, K., Oksanen, L. *et al.* (2003). Melanocortin-3-receptor gene variants in morbid obesity. *Int. J. Obes. Relat. Metab. Disord.* **27**, 70–4.

Seeley, R. J., Drazen, D. L. & Clegg, D. J. (2004). The critical role of the melanocortin system in the control of energy balance. *Annu. Rev. Nutr.* **24**, 133–49.

Shiri-Sverdlov, R., Custers, A., van Vliet-Ostaptchouk, J. V. *et al.* (2006). Identification of TUB as a novel candidate gene influencing body weight in humans. *Diabetes* **55**, 385–9.

Sleeman, M. W., Anderson, K. D., Lambert, P. D., Yancopoulos, G. D. & Wiegand, S. J. (2000). The ciliary neurotrophic factor and its receptor, CNTFR alpha. *Pharm. Acta. Helv.* **74**, 265–72.

Slominski, A., Fischer, T. W., Zmijewski, M. A. *et al.* (2005). On the role of melatonin in skin physiology and pathology. *Endocrine* **27**, 137–48.

Sorensen, T. I. (1995). The genetics of obesity. *Metabolism* **44**, 4–6.

Srinivasan, S., Lubrano-Berthelier, C., Govaerts, C. *et al.* (2004). Constitutive activity of the melanocortin-4 receptor is maintained by its N-terminal domain and plays a role in energy homeostasis in humans. *J. Clin. Invest.* **114**, 1158–64.

Strobel, A., Issad, T., Camoin, L., Ozata, M. & Strosberg, A. D. (1998). A leptin missense mutation associated with hypogonadism and morbid obesity. *Nat. Genet.* **18**, 213–15.

Stutz, A. M., Morrison, C. D. & Argyropoulos, G. (2005). The Agouti-related protein and its role in energy homeostasis. *Peptides* **26**, 1771–81.

Suviolahti, E., Ridderstrale, M., Almgren, P. *et al.* (2003). Pro-opiomelanocortin gene is associated with serum leptin levels in lean but not in obese individuals. *Int. J. Obes. Relat. Metab. Disord.* **27**, 1204–11.

Swarbrick, M. M., Waldenmaier, B., Pennacchio, L. A. *et al.* (2005). Lack of support for the association between GAD2 polymorphisms and severe human obesity. *PLoS Biol.* **3**, E315.

Tao, Y. X. (2005). Molecular mechanisms of the neural melanocortin receptor dysfunction in severe early onset obesity. *Mol. Cell Endocrinol.* **239**, 1–14.

Tartaglia, L. A., Dembski, M., Weng, X. *et al.* (1995). Identification and expression cloning of a leptin receptor, OB-R. *Cell* **83**, 1263–71.

Tiwari, H. K. & Allison, D. B. (2003). Do allelic variants of SLC6A14 predispose to obesity? *J. Clin. Invest.* **112**, 1633–6.

Vaisse, C., Clement, K., Guy-Grand, B. & Froguel, P. (1998). A frameshift mutation in human MC4R is associated with a dominant form of obesity. *Nat. Genet.* **20**, 113–14.

Vaisse, C., Clement, K., Durand, E., Hercberg, S., Guy-Grand, B. & Froguel, P. (2000). Melanocortin-4 receptor mutations are a frequent and heterogeneous cause of morbid obesity. *J. Clin. Invest.* **106**, 253–62.

Verdich, C., Clement, K. & Sorensen, T. I. (2004). Nutrient-gene interactions in the control of obesity. *Funct. Foods Aging Degenerat. Dis.* **10**, 219–59.

Williamson, D. A., Ravussin, E., Wong, M. L. *et al.* (2005). Microanalysis of eating behavior of three leptin deficient adults treated with leptin therapy. *Appetite* **45**, 75–80.

Xu, B., Goulding, E. H., Zang, K. *et al.* (2003). Brain-derived neurotrophic factor regulates energy balance downstream of melanocortin-4 receptor. *Nat. Neurosci.* **6**, 736–42.

Yeo, G. S., Farooqi, I. S., Aminian, S., Halsall, D. J., Stanhope, R. G. & O'Rahilly, S. (1998). A frameshift mutation in MC4R associated with dominantly inherited human obesity. *Nat. Genet.* **20**, 111–12.

Yeo, G. S., Lank, E. J., Farooqi, I. S., Keogh, J., Challis, B. G. & O'Rahilly, S. (2003). Mutations in the human melanocortin-4 receptor gene associated with severe familial obesity disrupts receptor function through multiple molecular mechanisms. *Hum. Mol. Genet.* **12**, 561–74.

Yeo, G. S., Connie Hung, C. C., Rochford, J. *et al.* (2004). A de novo mutation affecting human TrkB associated with severe obesity and developmental delay. *Nat. Neurosci.* **7**, 1187–9.

Yiannakouris, N., Melistas, L., Kontogianni, M., Heist, K. & Mantzoros, C. S. (2004). The Val81 missense mutation of the melanocortin 3 receptor gene, but not the 1908C/T nucleotide polymorphism in lamin A/C gene, is associated with hyperleptinaemia and hyperinsulinaemia in obese Greek caucasians. *J. Endocrinol. Invest.* **27**, 714–20.

Zhang, Y., Proenca, R., Maffei, M., Barone, M., Leopold, L. & Friedman, J. M. (1994). Positional cloning of the mouse obese gene and its human homologue. *Nature* **372**, 425–32.

3
_____

Hypothalamic control of energy homeostasis

NEEL S. SINGHAL AND REXFORD S. AHIMA

1. Introduction

The hypothalamus is a critical integrator of peripheral and central signals that mediate energy homeostasis. Over the last two decades, substantial progress has been made in elucidating the details of how neural, hormonal and nutrient signals from the gut and adipose tissue act on specific hypothalamic pathways to control energy balance and various physiologic processes. These hypothalamic circuits affect not only appetite, but through their diverse projections to the autonomic nervous system, brainstem and higher centers also influence motivational and motor function, and the endocrine system via the pituitary gland. Although the details of the interacting factors and effector mechanisms remain an area of active research, it is clear that neuropeptides at the level of the hypothalamus modulate key aspects of feeding behavior, energy expenditure and neuroendocrine function (Grill & Kaplan, 2002). In this chapter, we provide an overview of the hypothalamic circuitry within a framework for understanding its role as a sensor, integrator and effector of energy homeostasis and diverse physiologic processes.

2. Classical role of the hypothalamus in feeding regulation

A crucial involvement of the base of the diencephalon in energy homeostasis was first suggested by clinical observations in patients with

Neurobiology and Obesity, ed. Jenni Harvey and Dominic J. Withers. Published by Cambridge University Press. © Cambridge University Press 2008

pituitary tumors associated with excessive fat deposition and hypogonadism (Bramwell, 1888; Frolich, 1901). Several animal studies confirmed the importance of this region in body weight regulation, but it was not until the experiments of Hetherington and Ranson that the role of the hypothalamus rather than that of the pituitary gland was firmly established. In their classic study, large bilateral electrolytic lesions spanning the optic chiasm to the mammillary body (rostral-caudal), and into the lateral hypothalamic area and third ventricle (lateral-medial) were performed in rats. Remarkably, these lesions resulted in up to a doubling in body weight and marked lipid accumulation and fatty infiltration of tissues. The authors commented that, "symmetrical destruction of the ventral portion of this area, including the nuclei and possibly other structures near the base, seems to be more important than injury to the more dorsal structures for the production of maximum adiposity." Several studies also reported that lesions in the adjacent lateral hypothalamic areas could lead to a decrease in food intake (Clark et al., 1939; Hetherington & Ranson, 1940). Further pursuing these initial findings, Anand and Brobeck found that bilateral destruction of the lateral hypothalamus led to an abolishment of spontaneous eating, which prompted the designation of the lateral hypothalamus as a "feeding center" (Anand & Brobeck, 1951). From these observations arose the dual center model of neural regulation of feeding (Stellar, 1954), with the feeding center in the lateral hypothalamus and a satiety center in the ventromedial nucleus. While this model was influential in guiding investigation on feeding regulation, more refined experimental methodology and further analysis of the extent of lesions created in the initial studies led investigators to revise and challenge the dual center model (Ungerstedt, 1970; Gold, 1973). Modern cell biological techniques and the discovery of the adipocyte hormone, leptin and its receptors, led to the elucidation of a network of hypothalamic nuclei involved in feeding, satiety, and energy expenditure. Although substantial advances have made it clear that the regulation of energy balance is much more complex that the dual center model suggested by early research, many of the details of how peripheral and central signals specifically interact with hypothalamic and extra-hypothalamic circuits to regulate energy balance remain an area of active investigation.

3.   The hypothalamus mediates metabolic adaptations

The homeostatic systems regulating body weight display remarkable stability over long periods of time in spite of day-to-day variations in caloric intake and energy expenditure. To achieve long-term constancy of weight, coordinated networks of regulatory systems have evolved which allow for an

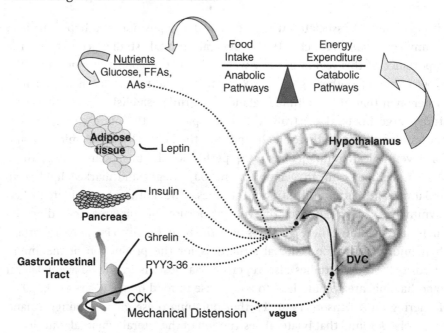

Figure 3.1 Brain-gut-adipose interactions in energy homeostasis. Nutrient, hormonal and neural signals act directly or indirectly on the hypothalamus. Hypothalamic nuclei coordinate metabolic adaptations which favor energy storage or expenditure. AAs, amino acids; CCK, cholecystokinin; DVC, dorsal vagal complex; FFAs, free fatty acids; PYY, peptide Y Y.

individual to appropriately balance food intake and energy expenditure. During the post-absorptive state of energy sufficiency, changes in specific peripheral signals sensitive to nutrient status engage hypothalamic circuits, which via central, peripheral, and neuroendocrine targets coordinate metabolic, behavioral, and cognitive states that allow for energy expenditure and reduce food intake. Conversely, during fasting, altered concentrations of various peripheral signals activate hypothalamic circuitry involved in stimulating anabolic metabolic pathways as well as energy-conserving and food-seeking responses (Figure 3.1). Thus, although food availability and energy expenditure demands vary greatly in the short term, body weight can be stably maintained over long periods.

4.   Overview of hypothalamic circuits controlling energy balance

As demonstrated by early lesion studies and supported by a diverse array of modern approaches, regulation of the metabolic processes maintaining

Table 3.1 *Peripheral factors involved in energy homeostasis.*

Adipokines	Pancreatic hormones	Other signals
Leptin	Insulin	Urocortin
Tumor necrosis factor-*α*	Amylin	IGF
Interleukin-6	Glucagon	Galanin-like peptide
? Adiponectin	Other hormones	
? Resistin	Glucocorticoids	
Gut hormones	Thyroid hormone	
Cholecystokinin	Gonadal steroids	
Ghrelin	Nutrients	
Glucagon-like peptide 1 and 2	Glucose, Pyruvate	
Gastric inhibitory polypeptide	Lactate	
Oxyntomodulin	Free fatty acids	
Peptide-YY	Amino acids	
Vasoactive intestinal peptide		

energy balance requires intact hypothalamic function. However, rather than specific hunger and satiety centers located in discrete hypothalamic nuclei as suggested by early research, energy homeostasis is regulated by interconnected and redundant neuronal circuits which signal via various neuropeptides as well as classical neurotransmitters. The hypothalamus coordinates metabolic responses in large part through sensing of peripheral signals sensitive to metabolic status, such as leptin and insulin (Table 3.1). The arcuate nucleus of the hypothalamus (ARC) contains receptors for leptin, insulin and various peptides and is able to integrate the metabolic information they provide, although other hypothalamic as well as extra-hypothalamic areas contain receptors for numerous peripheral signals (Figures 3.1, 3.2, 3.3). Utilizing a network of neuropeptides and neurotrans-mitters, the ARC relays this information to second-order hypothalamic sites such as the paraventricular nucleus (PVN), lateral hypothalamus/perifornical area (LHA), dorsomedial nucleus (DMN), and ventromedial nucleus (VMN) (Table 3.2; Figure 3.3). These second-order neurons also allow for an additional point of regulation prior to activation of third-order projections to extra-hypothalamic areas.

Three major effector mechanisms, which are not entirely independent, are utilized by the hypothalamus to appropriately modulate energy balance: (1) control of appetite, (2) endocrine modulation of thermogenesis and (3) auto-nomic/involuntary modulation of energy expenditure (Figure 3.3). The ability of

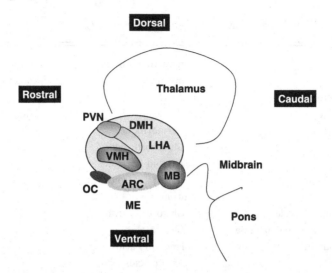

Figure 3.2 Hypothalamic nuclei involved in energy homeostasis. ARC, arcuate nucleus; DMH, dorsomedial hypothalamus; LHA, lateral hypothalamic area; MB, mammillary body; ME, median eminence; OC, optic chiasm; PVN, paraventricular nucleus; VMH, ventromedial hypothalamus.

the hypothalamus to respond to changes in peripheral signals and control appetite has been well established; however, the details of how hypothalamic nuclei and their downstream projections lead to a reduction in appetite and cessation of feeding remain an area of active investigation. Equally as important as the control of appetite, the hypothalamus is also able to modulate thermogenesis via endocrine modulation of peripheral targets such as the thyroid gland and adrenal gland. This is accomplished primarily by neurons of the PVN which can modulate release of stimulatory hormones by the pituitary gland. The third mechanism which the hypothalamus utilizes to alter energy expenditure involves downstream projections to nuclei critical to regulating autonomic output as well as those controlling involuntary motor behaviors. Second-order hypothalamic regions such as the PVN and LHA are a source of preganglionic autonomic projections, which can alter metabolism and energy expenditure by shifting the balance between sympathetic and parasympathetic nervous output to skeletal muscle and other targets such as brown adipose tissue. In adult humans, who lack brown adipose tissue, more important may be the ability of the hypothalamus to drive involuntary movements such as fidgeting which is associated with non-exercise activity thermogenesis, a key determinant of energy expenditure in humans (Levine, 2002).

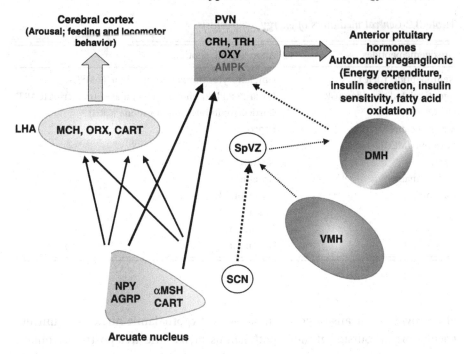

Figure 3.3 Hypothalamic neuronal circuitry. PVN, paraventricular nucleus; ORX, orexins; OXY, oxytocin; SpVZ, subparaventricular zone; SCN, suprachiasmatic nucleus; AMPK, AMP-activated protein kinase; AGRP, agouti-related protein; CART, cocaine- and amphetamine-regulated transcript; CRH, corticotropin releasing hormone; DMH, dorsomedial hypothalamus; LHA, lateral hypothalamic area; MCH, melanin-concentrating hormone; NPY, neuropeptide Y; TRH, thyrotropin-releasing hormone; VMH, ventromedial hypothalamus.

5. Peripheral nutrient-related signals and vagal inputs inuence hypothalamic output

The arcuate nucleus (ARC) in particular is essential to integrating the numerous peripheral signals that allow for the fine control of appetite and energy expenditure. Peripheral signals access the ARC and other hypothalamic nuclei via two mechanisms: (i) transport mechanisms across the blood–brain barrier (BBB) or (ii) diffusion through the fenestrated capillaries present at circumventricular organs (CVO) such as the median eminence (Broadwell & Brightman, 1976). Specific, saturable transport mechanisms across the BBB have been characterized for insulin and leptin (Banks *et al.*, 1996), while other peripheral hormones such as peptide YY and glucagon-like peptide 1 (GLP-1), are able to cross the BBB via a non-saturable mechanism (Kastin *et al.*, 2002). Diffusion of peripheral hormones through CVOs like the median eminence

Table 3.2 *Central mediators of energy homeostasis.*

Orexigenic peptides	Anorexigenic peptides
Neuropeptide Y (NPY)	a-melanocyte-stimulating hormone (a-MSH)
Agouti-related peptide (AGRP)	Cocaine and amphetamine-regulated transcript (CART)
Orexin A/B	Corticotropin-releasing hormone (CRH)
Melanin-concentrating hormone (MCH)	Urocortin
Opioids	Neurotensin
Endocannabinoids	Ghrelin
Galanin	Glucagon-like peptide 1 (GLP-1)
	Glucagon
	Bombesin
	Histamine

also provides a means of access to adjacent hypothalamic nuclei. Circumventricular organs outside of the hypothalamus such as the area postrema contain receptors for many of these peripheral signals which also contribute to their effects on energy regulation.

Much of what is currently known about the details of the hypothalamic circuitry controlling food intake and energy expenditure comes from examination of the neural mediators of leptin action. However, as shown in Table 3.1, a myriad of other hormones, gut-derived peptides and nutrients also shape the output of the hypothalamic circuitry regulating energy homeostasis. One of the first peripherally synthesized hormones found to alter energy homeostasis was insulin. Similar to leptin, centrally administered insulin decreases food intake by acting on specific receptors expressed in the arcuate nucleus. Other adipocyte-derived factors including adiponectin as well as gut-derived peptides such as cholecystokinin, ghrelin, proglucagon products, and the PP-fold peptides also appear to play a role in the regulation of food intake and/or energy expenditure in part by acting on the arcuate nucleus (Elias *et al.*, 1999).

The vagus nerve is another important afferent signal regulating energy balance. Vagal nerve sensory afferents from the upper-gastrointestinal tract project in a viscerotopic manner to the nucleus of the solitary tract (NTS). These afferents relay information about luminal distension, nutritional content, and are also sensitive to locally released gut peptides and neurotransmitters. Although integration of these signals at NTS is sufficient to partially modulate meal size, second-order vagal afferents terminate in regions of the basal forebrain which relay information critical to energy balance regulation.

6.   Integration of peripheral signals by the arcuate nucleus

Within the hypothalamus, attention has focused on the ARC as the key site of integration of peripheral metabolic cues (Figure 3.3). Neurons of the ARC express an assortment of receptors for various metabolically active peripheral factors. Thus, by responding dynamically to multiple hormonal signals, the ARC acts as an integrator of metabolic information as well as a relay of this integrated metabolic information to other hypothalamic and neural regions which participate in initiating the appropriate metabolic response. The details of how the ARC and other hypothalamic areas participate in the processing of multiple peripheral signals is still an active area of investigation, however, substantial evidence indicates that integrative properties at both the circuit and single-neuron level play a critical role.

The ARC is located at the base of the hypothalamus immediately above the median eminence bordering the third cerebral ventricle and extending from the posterior edge of the optic chiasm to the mammillary bodies. The median eminence, a CVO, by virtue of its position near the third ventricle and proximity to the portal vasculature provides access to a wide range of hormonal and nutrient signals (Broadwell & Brightman, 1976). The ARC consists of two major subpopulations of neurons which express distinct sets of neuropeptides (Figure 3.3). Neurons located in the medial half of the ARC express both neuropeptide-Y (NPY) and agouti-related protein (AGRP), which are potent orexigens and also stimulate other relevant aspects of endocrine and autonomic function discussed in subsequent sections. The lateral half of the ARC contains neurons co-expressing the anorexigenic cocaine and amphetamine-regulated transcript (CART) and proopiomelanocortin gene (POMC), which is the precursor for both beta-endorphin and the melanocortin-3/4 receptor (MC3/4R) agonist, a-melanocyte-stimulating hormone (a-MSH). These opposing sets of neuronal populations in the ARC send projections to target regions within the hypothalamus including the PVN and LHA. These other hypothalamic sites then relay information to other hypothalamic areas as well as to cortical, brainstem and autonomic circuits involved in the execution of the appropriate metabolic response (Figure 3.3).

The discovery of leptin and its receptors in the hypothalamus has greatly aided our understanding of the neurocircuitry regulating feeding and energy expenditure. The anorexigenic actions of leptin stem from its effects on ARC neurons expressing the long form of the leptin receptor (LRb), which signals via the JAK/STAT-3 pathway to modulate gene expression (Tartaglia, 1997). Leptin receptor mRNA is highly expressed in the hypothalamus, including NPY- and POMC-containing cells of the ARC (Elmquist et al., 1998). Although both populations of ARC neurons contain LRb, leptin stimulates the transcription of the orexigenic peptides POMC/CART, while it inhibits transcription of the anorexigenic peptides NPY/AGRP. The details of this differential regulation remain to be determined but likely involve activation of distinct intracellular targets downstream of JAK/STAT-3 in NPY and POMC cells such as suppressor of cytokine signaling-3 (SOCS-3) (Elias *et al.*, 1999), PI3K (Niswender & Schwartz, 2003), or FoxO1 (Kitamura *et al.*, 2006). Thus, by repressing NPY/AGRP expression and increasing that of POMC/CART, leptin promotes satiety and increases energy expenditure. The differential regulation of POMC/CART as compared to NPY/AGRP induces hyperphagia and energy conservation during fasted states when leptin levels are reduced. In contrast, the divergent effects of leptin on NPY/AGRP and POMC/CART increase energy expenditure and induce satiety in post-absorptive states when leptin levels are elevated.

The ARC also contains a dense concentration of insulin and ghrelin receptors (growth hormone secretagogue receptor: GHS-R) (Tannenbaum *et al.*, 1998). Similar to leptin, insulin inhibits NPY/AGRP while stimulating POMC/CART, resulting in appetite suppression and increased energy expenditure (Schwartz *et al.*, 2000). Ghrelin, on the other hand, increases expression of NPY, leading to an increase in food intake (Nakazato *et al.*, 2001). Other metabolically relevant nutrients and hormones have been found to modulate expression of these peptides including oleic acid (Obici *et al.*, 2002a), PYY (Acuna-Goycolea & Van den Pol, 2005), and pancreatic amylin (Lutz, 2006; Table 3.1). Some of these signals are known to have receptors expressed in the ARC, however, the degree to which they participate in regulating neural circuits and intracellular signals overlapping with those of leptin and insulin requires further study.

This reciprocal regulation of ARC neurons by leptin has served as a model by which the orexigenic/anorexigenic actions of other hormones and peptides are evaluated. However, it is clear that several other peripheral and central factors continuously provide input to the ARC. Moreover, areas outside of the ARC are also responsible for integrating peripheral and central metabolic information adding an additional layer of complexity. Thus, regulation of hypothalamic circuits is a dynamic phenomenon, the output of which can be modulated by a multitude of inputs.

7.   Hypothalamic signal transduction

Further specificity and complexity in the hypothalamic regulation of energy balance also resides at the level of single neurons, where multiple metabolically active signals may converge to ultimately modulate common intracellular molecules. Although still currently an active area of investigation,

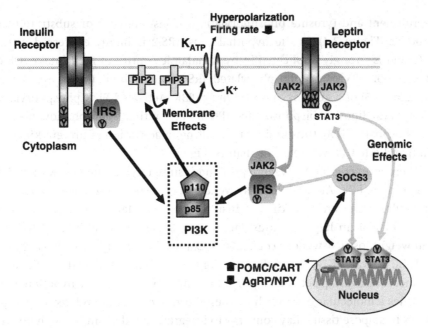

Figure 3.4 Leptin and insulin signal transduction in the hypothalamus. AGRP, agouti-related protein; CART, cocaine- and amphetamine-regulated transcript; JAK2, janus kinase-2; K-ATP, ATP-sensitive potassium channel; IRS, insulin receptor substrate; NPY, neuropeptide Y; PI3K, phosphatidylinositol-3-OH-kinase; PIP2, phosphatidylinositol-bisphosphate; PIP3, phosphatidylinositol-trisphosphate; POMC, proopiomelanocortin; SOCS3, suppressor of cytokine signaling-3; STAT3, signal transducer and activator of transcription-3.

candidate molecules that may be important integrators of multiple metabolic signals such as leptin and insulin include phosphatidylinositol-3-OH-kinase (PI3K), AMP-activated protein kinase (AMPK), and ATP-sensitive potassium (K-ATP) channels (Figure 3.4). Leptin activates the JAK-STAT pathway (Tartaglia, 1997). Jaks associate constitutively with conserved box 1 and 2 motifs in the intracellular domain of LRb. Binding of leptin to the LRb extracellular domain results in autophosphorylation of JAK2, phosphorylation of tyrosine residues on the LRb cytoplasmic domain, and activation of downstream transcription factors, named STATs. LRb has three conserved tyrosine residues, Y985, Y1077 and Y1138, in the intracellular domain. Leptin phosphorylates Y1138 recruiting STAT3 via its SH2 domain. Tyrosyl-phosphorylated STAT3 then undergoes homodimerization, is translocated into the nucleus and regulates transcription of neuropeptide and various mediators of leptin (Figure 3.4).

As in peripheral tissues, neuronal activation of the insulin receptor, a tyrosine kinase and member of the growth factor receptor family, induces the recruitment and tyrosine phosphorylation of insulin-receptor substrate (IRS) proteins (Figure 3.4). In the hypothalamus, IRS-2 is highly expressed in the ARC and is strongly implicated in hypothalamic control of food intake (Obici et al., 2002). Tyrosine phosphorylated IRS proteins bind to the regulatory domain (p85) of a key enzyme known as PI3K. Activated PI3K phosphorylates phosphatidylinositol-bisphosphate (PIP2) generating phosphatidylinositol-trisphosphate (PIP3), thus indirectly resulting in activation of protein kinase B (Akt) and other downstream mediators (Figure 3.4).

There is an overlap between leptin and insulin targets, such as IRS-1 and 2, MAP kinase, ERK, Akt and PI3K (Niswender et al., 2004; Morton et al., 2005). Of particular importance, leptin and insulin both stimulate IRS-2-mediated activation of PI3K in hypothalamus (Figure 3.4), leading to inhibition of feeding and weight loss (Niswender et al., 2004). Conversion of PIP2 to PIP3, catalyzed by PI3K, activates K_{ATP} channels, which are also important regulators of energy balance. The overlap between leptin and insulin signaling in the hypothalamus provides a molecular basis for how these hormones that are related to energy stores in adipose tissue may converge to integrate metabolism. Though not yet well-examined, it is possible that other peripheral hormones related to energy stores and gut function signal in the hypothalamus through similar intracellular signaling mechanisms as leptin and insulin.

AMP-activated protein kinase (AMPK) acts a sensor of cellular energy stores. Increasing evidence suggests that this pathway plays a crucial role in the hypothalamic coordination of metabolic responses (Kahn et al., 2005). AMPK in the hypothalamus is phosphorylated and activated by fasting, hypoglycemia, AGRP and ghrelin. Conversely, feeding, hyperglycemia, insulin, leptin and melanocortin agonists suppress AMPK (McCrimmon et al., 2004; Minokoshi et al., 2004). Likewise, inhibitors of fatty acid synthase or carnitine palmitoyl transferase (CPT)-1 suppress hypothalamic AMPK (Obici et al., 2003; Landree et al., 2004). Thus, regulation of hypothalamic AMPK activity appears to be coupled to the status of energy balance, leading to alterations in feeding, thermogenesis and weight. It is plausible that AMPK activation mediates differential changes in the levels of orexigenic versus anorexigenic peptides; however, the specific neuronal circuits are yet to be delineated.

ATP-sensitive K+ channels (K_{ATP}) belong to the family of inward rectifier (Kir) channels, which are important stabilizers of membrane potential (Nichols, 2006). K_{ATP} channels are found in various tissues throughout the body, including the pancreas and hypothalamus. High ATP concentrations inhibit the K_{ATP} channel, while decreasing ATP concentrations allow the channel to open. Thus, these channels act as sensors of cellular metabolism. In the pancreatic islets, the presence of glucose leads to increased ATP and cell depolarization which causes insulin to be released. Spanswick and colleagues first demonstrated that hypothalamic K_{ATP} channels open in response to peripheral signals such as leptin and insulin in normal rats leading to neuronal hyperpolarization (Spanswick *et al.*, 1997). Obese Zucker rats have defective LRb and K_{ATP} channel (Spanswick *et al.*, 1997, 2000). The activation of K_{ATP} channels stems from the effects of leptin and insulin on increasing PIP3 via PI3K activity (Shyng & Nichols, 1998; Plum *et al.*, 2006; Figure 3.4). While the specific means whereby leptin and insulin exert their hyperpolarizing effects are unclear, most ARC NPY cells contain Kir6.2, a subunit of the K_{ATP} channel, suggesting this may be a potential target. Recent studies have also found that free fatty acids, lactate and pyruvate can modify the activity of K_{ATP} channels, which leads to alterations in food intake as well as glucose homeostasis (Obici *et al.*, 2002a; Lam *et al.*, 2005). Thus, K_{ATP} represents another molecule on which hormones and nutrient signals may converge (Figure 3.4).

Leptin and insulin both induce suppressor of cytokine signaling (SOCS)-3 in hypothalamic neurons. SOCS-3 is a member of a family of proteins which inhibits JAK-STAT signaling and acts as a negative regulator of leptin and insulin signaling (Figure 3.4). As predicted, haploinsufficiency of SOCS-3 and, in particular, neuronal deletion of SOCS-3 led to enhancement of leptin-induced hypothalamic STAT3 phosphorylation, an increase in POMC levels in the hypothalamus, and reductions in food intake and body weight (Howard *et al.*, 2004; Mori *et al.*, 2004). The increase in leptin sensitivity in SOCS-3 deficiency was associated with enhancement of insulin sensitivity (Mori *et al.*, 2004).

Direct sensing of nutrients, especially glucose, has long been thought to be critical to initiating food-seeking responses. Glucose is the primary fuel utilized by the brain, and as even a few minutes of glucose deprivation will cause irreversible damage, the brain is especially sensitive to hypoglycemia. As such several biochemical processes have evolved that help maintain glucose at nearly constant physiological concentrations, even after longer periods of fasting. Nevertheless, to prevent hypoglycemia the brain must be able to sense falling serum glucose levels and coordinate the appropriate metabolic and behavioral responses. Glucose-sensing neurons are specialized cells located in the hypothalamus (Oomura *et al.*, 1969) and brainstem (DiRocco & Grill, 1979), which respond to changes in extracellular glucose by altering their firing rate. Within the hypothalamus, the glucose-sensing properties of VMN cells have received the most attention, although it is now also apparent that the orexin- and MCH-containing cells in the LH also display alterations in electrophysiological properties under conditions of varying glucose concentration (Burdakov *et al.*, 2005).

Subpopulations of neurons within the VMN are thought to be particularly important in sensing falls in glucose and initiating autonomic and endocrine responses such as increased sympathetic outflow and the release of glucagon, epinephrine and corticosterone which facilitates an increase in serum glucose (Borg et al., 1997). Elevations in extracellular glucose levels in a physiological range increases firing rate of a subpopulation of glucose-responsive VMN neurons, while decreasing the action potential frequency of glucose-sensitive neurons (Routh, 2003). Local stimulation or glucose deprivation in the VMN (Borg et al., 1995) results in activation of counter-regulatory responses, while lesions of VMN lead to increased parasympathetic tone (Yoshimatsu et al., 1984), further supporting a role for this region in responding to glucose levels and coordinating the appropriate metabolic response. While the details of how changes in extracellular glucose result in altered neuronal electrical activity are not fully understood, glucose-responsive neurons, like pancreatic β-cells, may utilize glucokinase to sense physiological changes in glucose concentrations (Routh et al., 2002).

Several reports have suggested that fatty acids' permeability across the blood–brain barrier is very high (Miller et al., 1987; Rapoport, 1999). In addition, several hypothalamic nuclei express enzymes involved in fatty acid metabolism including fatty acid synthase (FAS), acetyl coenzyme A carboxylase (ACC), CPT1, and malonyl-CoA decarboxylase (MCD; Kim et al., 2000). Recent studies have suggested that intraneural accumulation of long-chain fatty acyl CoA (FACoA) molecules via central infusion of oleic acid or inhibitors of CPT1 or FAS, leads to sustained anorexia, weight loss, and inhibition of hypothalamic NPY gene expression (Loftus et al., 2000; Obici et al., 2002b, 2003). While these studies link changes in neuronal fat metabolism to alterations in feeding and neuropeptide expression, further clarification of the regulation of neuronal FACoA content in physiological conditions and the mechanism by which it alters neuronal function are needed for a more complete understanding of this nutrient-sensing system in energy homeostasis.

8.   Electrophysiological responses of hypothalamic neurons to energy fluxes

While alterations in the expression levels of neuropeptides in response to peripheral metabolic cues are critical to initiating metabolic responses, as in other neural circuits, it is important to consider the rapid electrophysiological responses of hypothalamic cells to metabolic cues. In normal mice, fasting induces a rapid increase in action potential frequency in NPY/AGRP neurons (Takahashi & Cone, 2005). $Lep^{ob/ob}$ and $Lepr^{db/db}$ mice have higher action potential frequency in NPY/AGRP neurons, and they display no further increase during fasting (Takahashi & Cone, 2005). Interestingly, leptin treatment reduces the action potential frequency in fasted and $Lep^{ob/ob}$ mice, demonstrating that leptin is an important modulator of neurotransmission in these cells.

Recordings in hypothalamic slice preparations taken from mice genetically engineered to express fluorescent proteins in specific cell types have demonstrated that leptin acutely increases action potential frequency in POMC neurons, directly by leading to the opening of non-specific cation channels and indirectly by decreasing inhibitory GABA-mediated tone from local ARC NPY-expressing neurons (Cowley et al., 2001). Leptin also hyperpolarizes and decreases action potential firing in NPY/AGRP neurons, although the mechanism has not been characterized. Insulin is known to produce changes similar to leptin in hypothalamic neuropeptide expression, but it is not currently known whether it causes similar electrophysiological effects.

Ghrelin, which stimulates feeding and NPY expression in the ARC, has been found to dose-dependently stimulate action potential firing in a large proportion of cells that leptin inhibits (Van den Top et al., 2004). Bath application of ghrelin to hypothalamic slices increases spontaneous action potentials in NPY/AGRP neurons. Ghrelin was found to increase burst firing in NPY/AGRP neurons, which is a more effective stimuli for neuropeptide/neurotransmitter release. Contrary to leptin action, ghrelin decreases spontaneous activity in POMC neurons, which is dependent on the presynaptic activation of NPY/AGRP neurons. Calcium imaging studies also support a role for ghrelin in increasing activity of NPY neurons (Kohno et al., 2003).

9.   Role for hypothalamic plasticity in energy balance?

Leptin-deficient $Lep^{ob/ob}$ mice differ from wild-type mice by having greater excitatory than inhibitory synapses in NPY and POMC neurons (Pinto et al., 2004). This difference is reversed by leptin treatment and precedes the inhibition of feeding (Pinto et al., 2004). This suggests that hypothalamic circuits exhibit some degree of plasticity in response to adiposity signals such as leptin. Leptin is known to have a crucial role in brain development based on earlier reports of smaller brains in $Lep^{ob/ob}$ and $Lepr^{db/db}$ mice (Sena et al., 1985; Ahima et al., 1999), and more importantly, leptin treatment also reverses structural deficits in the brains of genetically leptin-deficient patients (Matochik et al., 2005). Neurotrophic actions of leptin have been demonstrated in vivo and in vitro. $Lep^{ob/ob}$ mice manifest a delay in maturation of the arcuate-PVN projection, which is corrected by leptin treatment during the postnatal period (Bouret et al., 2004). Leptin may also play a role in neuronal survival by preventing apoptosis (Russo et al., 2004). A neonatal leptin surge has been implicated in obesity and insulin resistance during adulthood (Yura *et al.*, 2005). These results in conjunction with the close correlation between the ontogeny of hypothalamic neuropeptides and timing of leptin's effects on thermogenesis and feeding, suggest that leptin may be involved in obesity by controlling neuronal structure and function (Ahima *et al.*, 1999; Bouret *et al.*, 2004).

Recently, brain-derived neurotrophic factor (BDNF), a neurotrophin that is critical for brain development and neuroplasticity in mature neurons, has been implicated as an important modulator of energy status. Central infusion of BDNF reduces food intake (Lapchak & Hefti, 1992). In addition, mice lacking the BDNF gene or its receptor, trkB, are hyperphagic and demonstrate excessive weight gain on a high-fat diet (Rios *et al.*, 2001; Xu *et al.*, 2003). BDNF is expressed throughout the hypothalamus, however, its expression in the VMN appears to be specifically regulated by nutritional status, leptin administration, and melanocortin signaling (Xu *et al.*, 2003). The mechanism by which BDNF/trkB signaling leads to reduced food intake and the extent to which the effect results from altered neuropeptide synthesis and release remains to be determined.

10.   Neuropeptide and neurotransmitter mediators of energy balance

Table 3.2 shows a list of hypothalamic and other CNS factors which inhibit feeding and decrease weight and fat content (anorexigenic), or stimulate feeding and weight gain (orexigenic).

10.1   *Arcuate nucleus*

Neuropeptide Y

Neuropeptide Y (NPY) is one of the most abundant neuropeptides and is widely expressed throughout the brain (Adrian *et al.*, 1983). In spite of its diffuse expression, NPY is a potent stimulator of feeding (Stanley & Leibowitz, 1985), an effect which appears to be specific to the hypothalamus. In the hypothalamus, NPY is expressed in the medial arcuate nucleus and released in the PVN and LHA. Neuropeptide Y expression and release in the hypothalamus increases with fasting and decreases with feeding (Kalra *et al.*, 1991). Neuropeptide Y administration in the brain reduces energy expenditure through suppression of brown adipose tissue thermogenesis (Billington *et al.*, 1991), inhibition of the thyroid axis (Fekete *et al.*, 2002) and reduced sympathetic nerve activity (Egawa *et al.*, 1991). While these data support NPY's role as an important orexigenic signal, genetic experiments have produced conflicting results. Mice lacking NPY from birth have normal body weight, but have a blunted hyperphagic response to fasting and hypoglycemia (Bannon et al., 2000). In contrast, leptin-deficient mice lacking NPY are less hyperphagic and have a milder obesity phenotype (Erickson et al., 1996).

Detailed pharmacological and genetic studies by Herzog and colleagues have found much of the orexigenic effect of NPY to be mediated by stimulation of a synergistic response in multiple NPY receptor types (Lin et al., 2004). Postsynaptic NPY Y1 receptors may be particularly important for increasing appetite. The most potent orexigenic actions of NPY are seen with micro-injection in the perifornical area and LHA. It has been suggested that NPY stimulates appetitive rather than consummatory behavior in the LHA, presumably through interaction with neurons expressing MCH and orexins (Ammar et al., 2000).

Melanocortins

Proopiomelanocortin (POMC) is expressed by neurons in the medial arcuate nucleus and gives rise to several bioactive peptides, including a- and γ-melanocyte-stimulating hormone, which have been shown to have potent anorexigenic effects when administered centrally. POMC mRNA and a-MSH levels are reduced in the fasted animal and increased by feeding (Schwartz et al., 1997). The effects of these peptides are mediated by MC3/4 receptors, which are expressed in the ARC, VMN, and PVN (Mountjoy et al., 1994). The critical role of melanocortin signaling is evident as mice lacking POMC or MC4R develop early-onset obesity. In addition, mutations in the POMC and MC4R have been associated with morbid obesity in humans (Krude et al., 1998; Farooqi et al., 2000). MC4R and to some extent MC3R mediate the thermogenic effect of a-MSH by increasing sympathetic nerve activity in brown adipose tissue and stimulating the thyroid axis (Kim et al., 2000). These actions are opposed by AGRP co-expressed in NPY neurons in the arcuate nucleus. AGRP is released in the PVN and other hypothalamic areas and acts as an endogenous antagonist of a-MSH at the MC3/4R, leading to hyperphagia (Kim et al., 2000). AGRP also decreases energy expenditure by reducing TRH expression and brown adipose thermo-genesis (Small et al., 2003). In contrast to the short action of a-MSH, these responses to AGRP can persist for up to one week, possibly due to interaction with syndecans (Rossi et al., 1998).

Cocaine and amphetamine-regulated transcript

Cocaine and amphetamine-regulated transcript (CART) was identified in rat hypothalamus as a transcript acutely regulated by cocaine and amphetamine administration (Douglass *et al.*, 1995). CART is highly conserved between rodents and humans. It is widely expressed in the brain, but is particularly abundant in the hypothalamus including LH, VMN, PVN, supraoptic nucleus, DMN, and ARC, where it is co-expressed with α-MSH (Kristensen *et al.*, 1998). Alternative splicing yields four CART transcripts, and a majority of studies on its role in energy balance have focused on $CART_{55-102}$, the putatively active form. Although the CART receptor has not been identified, CART immunoreactivity has been demonstrated in dendritic dense core vesicles and CART release in hypothalamic explants is calcium-dependent (Murphy *et al.*, 2000).

Similar to POMC, CART mRNA expression within the ARC is stimulated by feeding and leptin, and decreased by fasting (Kristensen *et al.*, 1998). Antibodies against CART peptide fragments administered in the cerebral ventricle or the ARC and VMN increase feeding (Kristensen *et al.*, 1998). Third ventricle administration of CART inhibits feeding in 24-hr fasted rats as well as suppressing NPY-induced feeding (Kristensen *et al.*, 1998; Vrang *et al.*, 1999). Some hypothalamic regions demonstrate increased CART immunoreactivity following fasting (Wang *et al.*, 2000). CART increases release of NPY and AGRP, and reduces the release of α-MSH from hypothalamic explants (Lambert *et al.*, 1998; Stanley *et al.*, 2001). Similar to α-MSH, CART increases brown adipose thermogenesis (Wang *et al.*, 2000), and is also able to modulate the effects of TRH (Stanley *et al.*, 2001; Raptis *et al.*, 2004). While CART clearly has a role in energy homeostasis, whether these effects are its primary role remains to be seen (Kuhar *et al.*, 2005).

Endocannabinoids

Cannabinoids have long been suspected of playing a role in the regulation of appetite. However, only recently has the participation of endogenous cannabinoids, including anandamide and the more abundant 2-arachidonyl glycerol (2-AG), in the hypothalamic and peripheral regulation of energy balance been appreciated (Di Marzo *et al.*, 2001). Endogenous cannabinoids are lipid-related molecules derived from the hydrolysis of arachidonic acid. They function as the ligands for either of two cannabinoid receptors (CB1 and CB2). Endocannabinoids are synthesized in several neural regions including the ARC, and CB1 receptors are present in the hypothalamus, including LHA cells expressing MCH.

Consistent with a role in energy balance, leptin treatment lowers hypothalamic cannabinoid levels, whereas interventions that reduce leptin signaling have the opposite effect (Di Marzo *et al.*, 2001). Hypothalamic levels of 2-AG have also been found to vary with nutritional status as they increase with fasting and return to baseline levels when animals are refed (Kirkham *et al.*, 2002). Administration of CB1 antagonists or genetic deletion of CB1 receptors reduce body fat mass, increase leptin sensitivity, and attenuate both refeeding hyperphagia and diet-induced obesity (Ravinet Trillou & Matias, 2004; Di Marzo & Matias, 2005).

The mechanism of action of cannabinoids in the hypothalamus is still controversial, and many of its effects on appetite may also be related to rewarding properties of food (Harrold & Williams, 2003). Also of great interest are the potential peripheral actions of cannabinoids. CB1 receptors are present in numerous metabolically important tissues such as liver and adipose tissue. Intestinal anandamide content is closely related to nutritional status and its peripheral but not central administration promoted feeding in partially satiated rats (Gomez *et al.*, 2002). Thus, although further clarification on the mechanisms of action is required it can be concluded that both central and peripheral endocannabinoids are involved in regulation of appetite and energy balance.

10.2   *Paraventricular nucleus*

The PVN is located on either side of the dorsal border of the third ventricle and consists of a magnocellular and parvocellular division. The lateral magnocellular division consists predominantly of vasopressin- and oxytocin-containing neurosecretory cells which project to the posterior pituitary gland. The parvocellular region is located medially and can be further divided into anterior, medial, periventricular, ventral, dorsal and lateral subdivisions. Neurons of this region express a variety of peptides including TRH, CRH, enkephalin, somatostatin and VIP. Of particular importance to coordinating metabolic adaptations in response to input from the ARC as well as other regions are the hypophysiotropic TRH located neurons in the medial and periventricular PVN (Lechan & Fekete, 2006) and the hypophysiotropic CRH neurons located throughout the PVN (Masaki *et al.*, 2003). The PVN is a critical integration site of ARC projections as well as projections from the NTS and DMN (Sawchenko & Swanson, 1983). The parvocellular subdivision of the PVN receives dense afferent input from the NTS as well as the DMN and other catecholamine-containing nuclei in the dorsal and ventral medulla (Knigge & Scott, 1970).

Thyrotropin-releasing hormone

The majority of TRH neurons in the PVN receive afferent input from axons of the ipsilateral ARC. Both a-MSH- and AGRP-containing ARC neurons project to similar regions of the PVN, which highly express MC3/4Rs. In vivo and in vitro studies suggest that a-MSH input to the PVN activates hypophysiotropic

TRH neurons (Fekete *et al.*, 2000) via cAMP-dependent phosphorylation of the transcription factor, CREB (Sarkar *et al.*, 2002). In contrast to α-MSH, AGRP has potent inhibitory effects on these neurons, as central infusion of AGRP greatly reduces TRH mRNA in the PVN and consequently causes circulating thyroid hormone levels to fall (Fekete *et al.*, 2004). Administration of NPY counteracts the ability of α-MSH to induce CREB phosphorylation on TRH neurons (Fekete *et al.*, 2002), further suggesting an integrative role of PVN-TRH neurons in energy balance. In addition to hypothalamic input, approximately 20% of TRH neurons in the PVN receive medullary afferent input (Fekete *et al.*, 2005). Most of these axons contain catecholamines as well as CART (Wittmann *et al.*, 2004), however their functional role in regulation of the hypothalamic–pituitary–thyroid axis remains to be determined.

Corticotropin-releasing hormone

Corticotropin-releasing hormone-expressing cells are concentrated predominantly in the medial parvocellular region, a proportion of which also express MC4R (Lu *et al.*, 2003). When infused centrally, CRH and related peptides such as urocortin have anorectic actions and potently stimulate sympathetically mediated thermogenesis and lipolysis (Richard *et al.*, 2000). In addition, central infusion of melanotan (MTII), a melanocortin agonist at doses that suppress food intake, rapidly increases expression of CRH in the PVN (Lu *et al.*, 2003). Pre-treatment of rodents with a CRH receptor antagonist blunts but does not completely suppress the effect of MTII on food intake (Lu *et al.*, 2003), indicating that CRH is a downstream mediator of the effects of melanocortins on feeding. However, phosphorylation of CREB in CRH neurons has also been reported to be increased by the orexigenic peptide NPY (Sarkar & Lechan, 2003). While this may seem incompatible given that NPY and POMC have opposing effects on energy balance, it may indicate that distinct subpopulations of TRH and CRH neurons may be differentially regulated by similar metabolic states.

10.3   Dorsomedial nucleus

The DMN is implicated in a wide variety of physiological behaviors including the stress response, ingestive behaviors and energy balance, reproduction and circadian rhythms. Most inputs to the DMN arise from other hypothalamic regions (Thompson & Swanson, 1998), particularly the ARC. Recent studies suggest that the DMN may serve as an important additional integrator in between ARC neurons responding to peripheral signals and PVN neurons executing autonomic and neuroendocrine responses (Elmquist *et al.*,

1998b). The DMN itself is rich in leptin receptors as well as those for ARC neuropeptides such as MC4R, Y1 and Y5 receptors. Recent studies in rodents have also suggested the DMN may regulate sympathetic nerve activity in intrascapular brown adipose tissue, via the periaqueductal gray and medullary raphe (Yoshida et al., 2005). Interestingly, the DMN may also play a role in coordinating the circadian rhythm to feeding and energy expenditure as expression of c-fos as well as period genes are specifically enhanced during food-entrained periods (Gooley et al., 2006; Mieda et al., 2006) and discrete lesions of the DMN abolish food-entrainable circadian rhythms (Gooley et al., 2006).

10.4   Lateral hypothalamic and perifornical areas

As suggested by early lesion and glucoprivation studies, the LHA/ perifornical area is critical to mediating orexigenic responses. NPY, AGRP and a-MSH terminals are abundant in the LHA and are in contact with neurons expressing the orexigenic peptides, MCH- and orexin. Central orexin neurons also express NPY and leptin receptors and are thus able to integrate adiposity signals. Notably, the perifornical area is more sensitive to NPY-elicited feeding than the PVN (Stanley et al., 1993).

Fasting increases MCH mRNA, and repeated intracerebroventricular administration or transgenic overexpression of MCH increases food intake and results in mild obesity (Qu et al., 1996). Conversely, chronic administration of an antagonist to the MCH-1 receptor reduces feeding and results in a sustained reduction in body weight (Borowsky et al., 2002), whereas mice with a disruption of the MCH gene are hypophagic, lean and have increased energy expenditure, despite reduced ARC POMC and circulating leptin (Marsh et al., 2002). Furthermore, hyperphagia and obesity are attenuated in mice deficient in MCH and leptin (Segal-Lieberman et al., 2003).

Orexin A and B (or hypocretin 1 and 2) are peptide products of prepro-orexin. These peptides are produced in the LHA/perifornical area and zona incerta by neurons distinct from those which produce MCH (Broberger et al., 1998). Orexin neurons exert their effects via wide projections throughout the brain including the PVN, ARC, NTS and dorsal motor nucleus of the vagus (Peyron et al., 1998). The VMN contains a high concentration of the orexin-1 receptor, which has a much greater affinity for orexin A. PVN neurons highly express the orexin-2 receptor, which has similar affinity for both orexin A and B (Sakurai et al., 1998). Expression of prepro-orexin mRNA is increased during fasting and its central administration has been found to result in both orexigenic behavior and generalized arousal (Sakurai et al., 1998). Central administration of orexin A, but not orexin B, has a potent effect on feeding (Haynes *et al.*, 1999) and vagally mediated gastric acid secretion (Takahashi *et al.*, 1999). Although intra-cerebroventricular administration of orexin A increased daytime feeding, there was no overall change in 24-h food intake (Haynes *et al.*, 1999). Furthermore, chronic administration of orexin A alone did not increase body weight (Yamanaka *et al.*, 1999). Orexin plays an important and well-characterized role in arousal and attention, and together with its role in increasing daytime feeding indicates that in circumstances of starvation, the orexin neuropeptides may mediate an arousal and food-seeking behavior.

10.5   *Ventromedial nucleus*

The VMN has long been known to play a role in energy homeostasis and glucose-sensing. Bilateral VMN lesions produce hyperphagia and obesity. These earlier lesion studies also demonstrated its involvement in both regulation of food intake and energy expenditure, as even pair feeding fails to prevent VMN-lesion induced obesity. Although it is no longer thought of as a "satiety center," the VMN is a critical relay in hypothalamic circuits of energy homeostasis, by virtue of its afferent and efferent connections and expression of receptors for various neuropeptides. NPY and MC4R expression is upregulated in the VMN of obese rodents (Huang *et al.*, 2003). Recent work has also demonstrated that BDNF is highly expressed within the VMN, and is a critical downstream mediator of melanocortin signaling (Xu *et al.*, 2003). In addition to expressing receptors for NPY and melanocortin input from the ARC, VMN neurons also express receptors for histamine and monoamines as well as leptin and insulin. VMN neurons project to the nucleus tractus solitarius (NTS) and other brainstem areas to regulate energy balance, glucose homeostasis and secretomotor activity.

11.   Brainstem pathways

There are extensive reciprocal connections between the hypothalamus and brainstem, particularly the dorsal vagal complex (DVC), which includes the NTS and dorsal motor vagal nucleus (Swanson & Sawchenko, 1980). Like the ARC, the NTS is in close anatomical proximity to a CVO, the area postrema, and therefore is accessible to peripheral circulating signals. NPY levels within the NTS fluctuate with feeding, and NPY neurons from this region feedback on to the hypothalamus. The NTS, dorsal vagal nucleus, and associated brainstem nuclei are critical to executing several metabolically important autonomic responses including modulating hormonal release, brown adipose tissue thermogenesis and hepatic glucose production. Thus, coordinated feedback between hypothalamic and the DVC are critical to modulating peripheral metabolic responses.

12.   Cognitive and reward pathways

In addition to the homeostatic mechanisms that drive food intake and energy expenditure, we are all keenly aware of the cognitive mechanisms driving energy balance. The motivation to eat or abstain from eating is ultimately the result of the processing of sensory information, stored memories, and emotional state in addition to homeostatic information. Hypothalamic nuclei project to several areas involved in these 'higher order' phenomena including the ventral tegmental area, nucleus accumbens and cortical areas. Functionally, these projections may allow for energy status to influence the sensation of reward or motivational states. As one may predict, subjective palatability of food is altered in the fed as compared with the fasting state (Berridge, 1991). Interestingly, fasting enhances while leptin administration attenuates LHA self-stimulation (Fulton et al., 2000). This effect may be related to effects of leptin on neural circuits mediating reward, as dopamine release in the nucleus accumbens is altered by feeding or leptin administration (Krugel et al., 2003). Along these lines, in primates hunger alters electrophysiological properties of orbitofrontal cortex neurons in response to visual or olfactory cues (Critchley & Rolls, 1996). Recent studies also suggest that orexin neurons may modulate mesolimbic reward circuits (Harris & Aston-Jones, 2006). Thus, signals of energy status via the hypothalamus are important regulators of neural circuits involved in hedonic and motivational processes.

13.   Summary

Since the discovery of leptin over a decade ago, rapid progress has been made in uncovering the details of the hypothalamic control of energy balance. It is now clear that discrete as well as overlapping hypothalamic pathways are critical to sensing metabolic status and effecting the appropriate metabolic adaptations to ensure that body weight is maintained. Peripheral factors responsive to energy stores as well as circulating nutrients are dynamically integrated by the ARC, PVN and various hypothalamic nuclei. Together with input from cortical, subcortical and brainstem sites, the hypothalamus coordinates feeding behavior, and hormonal and autonomic components of energy homeostasis.

References

Acuna-Goycolea, C. & Van den Pol. A. N. (2005). Peptide YY(3–36) inhibits both anorexigenic proopiomelanocortin and orexigenic neuropeptide Y neurons: implications for hypothalamic regulation of energy homeostasis. *J. Neurosci.* **25**, 10510–19.

Adrian, T. E., Allen, J. M., Bloom, S. R. *et al.* (1983). Neuropeptide Y distribution in human brain. *Nature* **306**, 584–6.

Ahima, R. S., Bjorbaek, C., Osei, S. & Flier, J. S. (1999). Regulation of neuronal and glial proteins by leptin: implications for brain development. *Endocrinology* **140**, 2755–62.

Ammar, A. A., Sederholm, F., Saito, T. R., Scheurink, A. J., Johnson, A. E. & Sodersten, P. (2000). NPY-leptin: opposing effects on appetitive and consummatory ingestive behavior and sexual behavior. *Am. J. Physiol. Regul. Integr. Comp. Physiol.* **278**, R1627–33.

Anand, B. K. & Brobeck, J. R. (1951). Localization of a "feeding center" in the hypothalamus of the rat. *Proc. Soc. Exp. Biol. Med.* **77**, 323–4.

Banks, W. A., Kastin, A. J., Huang, W., Jaspan, J. B. & Maness, L. M. (1996). Leptin enters the brain by a saturable system independent of insulin. *Peptides* **17**, 305–11.

Bannon, A. W., Seda, J., Carmouche, M. *et al.* (2000). Behavioral characterization of neuropeptide Y knockout mice. *Brain Res.* **868**, 79–87.

Berridge, K. C. (1991). Modulation of taste affect by hunger, caloric satiety, and sensory-specific satiety in the rat. *Appetite* **16**, 103–20.

Billington, C. J., Briggs, J. E., Grace, M. & Levine, A. S. (1991). Effects of intracerebroventricular injection of neuropeptide Y on energy metabolism. *Am. J. Physiol.* **260**, R321–7.

Borg, M. A., Sherwin, R. S., Borg, W. P., Tamborlane, W. V. & Shulman, G. I. (1997). Local ventromedial hypothalamus glucose perfusion blocks counterregulation during systemic hypoglycemia in awake rats. *J. Clin. Invest.* **99**, 361–5.

Borg, W. P., Sherwin, R. S., During, M. J., Borg, M. A. & Shulman, G. I. (1995). Local ventromedial hypothalamus glucopenia triggers counterregulatory hormone release. *Diabetes* **44**, 180–4.

Borowsky, B., Durkin, M. M., Ogozalek, K. *et al.* (2002). Antidepressant, anxiolytic and anorectic effects of a melanin concentrating hormone-1 receptor antagonist. *Nat. Med.* **8**, 825–30.

Bouret, S. G., Draper, S. J. & Simerly, R. B. (2004). Trophic action of leptin on hypothalamic neurons that regulate feeding. *Science* **304**, 108–10.

Bramwell, B. (1888). *Intracranial Tumours*. Edinburgh: Pentland.

Broadwell, R. D. & Brightman, M. W. (1976). Entry of peroxidase into neurons of the central and peripheral nervous systems from extracerebral and cerebral blood. *J. Comp. Neurol.* **166**, 257–83.

Broberger, C., De Lecea, L., Sutcliffe, J. G. & Hokfelt, T. (1998). Hypocretin/orexin- and melanin-concentrating hormone-expressing cells form distinct populations in the rodent lateral hypothalamus: relationship to the neuropeptide Y and agouti gene-related protein systems. *J. Comp. Neurol.* **402**, 460–74.

Burdakov, D., Luckman, S. M. & Verkhratsky, A. (2005). Glucose-sensing neurons of the hypothalamus. *Philos. Trans. R. Soc. Lond. B. Biol. Sci.* **360**, 2227–35.

Clark, G., Magoun, H. W. & Ranson, S. W. (1939). Hypothalamic regulation of body temperature. *J. Neurophysiol.* **2**, 61–80.

Cowley, M. A., Smart, J. L., Rubinstein, M. *et al.* (2001). Leptin activates anorexigenic POMC neurons through a neural network in the arcuate nucleus. *Nature* **411**, 480–4.

Critchley, H. D. & Rolls, E. T. (1996). Hunger and satiety modify the responses of olfactory and visual neurons in the primate orbitofrontal cortex. *J. Neurophysiol.* **75**, 1673–86.

Di Marzo, V. & Matias, I. (2005). Endocannabinoid control of food intake and energy balance. *Nat. Neurosci.* **8**, 585–9.

Di Marzo, V., Goparaju, S. K., Wang, L. *et al.* (2001). Leptin-regulated endocannabinoids are involved in maintaining food intake. *Nature* **410**, 822–5.

DiRocco, R. J. & Grill, H. G. (1979). The forebrain is not essential for sympathoadrenal hyperglycemic response to glucoprivation. *Science* **204**, 1112–14.

Douglass, J., McKinzie, A. A. & Couceyro, P. (1995). PCR differential display identifies a rat brain mRNA that is transcriptionally regulated by cocaine and amphetamine. *J. Neurosci.* **15**, 2471–81.

Egawa, M., Yoshimatsu, H. & Bray, H. G. (1991). Neuropeptide Y suppresses sympathetic activity to interscapular brown adipose tissue in rats. *Am. J. Physiol.* **260**, R328–34.

Elias, C. F., Aschkenasi, C., Lee, C. *et al.* (1999). Leptin differentially regulates NPY and POMC neurons projecting to the lateral hypothalamic area. *Neuron* **23**, 775–86.

Elmquist, J. K., Ahima, R. S., Elias, C. F., Flier, J. S. & Saper, C. B. (1998a). Leptin activates distinct projections from the dorsomedial and ventromedial hypothalamic nuclei. *Proc. Natl. Acad. Sci. USA* **95**, 741–6.

Elmquist, J. K., Bjorbaek, C., Ahima, R. S., Flier, J. S. & Saper, C. B. (1998b). Distributions of leptin receptor mRNA isoforms in the rat brain. *J. Comp. Neurol.* **395**, 535–47.

Erickson, J. C., Hollopeter, G. & Palmiter, R. D. (1996). Attenuation of the obesity syndrome of ob/ob mice by the loss of neuropeptide Y. *Science* **274**, 1704–7.

Farooqi, I. S., Yeo, G. S., Keogh, J. M. *et al.* (2000). Dominant and recessive inheritance of morbid obesity associated with melanocortin 4 receptor deficiency. *J. Clin. Invest.* **106**, 271–9.

Fekete, C., Legradi, G., Mihaly, E. *et al.* (2000). Alpha-melanocyte-stimulating hormone is contained in nerve terminals innervating thyrotropin-releasing hormone-synthesizing neurons in the hypothalamic paraventricular nucleus and prevents fasting-induced suppression of prothyrotropin-releasing hormone gene expression. *J. Neurosci.* **20**, 1550–8.

Fekete, C., Sarkar, S., Rand, W. M. *et al.* (2002). Neuropeptide Y1 and Y5 receptors mediate the effects of neuropeptide Y on the hypothalamic-pituitary-thyroid axis. *Endocrinology* **143**, 4513–19.

Fekete, C., Marks, D. L., Sarkar, S. *et al.* (2004). Effect of agouti-related protein in regulation of the hypothalamic pituitary-thyroid axis in the melanocortin 4 receptor knockout mouse. *Endocrinology* **145**, 14 816–21.

Fekete, C., Sarkar, S. & Lechan, R. M. (2005). Relative contribution of brainstem afferents to the cocaine- and amphetamine-regulated transcript (CART) innervation of thyrotropin-releasing hormone synthesizing neurons in the hypothalamic paraventricular nucleus (PVN). *Brain Res.* **1032**, 171–5.

Frolich, A. (1901). Ein fall von tumor der hypophysis cerebri ohne akromegalie. *Rundsch* **15**, 883–6.

Fulton, S., Woodside, B. & Shizgal, P. (2000). Modulation of brain reward circuitry by leptin. *Science* **287**, 125–8.

Gold, R. M. (1973). Hypothalamic obesity: the myth of the ventromedial nucleus. *Science* **182**, 488–90.

Gomez, R., Navarro, M., Ferrer, B. *et al.* (2002). A peripheral mechanism for CB1 cannabinoid receptor-dependent modulation of feeding. *J. Neurosci.* **22**, 9612–17.

Gooley, J. J., Schomer, A. & Saper, C. B. (2006). The dorsomedial hypothalamic nucleus is critical for the expression of food-entrainable circadian rhythms. *Nat. Neurosci.* **9**, 398–407.

Grill, H. J. & Kaplan, J. M. (2002). The neuroanatomical axis for control of energy balance. *Front. Neuroendocrinol.* **23**, 2–40.

Harris, G. C. & Aston-Jones, G. (2006). Arousal and reward: a dichotomy in orexin function. *Trends Neurosci.* **29**, 571–7.

Harrold, J. A. & Williams, G. (2003). The cannabinoid system: a role in both the homeostatic and hedonic control of eating? *Br. J. Nutr.* **90**, 729–34.

Haynes, A. C., Jackson, B., Overend, P. *et al.* (1999). Effects of single and chronic intracerebroventricular administration of the orexins on feeding in the rat. *Peptides* **20**, 1099–105.

Hetherington, A. W. & Ranson, S. W. (1940). Hypothalamic lesions and adiposity in the rat. *Anat. Rec.*, **78**, 149–72.

Howard, J. K., Cave, B. J., Oksanen, L. J., Tzameli, I., Bjorbaek, C. & Flier, J. S. (2004). Enhanced leptin sensitivity and attenuation of diet-induced obesity in mice with haploinsufficiency of Socs3. *Nat. Med.* **10**, 734–8.

Huang, X. F., Han, M., South, T. & Storlien, L. (2003). Altered levels of POMC, AgRP and MC4 R mRNA expression in the hypothalamus and other parts of the limbic system of mice prone or resistant to chronic high energy diet-induced obesity. *Brain Res.* **992**, 9–19.

Kahn, B. B., Alquier, T., Carling, D. & Hardie, D. G. (2005). AMP-activated protein kinase: ancient energy gauge provides clues to modern understanding of metabolism. *Cell Metab.* **1**, 15–25.

Kalra, S. P., Dube, M. G., Sahu, A., Phelps, C. P. & Kalra, P. S. (1991). Neuropeptide Y secretion increases in the paraventricular nucleus in association with increased appetite for food. *Proc. Natl. Acad. Sci. USA*, **88**, 10931–5.

Kastin, A. J., Akerstrom, V. & Pan, W. (2002). Interactions of glucagon-like peptide-1 (GLP-1) with the blood–brain barrier. *J. Mol. Neurosci.* **18**, 7–14.

Kim, M. S., Small, C. J., Stanley, S. A. *et al.* (2000). The central melanocortin system affects the hypothalamo-pituitary thyroid axis and may mediate the effect of leptin. *J. Clin. Invest.* **105**, 1005–11.

Kirkham, T. C., Williams, C. M., Fezza, F. & Di Marzo, V. (2002). Endocannabinoid levels in rat limbic forebrain and hypothalamus in relation to fasting, feeding and satiation: stimulation of eating by 2-arachidonoyl glycerol. *Br. J. Pharmacol.* **136**, 550–7.

Kitamura, T., Feng, Y., Kitamura, Y. I. *et al.* (2006). Forkhead protein FoxO1 mediates Agrp-dependent effects of leptin on food intake. *Nat. Med.* **12**, 534–40.

Knigge, K. M. & Scott, D. E. (1970). Structure and function of the median eminence. *Am. J. Anat.* **129**, 223–43.

Kohno, D., Gao, H. Z., Muroya, S., Kikuyama, S. & Yada, T. (2003). Ghrelin directly interacts with neuropeptide-Y-containing neurons in the rat arcuate nucleus: Ca2+ signaling via protein kinase A and N-type channel-dependent mechanisms and cross-talk with leptin and orexin. *Diabetes* **52**, 948–56.

Kristensen, P., Judge, M. E., Thim, L. *et al.* (1998). Hypothalamic CART is a new anorectic peptide regulated by leptin. *Nature* **393**, 72–6.

Krude, H., Biebermann, H., Luck, W., Horn, R., Brabant, G. & Gruters, A. (1998). Severe early onset obesity, adrenal insufficiency and red hair pigmentation caused by POMC mutations in humans. *Nat. Genet.* **19**, 155–7.

Krugel, U., Schraft, T., Kittner, H., Kiess, W. & Illes, P. (2003). Basal and feeding-evoked dopamine release in the rat nucleus accumbens is depressed by leptin. *Eur. J. Pharmacol.* **482**, 185–7.

Kuhar, M. J., Jaworski, J. N., Hubert, G. W., Philpot, K. B. & Dominguez, G. (2005). Cocaine- and amphetamine-regulated transcript peptides play a role in drug abuse and are potential therapeutic targets. *AAPS J.* **7**, E259–65.

Lam, T. K., Gutierrez-Juarez, R., Pocai, A. & Rossetti, L. (2005). Regulation of blood glucose by hypothalamic pyruvate metabolism. *Science* **309**, 943–7.

Lambert, P. D., Couceyro, P. R., McGirr, K. M., Dall Vechia, S. E., Smith, Y. & Kuhar, M. J. (1998). CART peptides in the central control of feeding and interactions with neuropeptide Y. *Synapse* **29**, 293–8.

Landree, L. E., Hanlon, A. L., Strong, D. W. *et al.* (2004). C75, a fatty acid synthase inhibitor, modulates AMP-activated protein kinase to alter neuronal energy metabolism. *J. Biol. Chem.* **279**, 3817–27.

Lapchak, P. A. & Hefti, F. (1992). BDNF and NGF treatment in lesioned rats: effects on cholinergic function and weight gain. *Neuroreport* **3**, 405–8.

Lechan, R. M. & Fekete, C. (2006). Chapter 12: The TRH neuron: a hypothalamic integrator of energy metabolism. *Prog. Brain Res.* **153C**, 209–35.

Levine, J. A. (2002). Non-exercise activity thermogenesis (NEAT). *Best Pract. Res. Clin. Endocrinol. Metab.* **16**, 679–702.

Lin, S., Boey, D. & Herzog, H. (2004). NPY and Y receptors: lessons from transgenic and knockout models. *Neuropeptides* **38**, 189–200.

Loftus, T. M., Jaworsky, D. E., Frehywot, G. L. *et al.* (2000). Reduced food intake and body weight in mice treated with fatty acid synthase inhibitors. *Science* **288**, 2379–81.

Lu, X. Y., Barsh, G. S., Akil, H. & Watson, S. J. (2003). Interaction between alpha-melanocyte stimulating hormone and corticotropin-releasing hormone in the regulation of feeding and hypothalamo-pituitary-adrenal responses. *J. Neurosci.* **23**, 7863–72.

Lutz, T. A. (2006). Amylinergic control of food intake. *Physiol. Behav.* doi:10.1016/j.physbeh.2006.04.001.

Marsh, D. J., Weingarth, D. T., Novi, D. E. *et al.* (2002). Melanin-concentrating hormone 1 receptor-deficient mice are lean, hyperactive, and hyperphagic and have altered metabolism. *Proc. Natl. Acad. Sci. USA*, **99**, 3240–5.

Masaki, T., Yoshimichi, G., Chiba, S. *et al.* (2003). Corticotropin-releasing hormone-mediated pathway of leptin to regulate feeding, adiposity, and uncoupling protein expression in mice. *Endocrinology* **144**, 3547–54.

Matochik, J. A., London, E. D., Yildiz, B. O. *et al.* (2005). Effect of leptin replacement on brain structure in genetically leptin deficient adults. *J. Clin. Endocrinol. Metab.* **90**, 2851–4.

McCrimmon, R. J., Fan, X., Ding, Y., Zhu, W., Jacob, R. J. & Sherwin, R. S. (2004). Potential role for AMP-activated protein kinase in hypoglycemia sensing in the ventromedial hypothalamus. *Diabetes* **53**, 1953–8.

Mieda, M., Williams, S. C., Richardson, J. A., Tanaka, K. & Yanagisawa, M. (2006). The dorsomedial hypothalamic nucleus as a putative food-entrainable circadian pacemaker. *Proc. Natl. Acad. Sci. USA*, **103**, 12 150–5.

Miller, J. C., Gnaedinger, J. M. & Rapoport, S. I. (1987). Utilization of plasma fatty acid in rat brain: distribution of [14C]palmitate between oxidative and synthetic pathways. *J. Neurochem.* **49**, 1507–14.

Minokoshi, Y., Alquier, T., Furukawa, N. *et al.* (2004). AMP-kinase regulates food intake by responding to hormonal and nutrient signals in the hypothalamus. *Nature* **428**, 569–74.

Mori, H., Hanada, R., Hanada, T. *et al.* (2004). Socs3 deficiency in the brain elevates leptin sensitivity and confers resistance to diet-induced obesity. *Nat. Med.* **10**, 739–43.

Morton, G. J., Gelling, R. W., Niswender, K. D., Morrison, C. D., Rhodes, C. J. & Schwartz, M. W. (2005). Leptin regulates insulin sensitivity via phosphatidylinositol-3-OH kinase signaling in mediobasal hypothalamic neurons. *Cell Metab.* **2**, 411–20.

Mountjoy, K. G., Mortrud, M. T., Low, M. J., Simerly, R. B. & Cone, R. D. (1994). Localization of the melanocortin-4 receptor (MC4-R) in neuroendocrine and autonomic control circuits in the brain. *Mol. Endocrinol.* **8**, 1298–308.

Murphy, K. G., Abbott, C. R., Mahmoudi, M. *et al.* (2000). Quantification and synthesis of cocaine- and amphetamine-regulated transcript peptide (79–102)-like immunoreactivity and mRNA in rat tissues. *J. Endocrinol.* **166**, 659–68.

Nakazato, M., Murakami, N., Date, Y. *et al.* (2001). A role for ghrelin in the central regulation of feeding. *Nature* **409**, 194–8.

Nichols, C. G. (2006). KATP channels as molecular sensors of cellular metabolism. *Nature* **440**, 470–6.

Niswender, K. D. & Schwartz, M. W. (2003). Insulin and leptin revisited: adiposity signals with overlapping physiological and intracellular signaling capabilities. *Front. Neuroendocrinol.* **24**, 1–10.

Niswender, K. D., Baskin, D. G. & Schwartz, M. W. (2004). Insulin and its evolving partnership with leptin in the hypothalamic control of energy homeostasis. *Trends Endocrinol. Metab.* **15**, 362–9.

Obici, S., Feng, Z., Morgan, K., Stein, D., Karkanias, G. & Rossetti, L. (2002a). Central administration of oleic acid inhibits glucose production and food intake. *Diabetes* **51**, 271–5.

Obici, S., Feng, Z., Karkanias, G., Baskin, D. G. & Rossetti, L. (2002b). Decreasing hypothalamic insulin receptors causes hyperphagia and insulin resistance in rats. *Nat. Neurosci.* **5**, 566–72.

Obici, S., Feng, Z., Arduini, A., Conti, R. & Rossetti, L. (2003). Inhibition of hypothalamic carnitine palmitoyltransferase-1 decreases food intake and glucose production. *Nat. Med.* **9**, 756–61.

Oomura, Y., Ono, T., Ooyama, H. & Wayner, M. J. (1969). Glucose and osmosensitive neurones of the rat hypothalamus. *Nature* **222**, 282–4.

Peyron, C., Tighe, D. K., van den Pol, A. N. *et al.* (1998). Neurons containing hypocretin (orexin) project to multiple neuronal systems. *J. Neurosci.* **18**, 9996–10015.

Plum, L., Ma, X., Hampel, B. *et al.* (2006). Enhanced PIP3 signaling in POMC neurons causes KATP channel activation and leads to diet-sensitive obesity. *J. Clin. Invest.* **116**, 1886–901.

Pinto, S., Roseberry, A. G., Liu, H. *et al.* (2004). Rapid rewiring of arcuate nucleus feeding circuits by leptin. *Science* **304**, 110–15.

Qu, D., Ludwig, D. S., Gammeltoft, S. *et al.* (1996). A role for melanin-concentrating hormone in the central regulation of feeding behaviour. *Nature* **380**, 243–7.

Rapoport, S. I. (1999). In vivo fatty acid incorporation into brain phospholipids in relation to signal transduction and membrane remodeling. *Neurochem. Res.* **24**, 1403–15.

Raptis, S., Fekete, C., Sarkar, S. *et al.* (2004). Cocaine- and amphetamine-regulated transcript co-contained in thyrotropin-releasing hormone (TRH) neurons of the hypothalamic paraventricular nucleus modulates TRH-induced prolactin secretion. *Endocrinology* **145**, 1695–9.

Ravinet Trillou, C., Delgorge, C., Menet, C., Arnone, M. & Soubrie, P. (2004). CB1 cannabinoid receptor knockout in mice leads to leanness, resistance to diet-induced obesity and enhanced leptin sensitivity. *Int. J. Obes. Relat. Metab. Disord.* **28**, 640–8.

Richard, D., Huang, Q. & Timofeeva, E. (2000). The corticotropin-releasing hormone system in the regulation of energy balance in obesity. *Int. J. Obes. Relat. Metab. Disord.* **24 (Suppl. 2)**, S36–9.

Rios, M., Fan, G., Fekete, C. *et al.* (2001). Conditional deletion of brain-derived neurotrophic factor in the postnatal brain leads to obesity and hyperactivity. *Mol. Endocrinol.* **15**, 1748–57.

Rossi, M., Kim, M. S., Morgan, D. G. *et al.* (1998). A C-terminal fragment of Agouti-related protein increases feeding and antagonizes the effect of alpha-melanocyte stimulating hormone in vivo. *Endocrinology* **139**, 4428–31.

Routh, R. E., Johnson, J. H. & McCarthy, K. J. (2002). Troglitazone suppresses the secretion of type I collagen by mesangial cells in vitro. *Kidney Int.* **61**, 1365–76.

Routh, V. H. (2003). Glucosensing neurons in the ventromedial hypothalamic nucleus (VMN) and hypoglycemia-associated autonomic failure (HAAF). *Diabetes Metab. Res. Rev.* **19**, 348–56.

Russo, V. C., Metaxas, S., Kobayashi, K., Harris, M. & Werther, G. A. (2004). Antiapoptotic effects of leptin in human neuroblastoma cells. *Endocrinology* **145**, 4103–12.

Sakurai, T., Amemiya, A., Ishii, M. *et al.* (1998). Orexins and orexin receptors: a family of hypothalamic neuropeptides and G protein-coupled receptors that regulate feeding behavior. *Cell* **92**, 573–85.

Sarkar, S. & Lechan, R. M. (2003). Central administration of neuropeptide Y reduces alpha melanocyte-stimulating hormone-induced cyclic adenosine 5'-monophosphate response element binding protein (CREB) phosphorylation in pro-thyrotropin-releasing hormone neurons and increases CREB phosphorylation in corticotropin-releasing hormone neurons in the hypothalamic paraventricular nucleus. *Endocrinology* **144**, 281–91.

Sarkar, S., Legradi, G. & Lechan, R. M. (2002). Intracerebroventricular administration of α-melanocyte stimulating hormone increases phosphorylation of CREB in TRH- and CRH-producing neurons of the hypothalamic paraventricular nucleus. *Brain Res.* **945**, 50–9.

Sawchenko, P. E. & Swanson, L. W. (1983). The organization of forebrain afferents to the paraventricular and supraoptic nuclei of the rat. *J. Comp. Neurol.* **218**, 121–44.

Schwartz, M. W., Seeley, R. J., Woods, S. C. *et al.* (1997). Leptin increases hypothalamic pro-opiomelanocortin mRNA expression in the rostral arcuate nucleus. *Diabetes* **46**, 2119–23.

Schwartz, M. W., Woods, S. C., Porte, D. Jr, Seeley, R. J. & Baskin, D. G. (2000). Central nervous system control of food intake. *Nature* **404**, 661–71.

Segal-Lieberman, G., Bradley, R. L., Kokkotou, E. *et al.* (2003). Melanin-concentrating hormone is a critical mediator of the leptin-deficient phenotype. *Proc. Natl. Acad. Sci. USA* **100**, 10 085–90.

Sena, A., Sarlieve, L. L. & Rebel, G. (1985). Brain myelin of genetically obese mice. *J. Neurol. Sci.* **68**, 233–43.

Shyng, S. L. & Nichols, C. G. (1998). Membrane phospholipid control of nucleotide sensitivity of KATP channels. *Science* **282**, 1138–41.

Small, C. J., Liu, Y. L., Stanley, S. A. *et al.* (2003). Chronic CNS administration of Agouti-related protein (Agrp) reduces energy expenditure. *Int. J. Obes. Relat. Metab. Disord.* **27**, 530–3.

Spanswick, D., Smith, M. A., Groppi, V. E., Logan, S. D. & Ashford, M. L. (1997). Leptin inhibits hypothalamic neurons by activation of ATP-sensitive potassium channels. *Nature* **390**, 521–5.

Spanswick, D., Smith, M. A., Mirshamsi, S., Routh, V. H. & Ashford, M. L. (2000). Insulin activates ATP-sensitive K+ channels in hypothalamic neurons of lean, but not obese rats. *Nat. Neurosci.* **3**, 757–8.

Stanley, B. G. & Leibowitz, S. F. (1985). Neuropeptide Y injected in the paraventricular hypothalamus: a powerful stimulant of feeding behavior. *Proc. Natl. Acad. Sci. USA* **82**, 3940–3.

Stanley, B. G., Magdalin, W., Seirafi, A., Thomas, W. J. & Leibowitz, S. F. (1993). The perifornical area: the major focus of (a) patchily distributed hypothalamic neuropeptide Y sensitive feeding system(s). *Brain Res.* **604**, 304–17.

Stanley, S. A., Small, C. J., Murphy, K. G. *et al.* (2001). Actions of cocaine- and amphetamine-regulated transcript (CART) peptide on regulation of appetite and hypothalamo-pituitary axes in vitro and in vivo in male rats. *Brain Res.* **893**, 186–94.

Stellar, E. (1954). The physiology of motivation. *Psychol. Rev.* **61**, 5–22.

Swanson, L. W. & Sawchenko, P. E. (1980). Paraventricular nucleus: a site for the integration of neuroendocrine and autonomic mechanisms. *Neuroendocrinology* **31**, 410–17.

Takahashi, K. A. & Cone, R. D. (2005). Fasting induces a large, leptin-dependent increase in the intrinsic action potential frequency of orexigenic arcuate nucleus neuropeptide Y/Agouti-related protein neurons. *Endocrinology* **146**, 1043–7.

Takahashi, N., Okumura, T., Yamada, H. & Kohgo, Y. (1999). Stimulation of gastric acid secretion by centrally administered orexin-A in conscious rats. *Biochem. Biophys. Res. Commun.* **254**, 623–7.

Tannenbaum, G. S., Lapointe, M., Beaudet, A. & Howard, A. D. (1998). Expression of growth hormone secretagogue-receptors by growth hormone-releasing hormone neurons in the mediobasal hypothalamus. *Endocrinology* **139**, 4420–3.

Tartaglia, L. A. (1997). The leptin receptor. *J. Biol. Chem.* **272**, 6093–6.

Thompson, R. H. & Swanson, L. W. (1998). Organization of inputs to the dorsomedial nucleus of the hypothalamus: a reexamination with Fluorogold and PHAL in the rat. *Brain Res. Rev.* **27**, 89–118.

Ungerstedt, U. (1970). Is interruption of the nigro-striatal dopamine system producing the "lateral hypothalamus syndrome"? *Acta Physiol. Scand.* **80**, 35A–6A.

van den Top, M., Lee, K., Whyment, A. D., Blanks, A. M. & Spanswick, D. (2004). Orexigen sensitive NPY/AgRP pacemaker neurons in the hypothalamic arcuate nucleus. *Nat. Neurosci.* **7**, 493–4.

Vrang, N., Tang-Christensen, M., Larsen, P.J. & Kristensen, P. (1999). Recombinant CART peptide induces c-Fos expression in central areas involved in control of feeding behaviour. *Brain Res.* **818**, 499–509.

Wang, C., Billington, C.J., Levine, A.S. & Kotz, C.M. (2000). Effect of CART in the hypothalamic paraventricular nucleus on feeding and uncoupling protein gene expression. *Neuroreport* **11**, 3251–5.

Wittmann, G., Liposits, Z., Lechan, R.M. & Fekete, C. (2004). Medullary adrenergic neurons contribute to the cocaine- and amphetamine-regulated transcript-immunoreactive innervation of thyrotropin-releasing hormone synthesizing neurons in the hypothalamic paraventricular nucleus. *Brain Res.* **1006**, 1–7.

Xu, B., Goulding, E.H., Zang, K. *et al.* (2003). Brain-derived neurotrophic factor regulates energy balance downstream of melanocortin-4 receptor. *Nat. Neurosci* **6**, 736–42.

Yamanaka, A., Sakurai, T., Katsumoto, T., Yanagisawa, M. & Goto, K. (1999). Chronic intracerebroventricular administration of orexin-A to rats increases food intake in daytime, but has no effect on body weight. *Brain Res.* **849**, 248–52.

Yoshida, K., Konishi, M., Nagashima, K., Saper, C.B. & Kanosue, K. (2005). Fos activation in hypothalamic neurons during cold or warm exposure: projections to periaqueductal gray matter. *Neuroscience* **133**, 1039–46.

Yoshimatsu, H., Niijima, A., Oomura, Y., Yamabe, K. & Katafuchi, T. (1984). Effects of hypothalamic lesion on pancreatic autonomic nerve activity in the rat. *Brain Res.* **303**, 147–52.

Yura, S., Itoh, H., Sagawa, N. *et al.* (2005). Role of premature leptin surge in obesity resulting from intrauterine undernutrition. *Cell Metab.* **1**, 371–8.

4
_____

Leptin and insulin as adiposity signals

KEVIN D. NISWENDER

1.   Summary

Obesity is an epidemic in the USA and worldwide. Despite a rapid increase in the burden of obesity, scientific evidence indicates that body adiposity is a tightly regulated physiological variable. Current models implicate a classical endocrine feedback loop in the process termed energy homeostasis. Both the pancreatic β cell-derived hormone insulin and the adipocyte-derived hormone leptin are secreted in proportion to fat mass and, thus, signal the status of body energy stores to the hypothalamus. Key hypothalamic nuclei contain neurons that respond directly to insulin and leptin and integrate these and other signals in order to regulate food intake and energy homeostasis through a series of complex neuronal circuits.

Although the personal, societal and economic costs of obesity are staggering, the medical research community has yet to develop definitive therapies. Recent advances in our understanding of the interactions of insulin and leptin with hypothalamic target neurons has shed light upon potential pathophysiological mechanisms and therefore therapeutic targets. In this chapter, basic mechanisms of energy homeostasis will be presented in the context of an adiposity negative feedback model with the hormones insulin and leptin serving an important role. This model will then be extended and discussed in the context of the pathophysiology of obesity.

Neurobiology and Obesity, ed. Jenni Harvey and Dominic J. Withers. Published by Cambridge University Press. © Cambridge University Press 2008

2.   Introduction

Obesity is an international health epidemic (Kopelman, 2000; Mokdad et al., 2001) afflicting 1.7 billion people worldwide (James, 2003) and has surpassed infectious disease and under-nutrition as the major threat to health in most parts of the world. Increased body fat mass increases relative risk for the development of cardiovascular disease, hypertension, diabetes mellitus, obstructive sleep apnea, degenerative joint disease, depression and other conditions that collectively combine to greatly increase morbidity and mortality (Willett et al., 1999). The health-related costs of obesity (Rosenbaum et al., 1997) and diabetes (Association, 2000) in the USA are estimated to exceed US$ 240 billion per year, and as such, these disorders and their comorbidities constitute a significant medical and financial burden.

The rapidity with which obesity has developed within so many populations is one of the most alarming aspects of this problem. United States Centers for Disease Control statistics document a dramatic increase in the prevalence of obesity over the last 15 years (Mokdad et al., 2001). Highly alarming is the relative rate of increase over the last several years (Control, 2003) and the increasing prevalence of obesity in children (Ogden et al., 2002) suggesting that current efforts at curbing the problem are wholly ineffective. The accelerating and seemingly self-perpetuating nature of this disorder has raised the concern of scientists, clinicians, epidemiologists and governmental agencies, whose collective response will ultimately determine our success in improving public health (Kopelman, 2000; Mokdad et al., 2001).

Unequivocally, an improved understanding of the neurobiology of energy homeostasis and pathophysiological mechanisms of obesity will be required to develop effective therapy. It could be argued that the relative lack of efficacy of currently approved drugs is due to a lack of understanding and therefore targeting of fundamentally relevant pathophysiology. This is despite an ever-increasing understanding of the critical roles of a number of molecular determinants and CNS circuits in energy homeostasis (Schwartz et al., 2000; Spiegelman & Flier, 2001).

The concept of adiposity negative feedback, wherein hormonal signals generated in proportion to fat mass and recent energy balance provide feedback to the brain (Figure 4.1) is fundamental to the biology of energy homeostasis (Schwartz et al., 2000; Spiegelman & Flier, 2001). This generally accepted model is the focus of this chapter, although it must be pointed out that other models have been proposed (Flier, 1998; Leibel, 2002; Speakman et al., 2002). In this chapter, the roles for insulin and leptin as adiposity signals in normal energy balance and in the context of the pathophysiology of obesity

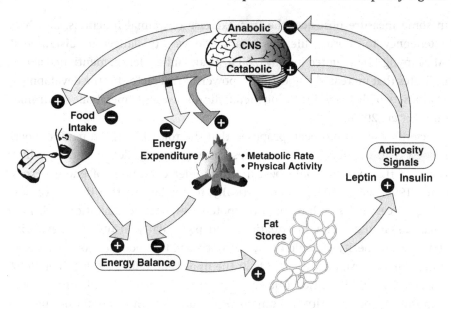

Figure 4.1 Insulin and leptin function as adiposity signals in an endocrine negative feedback loop to regulate energy balance. Insulin and leptin circulate in proportion to body fat stores and regulate the activity of key target neurons found in the mediobasal hypothalamus and elsewhere. Catabolic circuits are activated and anabolic circuits suppressed in response to increased insulin and leptin levels resulting in reduced food intake, increased energy expenditure, and restoration of body adipose stores.

will be discussed. Both historical and recent findings will be highlighted that support a key role for insulin, leptin and downstream signal transduction pathways in the central nervous system (CNS) regulation of energy homeostasis. Key unanswered questions will be highlighted and hypotheses for the pathophysiology of obesity proposed.

3.   Is obesity a disease?

Implicit in a discussion of the role of insulin and leptin in energy homeostasis is the concept that body adiposity is a regulated physiological variable and that obesity must represent a "pathophysiological" or "disease" process (Niswender *et al.*, 2004b; Schwartz & Niswender, 2004). Yet common public perception and, unfortunately, the perception of many medical practitioners is that obesity is a "disorder" of willpower, a character flaw or a cognitive choice. Intriguingly, predecessors of several centuries realized that "Corpulency, when in extraordinary degree, may be reckoned a disease, as it in some measure obstructs the free exercise of animal functions; and hath a tendency to shorten life, by paving the way to dangerous distempers" (M Flemyng 1760, quoted in Bray, 2003). Abundant evidence, mentioned above, indicates that increased adiposity is a powerful risk factor for the development of a variety of diseases, including metabolic disease and "metabolic syndrome" (Eckel *et al.*, 2005).

Scientifically, it has been proposed that the role of leptin in neuroendocrinology is to organize the potent response to energy deficit and that little effect of this system would be expected under conditions of energy excess (Flier, 1998; Leibel, 2002). Mechanistically, it may be true that the response to energy excess is less robust than the potent response to starvation (Schwartz *et al.*, 2003) under certain situations and particularly in obesity. Reviewing statistics on obesity, it could easily be concluded that body adipose mass is an unregulated physiological variable at the upper end (Flier, 1998; Leibel, 2002; Berthoud, 2004); increased caloric availability appears to result in increased adiposity in the majority of humans. A variation of this hypothesis suggests that humans evolved under conditions of chronic caloric deprivation and that individuals who could efficiently acquire and store energy in the form of fat would have a selective survival advantage and their genes positively selected over time. This concept is often termed the "thrifty genotype hypothesis" (Neel *et al.*, 1998; Neel, 1999).

Thus, whether body fat mass is regulated is a critical issue in our attempt to define research questions aimed at understanding the role of insulin and leptin as adiposity signals and of addressing the obesity epidemic. If obesity indeed represents the ultimate manifestation of thrifty genes exposed to caloric excess, then we may be destined for an ever-more obese existence. In this context, obesity could be viewed as the efficient and "normal" function of a regulatory system whose primary objective is to obtain and store energy or at the very least is not designed to efficiently respond to energy excess (Flier, 1998; Leibel, 2002; Schwartz *et al.*, 2003; Berthoud, 2004).

The counter hypothesis, to be discussed in this chapter, is that body weight in *normal* individuals is tightly regulated and that *pathological* changes in the regulatory system must occur in order to develop obesity. The role of insulin and leptin as key regulators of energy balance are fundamental to this hypothesis and will be discussed at length.

4.   Evidence in favor of tight regulation of energy balance

Firstly, the observation that not all individuals express an obese phenotype in today's sedentary and calorically dense milieu suggests that energy balance can be tightly regulated. Even accounting for age-associated weight gain, it is estimated that energy intake is balanced to within less than 0.2% of energy expenditure over time. Such precision in the matching of a caloric intake with expenditure seems implausible in the absence of a physiological system designed to perform this function (Weigle, 1994). Further, while it is elegantly argued that the neurohormonal response to energy deficit is potent (Flier, 1998; Leibel, 2002), numerous experimental systems have demonstrated a similarly potent response to "acute" overfeeding in "normal" volunteers. For example, in the "Experimental Obesity in Man" series of studies, volunteers were able to achieve significant weight gain when provided with sufficient external motivation (Sims et al., 1968, 1972, 1973; Saad et al., 1993). The caloric intake necessary to maintain the excess body weight was higher than the caloric intake necessary to maintain excess body weight in individuals expressing typical human obesity, implying that the "normal" volunteers exhibited markedly increased energy expenditure in the face of increased fat mass, i.e. exhibited responses that would be predicted if energy homeostasis was intact. Of course, once the external motivation to overfeed was discontinued the volunteers spontaneously consumed very few calories for many weeks, and caloric intake only approached pre-study intake when body weight dropped to the pre-study body weight. This set of observations had essentially been made 50 years prior, albeit in a far more crude fashion (Gulick, 1922).

Similarly vigorous responses have been observed in a unique series of observations made in Cameroonian society where male coming of age includes a "fattening ceremony" or "Guru Walla." In this culture, obesity is viewed as a positive social trait, eliminating such factors as confounders, and yet when observed after the period of inactivity, overfeeding and obesity, the individuals had returned to their initial body weight and body composition (Pasquet et al., 1992; Pasquet & Apfelbaum, 1994). Other, more sophisticated studies of less dramatic overfeeding in humans have generally confirmed these observations; i.e. that overfeeding results in adaptive responses including reduction in spontaneous food intake until excess adiposity is dissipated (Roberts et al., 1990).

Abundant evidence in a variety of animal models has also indicated the potential for potent responses to overfeeding. Whether it be monkeys (Wilson et al., 1990), or rodents (Bernstein et al., 1975), a period of forced over feeding by gavage or gastric catheter results in the absence of spontaneous food intake. When the gavage feeding is discontinued, spontaneous feeding does not occur until body fat mass returns to normal levels, a potent response reminiscent of those observed in humans just described. Thus, in a selected group of "normal" individuals, the catabolic or anorexic response to experimentally induced obesity is demonstrated to be both robust and accurate. The situation in humans expressing typical forms of obesity (i.e. non-monogenetic), or common human obesity, or similar rodent models of diet-induced obesity (DIO) are fundamentally different in that individuals are not externally motivated or experimentally forced to overfeed, rather obesity occurs in the setting of ad libitum feeding. Of course, human and rodent obesity typically develops over a different (longer) time-course than the forms of experimental obesity just discussed, and it would be interesting to determine whether long-term slight overfeeding results in typical obesity with maintenance of excess adiposity. Nonetheless, the remainder of this chapter will focus on the fundamental key question, what is different between the "experimental" obesities just mentioned and typical human obesity, and will do so in the context of the role of insulin and leptin as adiposity signals.

5.   Adiposity signals

Although the regulated nature of body adiposity has been recognized for over 100 years (Neumann, 1902; Gulick, 1922), our current understanding of body weight regulation, incorporating the notion of negative adiposity feedback signaling arose nearly 50 years ago in an insightful article by Gordon Kennedy entitled "The role of depot fat in the hypothalamic control of food intake in the rat" (Kennedy, 1953). Kennedy put forth the hypothesis that body adiposity is regulated by a feedback loop in which the status of body fat stores is sensed and a signal sent to the hypothalamus to regulate the intake of calories and the storage of energy in the form of fat. Of course, CNS lesioning experiments had identified the mediobasal hypothalamus as a key site for the regulation of energy balance (Brobeck et al., 1943; Marshall et al., 1955; Mayer et al., 1955). Thus, the basic structure of the systems involved in energy balance as understood today (Figure 4.1) were appreciated prior to the discovery of specific hormones that function as adiposity negative feedback signals. It took nearly 50 years for such a signal to be identified and widely appreciated; in 1994 the fat derived "adiposity" signal leptin was cloned and its critical role in body weight regulation established (Zhang et al., 1994). It should be noted, however, that work focusing on adipostatic signals occurred well before the discovery of leptin.

Although the cloning of leptin (Zhang et al., 1994) and elucidation of its critical role in energy homeostasis (Halaas et al., 1995) were clearly seminal events for energy homeostasis research, Woods and Porte demonstrated the existence of neural circuits that respond to insulin and regulate food intake and adipose mass many years prior (Woods & Porte, 1978; Woods et al., 1979; Woods & Seeley, 2001). Chronic infusion of insulin into the cerebral ventricles of baboons was noted to reduce food intake and body adiposity as far back as the 1970s and early 1980s (Woods et al., 1979). Coupled with evidence that insulin circulates in proportion to adiposity (Bagdade et al., 1967), this work provided crucial early evidence in support of the feedback loop model of energy homeostasis on which current models are based (Woods & Porte, 1978; Schwartz et al., 2000; Spiegelman & Flier, 2001).

6.   Adiposity signal definition

In a feedback loop model of energy homeostasis, an afferent "adiposity" signal to the CNS should meet several requisite criteria. Indeed, both insulin and leptin fulfill several requirements of such a signal. Both hormones are secreted and circulate in proportion to body fat mass (Bagdade et al., 1967; Considine et al., 1996). In particular, both fasting and integrated circulating insulin levels correlate well with adiposity (Bagdade et al., 1967). Next, receptors for both hormones are expressed on key neurons found in important regulatory centers in the brain and these hormones can be demonstrated to bind their receptors in these brain regions (Corp et al., 1986; Marks et al., 1990; Schwartz et al., 1996b). Experimentally, delivery of either hormone into the brain reduces food intake (Halaas et al., 1995; Sipols et al., 1995; Sindelar et al., 1999; Air et al., 2002) and deficiency of either hormone results in hyperphagia and/or obesity (Zhang et al., 1994; Sipols et al., 1995; Farooqi et al., 1999; Sindelar et al., 1999) both as one would predict for an adiposity signal. Finally, the hyperphagia due to insulin or leptin deficiency can be reversed by treatment with either hormone (Sipols et al., 1995; Farooqi et al., 1999; Sindelar et al., 1999). Thus, fundamental negative feedback principles are clearly met by both insulin and leptin supporting the concept that both hormones participate in energy homeostasis via roles as negative adiposity signals. After a brief description of the structure–function relationships in current models of energy homeostasis, the roles of insulin and leptin as adiposity signals will be elucidated further.

7.   Current model of energy homeostasis

A current and well-accepted model for the regulation of adipose tissue stores is reviewed in detail elsewhere (Schwartz et al., 2000; Spiegelman & Flier, 2001). The basics will be briefly presented here to provide context for the remaining discussion, and key features are summarized in Figures 4.1 and 4.2.

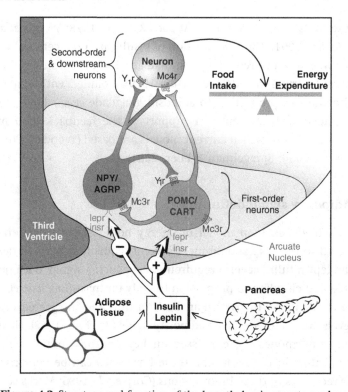

Figure 4.2 Structure and function of the hypothalamic arcuate nucleus. The arcuate nucleus is found in the mediobasal hypothalamus and is one important nucleus involved in energy balance. Neurons found in the arcuate nucleus express insulin and leptin receptors and respond directly to these hormones. The proopiomelanocortin (POMC) expressing neuron is catabolic in nature; when activated by insulin and leptin it releases a-MSH on downstream receptors to lower food intake and increase energy expenditure. The anabolic neuropeptide Y (NPY), agouti-related protein (AGRP) co-expressing neuron releases NPY and AGRP on downstream neurons when insulin and leptin levels are decreased robustly increasing food intake and lowering energy expenditure. It is this dual, coordinate regulation of NPY/AGRP and POMC neurons by insulin and leptin that, in part, generates robust counter-regulatory responses to changes in body energy stores.

In this basic model, both leptin, the adipocyte-derived hormone, and insulin, the pancreatic beta-cell-derived hormone, function as adiposity signals (criteria mentioned above) in the negative feedback regulation of adipose mass (Schwartz *et al.*, 2000; Spiegelman & Flier, 2001). Both hormones circulate in the bloodstream in proportion to adipose mass (Considine *et al.*, 1996; Bagdade *et al.*, 1967) and regulate the activity of neurons found in regions of the brain associated with body weight regulation. In particular, neurons found in the hypothalamic arcuate nucleus (ARC) express receptors for and bind both insulin and leptin (Marks *et al.*, 1990; Schwartz *et al.*, 1996b) and are increasingly well characterized as targets for both hormones (Spanswick *et al.*, 1997, 2000; Cone *et al.*, 2001) (Figure 4.2). The ARC is bilaterally located at the base (ventral) aspect of the hypothalamus on either side of the third ventricle and above the median eminence (Figure 4.2). Arcuate nucleus neurons project to many other key brain areas, including the paraventricular nucleus, lateral hypothalamic area, hindbrain and directly to the spinal cord, and are thought to function as primary neurons in a series of neural circuits that regulate food intake, energy expenditure, hypothalamic–pituitary function and sympathetic outflow. Intriguingly, insulin and leptin receptors are expressed in many of these other brain regions as well (Grill & Kaplan, 2002; Berthoud, 2004). Mechanisms by which insulin and leptin interact with these other neurons and how signaling from multiple brain areas is ultimately integrated into physiological output has yet to be fully understood, although compelling inroads have been made (Figlewicz *et al.*, 2001, 2003, 2004; Grill *et al.*, 2002, Faulconbridge *et al.*, 2003, 2005; Figlewicz, 2003b; Georgescu *et al.*, 2005; Dhillon *et al.*, 2006).

Discussion on the role of insulin and leptin will be limited to the ARC herein both for simplicity's sake and because most is known about their role in ARC (as above). Further, while other brain areas express insulin and leptin receptors, the activity of these brain regions are potentially modulatory in some sense and overlaid upon the signals from the "primary" and/or dominant neurons and neural circuits originating in the ARC (Schwartz *et al.*, 2000; Spiegelman & Flier, 2001). Situated in the ARC are at least two distinct neuronal cell types that respond to adiposity signals and exert opposing effects on energy balance; one being anabolic, while the other is catabolic in nature (Schwartz *et al.*, 2000; Cone *et al.*, 2001) (Figure 4.2). Anabolic neurons are those that, when activated by reduced insulin and leptin levels, promote increased food intake and decreased energy expenditure, leading to the storage of energy. In the ARC, these neurons co-express the orexigenic neuropeptides neuropeptide Y (NPY) and agouti-related protein (AGRP). NPY/AGRP neurons are inhibited by rising leptin and insulin levels, and this inhibition is believed to mediate a portion of the anorectic actions of these hormones. For example, insulin or leptin infusion directly into the third cerebral ventricle reduces NPY gene expression in fasted or STZ-diabetic rats or *ob/ob* mice in effect blocking the increase of NPY gene expression that would otherwise occur (Schwartz *et al.*, 1991, 1996a, 1996b). Antisense "knockdown" of hypothalamic insulin receptors increases both food intake and NPY and AGRP gene expression (Obici *et al.*, 2002a) and NPY and AGRP gene expression are elevated in *ob/ob* (Stephens *et al.*, 1995; Erickson *et al.*, 1996; Schwartz *et al.*, 1996a; Mizuno *et al.*, 1998), *db/db* (Mizuno *et al.*, 1998),

Zucker (Beck et al., 1990) and Koletsky rats (Keen Rhinehart et al., 2004), all genetic models of deficient leptin input to ARC neurons. These findings add neuropeptidergic significance to the observation that intracerebroventricular (icv) insulin or leptin reduces food intake (Woods et al., 1979; Foster et al., 1991; Campfield et al., 1995; Weigle et al., 1995; Air et al., 2002; Niswender et al., 2003b) by suggesting that the tonic action of leptin and insulin to inhibit the production and release of a potent orexigenic neuropeptide, NPY, normally constrains food intake (Niswender & Schwartz, 2003).

Further, in an isolated neuronal preparation, the firing rate (and thus release of neuropeptide) of a subset of ARC neurons hypothesized to be NPY/ AGRP neurons is reduced by insulin treatment and similar effects are induced by leptin (Spanswick et al., 1997, 2000). The effect of both insulin and leptin to hyperpolarize this population of hypothalamic neurons is dependent upon signaling through phosphatidylinositol 3-kinase (PI3K), a classic insulin signaling target, and upon the opening of ATP sensitive potassium channels (Spanswick et al., 1997, 2000). Thus, a portion of the effect of insulin and leptin to regulate energy homeostasis is based upon their ability to regulate NPY/ AGRP neuronal function.

Acting in opposition to the NPY/AGRP neuron is the catabolic proopiomelanocortin (POMC)-expressing neuron. According to current models, these cells release the anorexic neuropeptide, a-melanocyte stimulating hormone (a-MSH), when stimulated by insulin and leptin, and thereby promote decreases of food intake and body weight. Insulin, like leptin, increases POMC gene expression (Elias et al., 1999; Benoit et al., 2002), and activates downstream melanocortin "target" neurons (Benoit et al., 2002). Further, in all of the genetic obesity models mentioned above with deficient leptin input to ARC neurons, POMC gene expression is suppressed (in contrast to elevated NPY gene expression) (Mizuno et al., 1998; Kim et al., 2000; Keen Rhinehart et al., 2004). A great deal of genetic evidence is available in support of a primary role of the so-called "melanocortin" pathway in energy homeostasis, including the fact that mutations in the POMC gene and downstream melanocortin-3 (MC3R) and melanocortin-4 receptors (MC4R), cause obesity in rodents (Butler, 2006) and humans (Coll et al., 2004). Fundamental to insulin and leptin action in energy homeostasis, therefore, is their ability to activate POMC-expressing neurons.

Data such as those just summarized were utilized to develop the model (Figures 4.1, 4.2) of dual catabolic and anabolic neural circuits that are differentially regulated by insulin and leptin to control energy balance. Although presented as parallel circuits for the sake of simplicity, in point of fact, much cross-talk occurs and numerous other inputs enter these circuits at various levels. For example, AGRP, produced in the anabolic NPY/AGRP neuron functions as an endogenous antagonist of the catabolic pathway by antagonizing downstream MC4R (Ollmann *et al.*, 1997). Furthermore, important studies have identified intra-ARC innervation of POMC neurons by NPY neurons, utilizing both NPY and GABA neurotransmission. For instance, leptin depolarizes (activates) the POMC neuron, while hyperpolarizing the NPY cell body, in turn reducing inhibitory GABA release onto the POMC cell (Cowley *et al.*, 2001).

Another example of the complexity of this system is that ARC neurons respond to a number of additional stimuli besides insulin and leptin. Intriguingly, ARC neurons appear to receive input from nutritional signals (glucose, fatty acids, amino acids) and all of these inputs, of course, must be integrated to generate an efferent signal (Schuit *et al.*, 2001; Obici *et al.*, 2002b, 2002c; Lam *et al.*, 2005; Lopez *et al.*, 2005; He *et al.*, 2006; Pocai *et al.*, 2006), a concept termed metabolic sensing. A final example of the ultimate complexity of energy homeostasis arises from the fact that animals and humans feed for a variety of reasons, including for "reward" or "hedonism." Reward centers are found in the limbic system, and such nuclei clearly innervate and are capable of modulating the output of hypothalamic "homeostatic" nuclei (Berthoud, 2004). Interestingly, both insulin and leptin have also been implicated in the cognitive aspects of feeding (reward, learning and memory) via receptors in these cortico-limbic sites (Figlewicz, 2003a), an emerging area of interest that may be particularly pertinent to populations that become obese in association with consumption of highly palatable diets (Niswender *et al.*, 2004b). This concept will be discussed in more detail later.

The conceptualization of energy homeostasis as an endocrine negative feedback loop with insulin and leptin serving a primary role as adiposity signals both derives from ongoing observations and serves as an intellectual framework within which to develop and test new hypotheses. That it has survived 50 years and the recent explosion in our understanding of the molecular mechanisms of energy homeostasis is a testament to the insight of those who initially proposed and refined such an idea. Thus, this widely accepted negative adiposity feedback model of energy homeostasis will be used as a framework for further discussion, but, it should be again noted that other models and interpretations have been proposed (Flier, 1998; Leibel, 2002; Speakman *et al.*, 2002).

8.   Insulin as an adiposity signal: the catabolic nature of insulin action in the CNS

Before adding detail to a discussion of insulin and leptin action as key determinants of energy balance, further comment specific to insulin is warranted. Although leptin is recognized as a major regulator of fat mass, the concept that insulin functions as a catabolic "adiposity" negative-feedback signal through the regulation of key hypothalamic neurons is relatively less appreciated even though the strength of evidence in support of this hypothesis is robust (Niswender & Schwartz, 2003; Niswender *et al.*, 2004a). Confusion may surround the notion of insulin as a centrally acting catabolic hormone because of its well-recognized role as the prototypical anabolic (and glucoregulatory) hormone in peripheral tissues. For example, clinical administration of insulin can lead to hypoglycemia and counter-regulatory increases in food intake and, if repeated, can cause weight gain via this mechanism; i.e. "feeding the insulin" (Dryden *et al.*, 1998). Of course, insulin functions in the periphery to promote storage of energy in the forms of carbohydrate, protein and fat; it potently stimulates glucose uptake, protein synthesis, and lipogenesis and inhibits lipolysis. A combination of these factors likely explains the general clinical observation that insulin usage can lead to weight gain in patients with diabetes (Carlson & Campbell, 1993), rather than the weight loss predicted to occur with administration of an "adiposity signal." It has been further postulated, that as beta-cell function declines over the course of diabetes, relative insulin deficiency would yield a CNS signal of energy deficit, activate anabolic circuits, and potentially contribute to diabetes-associated weight gain (Schwartz & Porte, 2005). The idea that central insulin action is fundamentally catabolic (i.e. reduces food intake and body weight), whereas its peripheral actions are anabolic (i.e. increasing energy storage and potentially increasing body weight if a patient is over-insulinized), is ultimately consistent with and illustrative of the concept of an endocrine feedback loop in the control of energy stores (Schwartz *et al.*, 2000). Like many physiological systems, the peripheral and central actions of insulin are balanced to promote (i) euglycemia, (ii) optimal body composition and (iii) reproductive fitness.

A reversal of the situation just mentioned is evident in the condition known as diabetic hyperphagia, a prominent behavioral manifestation of uncontrolled human type I diabetes or experimental animal diabetes. When beta cells have been destroyed, an absolute lack of insulin results in hyperglycemia and an inability to store energy in peripheral tissues, ultimately causing a dramatic loss of body weight due to renal glucose wasting. The lack of catabolic insulin action in the brain coupled with decreased serum leptin levels that accompany weight loss, however, leads to dramatic increases in food intake that compensates in part for energy wasting and prevents a more rapid demise. Thus, if the "catabolic" tone of hypothalamic insulin and leptin action were not relieved by the absence of these hormones, weight loss would be more dramatic and death would occur more rapidly. In proof of "adiposity negative feedback" principles, either insulin or leptin given directly into the third cerebral ventricle of rats with streptozotocin-induced diabetes completely blocks this compensatory hyperphagia (Sipols et al., 1995; Sindelar et al., 1999) and results in more rapid weight loss. The observation that either hormone given alone can block diabetic hyperphagia is compelling evidence of the overlap in the function of insulin and leptin in the CNS as adiposity signals.

9.   Adiposity signal access to the CNS

Although not the focus of this chapter, a few words about CNS access of peripheral signals is warranted. The hypothesis that circulating insulin and leptin provides a physiological signal to brain areas involved in energy homeostasis implies either a mechanism whereby these peptides traverse the blood–brain barrier (BBB) to enter the brain or that key regulatory centers are located in brain regions without a rigorous blood–brain barrier. After intravenous insulin infusion, increases of plasma insulin are reflected by proportionate but smaller increases in cerebrospinal fluid insulin concentrations in animals (Woods & Porte, 1977) and humans (Wallum et al., 1987). Subsequent studies demonstrated that the insulin uptake process involves a saturable transport mechanism (Baura et al., 1993) and similar transport mechanisms have been identified and proposed for leptin access to the CNS (Banks et al., 1996). The observation that insulin and leptin transport into the brain is attenuated by consumption of a high-fat diet (Kaiyala et al., 2000; Banks & Farrell, 2003) raises the possibility that acquired reductions of brain insulin and leptin delivery would yield decreased hormone action and favor weight gain. However, the extent to which insulin and leptin access to key neuronal targets such as the ARC requires a regulated transport mechanism continues to be discussed (Kurrimbux et al., 2004). The ARC is situated adjacent to the median eminence, which lacks a BBB, and it is not yet clear whether ARC neurons are protected by the BBB (Krisch & Leonhardt, 1978; Merchenthaler, 1991). Capillary permeability may vary extensively across the ARC, being greater in its mediobasal than its lateral aspect (Shaver et al., 1992). Thus, either increased permeability to adiposity signals in the ARC or specific transport mechanisms explain insulin and leptin access to these key neurons and, of course, defects in these mechanisms may ultimately be involved in the pathophysiology of obesity as decreased exposure of target neurons to circulating insulin and leptin would translate into a neuroendocrine signal of energy deficit.

10.   Evolutionary basis of adiposity signaling

The hypothesis that insulin acts in the CNS to control energy homeo-stasis, first proposed in the 1970s, has enjoyed a resurgence of interest in response to several novel models of insulin action in the CNS. Interestingly, nematodes such as *Caenorhabditis elegans* express homologues of insulin, insulin receptors, and insulin signal transduction molecules (Wolkow *et al.*, 2000, 2002). Although *C. elegans* functionally regulate body fat stores, they do not express leptin-signaling homologues, suggesting that the insulin signaling system may be more primitively involved in energy homeostasis than leptin. An insulin receptor homologue null mutant, referred to as *Daf-2*, has increased fat storage in the intestine, increased longevity, and reduced reproductive function (Wolkow *et al.*, 2000, 2002). The "obesity" in this *C. elegans* mutant appears to reflect a role for insulin signaling in the nervous system where insulin action has the "catabolic" effect of limiting energy storage. It is also noteworthy that these primitive organisms do not appear to actively regulate carbohydrate flux, suggesting that insulin homologues played an important role in the control of energy balance, life cycle and reproduction prior to the evolution of its role in the regulation of glucose homeostasis (Wolkow *et al.*, 2000, 2002; Lee *et al.*, 2003). Likewise, the fruit fly, *Drosophila melanogaster*, expresses insulin-signaling homologues that may have a similar role in the regulation of energy metabolism and lifespan (Garofalo, 2002). Homologues of the leptin system have not been identified in such primitive organisms suggesting that it evolved later, after the evolutionary establishment of a mechanism to control energy balance. As dis-cussed later, leptin utilizes insulin signal transduction mechanisms (i.e. PI3K), in part, to control energy homeostasis in mammals. Since leptin and its signaling components are evolutionarily related to cytokine/immunity systems, it seems that a role in energy balance evolved as an "overlap" function in relation to insulin. This redundancy further implies significant evolutionary pressure for the phenotype of efficient control of energy balance such that two distinct hormonal systems have evolved to overlap in this function.

11.   Insulin as an adiposity signal: other evidence

Although nematodes and flies provide an intriguing evolutionary perspective, recently developed molecular genetics models in rodents have shed additional light on the role played by both insulin and leptin (next sec-tion) in both reproduction and energy balance. Both brain-specific knockouts of the insulin receptor and animals lacking insulin receptor substrate-2 (IRS-2; a key molecule linking activated insulin receptors to signal transduction via

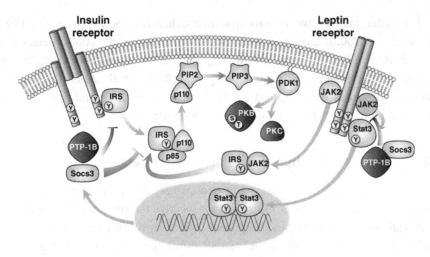

Figure 4.3 Insulin and leptin signal transduction and "cross-talk" in the activation and termination of signaling. Upon ligand binding and activation of its intrinsic tyrosine kinase, the insulin receptor couples to phosphatidylinositol 3-kinase (PI3K; p85 regulatory subunit, p110 catalytic subunit) for the majority of its physiological effects and does so via insulin receptor substrate (IRS) proteins. Downstream targets include 3-phosphoinositide-dependent kinase-1 (PDK1), glycogen synthase kinase-3 (GSK3), protein kinase B (PKB/Akt), and protein kinase C (PKC). The effects of insulin on food intake and membrane potential have been demonstrated to be PI3K dependent. Leptin, a cytokine family member, signals via a cytokine type receptor; after ligand binding and dimerization an extrinsic kinase (Janus kinase; JAK2) is recruited and phosphorylates the intracellular portion of the receptor. This creates a binding site for signal transducers and activators of transcription-3 (STAT3) that once phosphorylated translocates to the nucleus and induces gene transcription. Additionally, leptin has been shown to activate PI3K signaling in numerous cell types, perhaps via JAK2, a phenomenon referred to as "cross-talk." Both suppressor of cytokine signaling-3 (SOCS3) and protein tyrosine phosphatase-1B can terminate signaling by both insulin and leptin via dephosphorylation and targeting of signaling proteins for degradation. Of course, both insulin and leptin activate additional signal transduction mechanisms.

PI3K, Figure 4.3) exhibit a phenotype of obesity and reproductive dysfunction (Bruning *et al.*, 2000; Burks *et al.*, 2000). Similarly, knockdown of insulin receptor expression locally in the mediobasal hypothalamus using antisense technology (Obici *et al.*, 2002a) resulted in cumulative food intake of 152% and fat mass of 186% compared with nonsense treated controls (Obici *et al.*, 2002a). The consensus from a variety of molecular genetics approaches, therefore, is that insulin action in the hypothalamus plays an essential role in the regulation of energy homeostasis.

A broader perspective reveals that neurochemical (Schwartz *et al.*, 1991; Benoit *et al.*, 2002), electrophysiological (Spanswick *et al.*, 2000), behavioral (Woods *et al.*, 1979; Air *et al.*, 2002; Clegg *et al.*, 2003; Niswender *et al.*, 2003b) and molecular genetics (Bruning *et al.*, 2000; Burks *et al.*, 2000; Obici *et al.*, 2002a) approaches each support a role for insulin in the regulation of hypothalamic neurons and therein of energy homeostasis.

12.   Leptin as an adiposity signal: other evidence

The cloning of leptin (Zhang *et al.*, 1994) and its receptor (Lee *et al.*, 1996) and validation of their roles in the respective obesity phenotypes of *ob/ob* and *db/db* mice made obvious the potent role of leptin in energy balance. The discovery of leptin mutations in a small number of children with dramatic obesity syndromes (Montague *et al.*, 1997) validates the relevance of the leptin axis to energy balance in humans, but ultimately does not explain a significant proportion of human obesity. That the majority of leptin's actions on energy balance are mediated by the CNS are confirmed by studies in which deletion of leptin receptors specifically in neurons (Cohen *et al.*, 2001) recapitulates to a large extent the *db/db* phenotype and studies in which leptin receptors transgenically expressed specifically in neurons of *db/db* mice virtually completely rescues the phenotype (de Luca *et al.*, 2005). Similarly, treatment of morbidly obese, leptin-deficient children with recombinant leptin has largely reversed all of the neuroendocrine manifestations of leptin deficiency including hypogonadotropic hypogonadism (Farooqi *et al.*, 1999).

13.   Insulin and leptin signal transduction

Conceptualization of energy balance as a negative feedback loop involving insulin and leptin and specific neuronal subpopulations has allowed numerous specific hypotheses to be developed and tested. Yet much remains to be understood about the systems responsible for maintenance of energy balance. Relevant to an improved understanding of the pathophysiology of obesity, is determination of the mechanisms by which insulin and leptin receptor signaling couples to changes in neuronal function that are ultimately responsible for the adaptive response to changes in energy availability. Given the strength of evidence for their respective roles and similarities in their physiological actions in the hypothalamus, an exploration of the intracellular signal transduction mechanisms utilized by insulin and leptin in hypothalamus is warranted.

Although both function as adiposity signals, they are traditionally associated with divergent signal transduction pathways (Banks *et al.*, 2000; Kido *et al.*, 2001)

(Figure 4.3). The insulin receptor is a heterodimer of α and β subunits; ligand binding activates an intrinsic tyrosine kinase leading to the autophosphorylation of multiple tyrosine residues on the intracellular portion of the receptor. Receptor autophosphorylation, in turn, recruits one of a family of proteins known as insulin receptor substrate (IRS) molecules that are phosphorylated, activated and subsequently interact with the enzyme phosphatidylinositol 3-kinase (PI3K). A major isoform of PI3K (class IA (Vanhaesebroeck et al., 2005)) that is heavily involved in insulin action and metabolic control consists of a p85 regulatory subunit and p110 catalytic subunit. Binding of the p85 subunit by a phosphorylated IRS molecule results in the activation of the p110 subunit, which catalyzes the phosphorylation of membrane-localized phosphatidylinositol 4,5 bisphosphate (PIP2) to phosphatidylinositol 3,4,5 trisphosphate (PIP3). PIP3 serves as a cofactor and active signal transduction moiety leading to the activation of several downstream targets such as 3-phosphoinositide dependent kinase 1 (PDK1), glycogen synthase kinase 3 (GSK3) and protein kinase B, among others (PKB/Akt) (Kido et al., 2001; Saltiel & Pessin, 2002). Of course, PI3K is a ubiquitously expressed signal transduction mechanism utilized by multiple hormones and signaling systems (Katso et al., 2001; Vanhaesebroeck et al., 2005).

In contrast, leptin is a cytokine-like molecule and its receptor is homologous with the Type 1 cytokine receptor family (Banks et al., 2000). While multiple isoforms of the leptin receptor exist, the fully active signaling isoform is referred to as the long form or the B form (Myers, 2004). Leptin binding leads to the recruitment of a cytosolic tyrosine kinase known as Janus kinase 2 (JAK2). JAK2 tyrosine phosphorylates critical residues on the intracellular portion of the leptin receptor, resulting in the recruitment and subsequent activation of molecules known as signal transducer and activator of transcription 3 (STAT-3). STAT molecules are transcription factors that when activated by phosphorylation dimerize and translocate to the nucleus to regulate gene transcription. Both the leptin and insulin receptors also couple to additional signal transduction pathways (Banks et al., 2000; Saltiel & Pessin, 2002) although evidence is currently only available for the critical role of PI3K and JAK-STAT signaling. Because cross-talk, or modulation of one pathway by another, is increasingly described, it is likely that other critical signal transduction mediators of energy balance will be characterized in the coming years.

14.   Cross-talk between leptin and insulin action in hypothalamus

Most of our understanding of insulin and leptin signaling arose from studies in peripheral tissues and cell culture. In several of these models, leptin has the ability to activate both the JAK-STAT and the classically insulin-like PI3K pathway (Kellerer et al., 1997; Harvey et al., 2000; Zhao et al., 2000; Anderwald et al., 2002), a phenomenon referred to as "cross-talk" (Figure 4.3). Given the overlapping physiological effects of insulin and leptin in the hypothalamus, the hypothesis that signaling cross-talk occurs in key brain areas such as the ARC is attractive (Niswender & Schwartz, 2003). Addressing this possibility, Spanswick and Ashford performed a series of electrophysiological studies in hypothalamic slice preparations, and demonstrated that both leptin and insulin acutely regulate the membrane potential and firing rates of a specific subset of neurons (Spanswick et al., 1997, 2000). Interestingly, for both hormones, this effect was dependent upon signaling through PI3K (Spanswick et al., 1997, 2000), a clear demonstration of "cross-talk" in the CNS. These studies have intriguingly also demonstrated a requirement for cytoskeletal rearrangement in coupling the PI3K signal to membrane potential via the ATP sensitive potassium channel (Mirshamsi et al., 2004).

The behavioral overlap of CNS insulin and leptin signaling has further been explored in the in vivo context. We and others have demonstrated that insulin activates the IRS-PI3K signaling cascade in mediobasal hypothalamus of intact rats, and further, that PI3K signaling is required for inhibition of food intake by icv insulin (Carvalheira et al., 2003; Niswender et al., 2003b). Insulin activates PI3K signaling, as detected via an immunohistochemical stain for the PI3K catalyzed reaction product (PIP3) (Niswender et al., 2003a), in ARC neurons that co-express IRS-2, as predicted by current models of insulin signaling (Figure 4.3) (Niswender et al., 2003b). The hypothesis that at least a portion of the hypothalamic effects of leptin may be mediated by PI3K signaling was tested based on the rationale of their overlap in function, and that the acute effects of leptin observed in slice preparations occurred within minutes rather than hours as predicted from a wholly transcriptional mechanism (JAK-STAT). Like insulin, leptin activates PI3K in hypothalamic neurons and this activation is required for the ability of intracerebroventricular leptin to reduce food intake (Niswender et al., 2001), an observation that has been confirmed by other groups (Zhao et al., 2002). These findings in toto support a model in which activation of IRS-PI3K signaling in hypothalamic neurons is a critical event in the ability of adiposity signals to regulate energy homeostasis, or at least control food intake. As discussed before, insulin-related signaling in C. elegans and Drosophila also utilizes a pathway involving IRS and PI3K homologues and regulates energy homeostasis (Wolkow et al., 2000, 2002). The overlap in physiological function of insulin and leptin in the CNS and overlap in signal transduction mechanisms used importantly suggests potential common mechanisms for the development of CNS resistance to both insulin and leptin.

15.   Important unanswered questions: relative role of JAK-STAT vs. PI3K signaling

A number of important questions regarding hypothalamic adiposity signal function remain unanswered; three key issues will be mentioned here. First, what is the relative contribution of PI3K pathway vs. JAK-STAT signaling to insulin and leptin action and ultimately to integrated energy homeostasis? For example, leptin (*ob/ob*) or leptin receptor (*db/db*) mutant mice have a more severe obesity phenotype than the insulin signaling pathway mutants mentioned above suggesting a differential participation by insulin vs. leptin signaling in the processes underlying energy homeostasis. Some insight into this question is provided by a germ-line altered mutant leptin receptor mouse that is genetically defective specifically in its ability to activate STAT signaling (Bates *et al.*, 2003). The observation that these animals are hyperphagic and obese (more obese than insulin signaling mutants, but not as obese as *db/db* control mice) suggest an important role for JAK-STAT signaling in leptin-mediated control of body adiposity. Unlike *db/db* mice that lack all leptin receptor function, however, these mice do not have reproductive defects (hypogonadotropic hypogonadism) and have an attenuated diabetes phenotype (Bates *et al.*, 2003). The conclusion by inference is that STAT3 activation is necessary for some, but not all of leptin's signaling functions. As mentioned above, brain-specific knockouts of the insulin receptor and animals lacking insulin receptor substrate-2 exhibit a phenotype of milder obesity with reproductive impairment and glucose intolerance (Bruning *et al.*, 2000; Burks *et al.*, 2000). One interpretation of these data yields a model in which insulin/ PI3K signaling and reproduction may be "localized" predominantly to the NPY/ AGRP neuron/circuit in the ARC, whereas the control of energy expenditure, food intake and fat mass may rely more heavily on signaling via the POMC neuronal subtype (Myers, 2004). An alternative, but not mutually exclusive, hypothesis states that insulin and leptin neuronal signal transduction are intricately related and, for example, that defects in leptin signal transduction lead to insulin resistance, as is observed in the *db/db* mouse model (Niswender & Schwartz, 2003). Thus, current data have yet to clarify how *both* insulin and leptin input to a specific neuron is integrated in the control of either reproduction or energy homeostasis. A critical dissection of the individual contributions of physiological insulin vs. leptin and PI3K vs. JAK-STAT signaling in the hypothalamus will require novel approaches given the interrelatedness of these systems. Neuronal cell-type specific (i.e. NPY vs. POMC) modulation of insulin and leptin signaling will be required to address such questions, and models sufficient for addressing these questions are in development (Xu *et al.*, 2005).

16.   Differential coupling in anabolic (NPY) vs. catabolic (POMC) neurons

Another related and compelling basic question is whether PI3K or JAK-STAT signaling is required for the response of NPY/AGRP neurons, POMC neurons, or both sets of neurons to adiposity signals. Because POMC neurons are activated, whereas NPY/AGRP neurons are inhibited by insulin and leptin, it seems counterintuitive to suggest that both responses involve either a PI3K or JAK-STAT dependent mechanism given that signal transduction would have to couple to opposing membrane effects in these opposing cell types. What key difference might allow this regulation to occur in opposite directions in adjacent cell populations? For example the work of Spanswick and Ashford, conducted in a subset of glucose responsive neurons (presumably NPY/AGRP) suggests that PI3K activation by insulin and leptin couples to ATP sensitive potassium channel, membrane hyperpolarization and inhibition of firing (Spanswick et al., 1997, 2000). Several recent studies have shed new light upon this question.

Xu et al. (2005) utilized mice in which fluorescent probes for PI3K activation were targeted specifically to NPY/AGRP or POMC neurons and performed real-time "field" fluorescence microscopy of reporter fluorescence in slices treated with insulin or leptin. In these studies, insulin and leptin both activated PI3K signal transduction in POMC neurons which resulted in activation of neuronal firing as detected by calcium flux. The situation is more complex in the NPY/AGRP neuron where insulin also activates PI3K signaling but leptin inhibits, or decreases signaling, albeit indirectly. Despite the presence of leptin receptors on NPY/AGRP neurons, the effect of leptin to decrease PI3K signaling is dependent upon synaptic transmission perhaps via input from the POMC neuron. To be precise, leptin withdrawal activates PI3K signaling in the NPY/AGRP neuron. Further, these studies showed that leptin stimulation of PI3K signaling in POMC neurons is not dependent upon STAT3 signaling, as the effect is observed in STAT3 knock-out slices (Xu et al., 2005).

In a second comprehensive set of recent experiments, Mirshamshi et al. (2004) examined insulin and leptin signaling in rat ARC wedges in vitro. They observed that both insulin and leptin were capable of activating PI3K, MAPK, GSK3 and STAT3 signaling in this preparation and further that both insulin and leptin activation of PKB, GSK3 and MAPK were blocked by PI3K inhibition. This data set suggests that cross-talk is bidirectional with insulin likewise being able to activate leptin-like STAT3 signaling. Finally, and the most intriguing aspect of this work, is the fact that insulin and leptin coupling to ATP sensitive potassium channel activation is not only PI3K dependent, but dependent upon cytoskeletal rearrangement, as stabilizers of actin filaments prevent this coupling. While this work sheds significant light upon signal transduction mechanisms and on coupling to membrane potential, it does not address the neuronal phenotype in which these events occur (Mirshamsi *et al.*, 2004). As the basic structure and function of the systems regulating energy balance become better understood, studies such as those just described indicate increasing levels of complexity in the coupling of insulin and leptin membrane receptor activation to neuronal cellular responses.

17.   Termination of adiposity signaling

Negative feedback is a critical regulatory mechanism for many physiological and intracellular signaling pathways. Just as insulin and leptin provide negative feedback signals in organismal energy balance, mechanisms exist at the cellular level to provide negative feedback upon activation of insulin and leptin signal transduction. Inferred from the existence of such systems is the concept that adiposity signaling must ordinarily be tightly regulated given that it is subject to feedback regulation at several levels. Further, just as pathways involved in activation of adiposity signaling must be considered to be candidate targets for disruption in obesity, pathways involved in negative feedback to insulin and leptin signaling are also candidates for involvement in obesity pathogenesis.

Like activation of signaling pathways, overlap also exists in mechanisms for termination of signaling via insulin and leptin. Protein tyrosine phosphatase-1B (PTP-1B) is capable of terminating both leptin and insulin signal transduction by dephosphorylation of key tyrosine residues in molecules in the signaling cascade (e.g. insulin receptor, IRS, JAK2; Figure 4.3); molecules ordinarily activated by tyrosine phosphorylation. Consistent with this proposed role, PTP-1B knockout mice have increased sensitivity to both leptin and insulin (Elchebly *et al.*, 1999; Zabolotny *et al.*, 2002), indicating that this enzyme physiologically constrains adiposity signaling since the signals are magnified in its absence.

Suppressor of cytokine signaling-3 (SOCS3) is a second molecule implicated in the termination of cell signaling by both insulin and leptin (Bjorbaek *et al.*, 1999) (Figure 4.3). SOCS3 expression is transcriptionally induced via the JAK-STAT pathway in response to leptin or other cytokines, and it inhibits further signaling by binding to and inactivating key molecules such as JAK2 and IRS-2. Intriguingly, it appears that insulin also activates SOCS3 (Emanuelli *et al.*, 2000, 2001; Peraldi *et al.*, 2001) and that, importantly, SOCS3 dampens signaling by both the insulin receptor-IRS-PI3K pathway (Emanuelli *et al.*, 2000) as well as the JAK-STAT pathway (Figure 4.3). SOCS3 binds to phosphotyrosine residues on the insulin receptor and inhibits insulin-mediated tyrosine phosphorylation of IRS proteins (Ueki et al., 2004a) and also promotes ubiquitin-mediated degradation of IRS proteins (Rui et al., 2002). By way of example, overexpression of SOCS3 in liver causes marked insulin resistance and steatosis in mice (Ueki et al., 2004b). In further proof of this principle, mice with SOCS3 haploinsufficiency or neuron-specific SOCS3 deletion are both resistant to diet-induced obesity (DIO) and have increased sensitivity to insulin and leptin (Howard et al., 2004; Mori et al., 2004). This phenotype is similar to the PTP-1B deletion (Elchebly et al., 1999; Zabolotny et al., 2002) and similarly indicates a role for SOCS3 in the basal regulation of energy homeostasis.

That regulatory systems exist to dampen neuronal signal transduction by both insulin and leptin has potentially important implications for the pathophysiology of obesity. Since both proteins are expressed in key hypothalamic areas involved in energy homeostasis (Bjorbaek et al., 1998; Zabolotny et al., 2002), the data just mentioned suggest that SOCS3 and PTP-1B signaling regulate the amplitude of adiposity signal transduction in neuronal targets. Based upon these principles, over-activity of SOCS3 or PTP-1B would be predicted to cause neuronal resistance to both insulin and leptin. Thus, if either or both are induced during high-fat feeding, attenuated signal transduction via the JAK-STAT and IRS-PI3K pathways would be the expected outcome. Decreased signaling would favor increased food intake, decreased metabolic rate and weight gain and consistent with this rationale, elevated SOCS3 expression in the hypothalamus of diet-induced obese animals has been reported (Bjorbaek et al., 1998; Munzberg et al., 2004). It has been proposed that the markedly elevated leptin (and presumably insulin) levels associated with obesity would be sufficient, via JAK-STAT3 signaling, to over-induce SOCS3 resulting in phenotypical and biochemical leptin resistance (Munzberg & Myers, 2005). Given that inhibition of upstream insulin and leptin signaling in this model should, in turn, decrease SOCS3 stimulation, a different mechanism of sustained SOCS3 elevation should also be considered, such as inflammatory cytokines. Stimulation of SOCS3 expression by IL-6 or TNF-a, both known to be elevated in obesity, would dampen leptin (and insulin) signaling while stimulating and maintaining high levels of SOCS3 expression independent of insulin and leptin (Munzberg & Myers, 2005).

18.   Insulin and leptin as adiposity signals, energy homeostasis and obesity

To summarize the basic structure–function of this model (Schwartz et al., 2000), decreased body fat mass, as might occur in starvation, leads to

decreases in serum insulin and leptin levels, activation of "anabolic" NPY/
AGRP neurons and, simultaneously, suppression of "catabolic" POMC neurons
(Figure 4.1). Since AGRP is an endogenous antagonist of the downstream
receptor for the POMC derived catabolic peptide, a-MSH, activation of NPY/AGRP
neurons simultaneously increases "anabolic" tone and decreases "catabolic"
tone, resulting in a robust hyperphagic response to caloric deprivation.

Conversely, increased body fat mass increases serum insulin and leptin
levels in direct proportion with the increased fat mass (Bagdade *et al.*, 1967;
Considine *et al.*, 1996). In "normal" subjects, increases in insulin and leptin
levels function to inhibit NPY neurons and activate POMC neurons resulting in
decreased food intake, increased energy expenditure, and the loss of excess
body fat stores. Indeed, in the "Experimental Obesity in Man" and "Guru
Walla" subjects, this is exactly the response that was observed in the setting of
overfeeding and obesity. However, it is evident that the compensatory
responses to these signals are blunted or absent in typical human obese individuals who have markedly elevated serum insulin and leptin levels, but
nonetheless remain hyper- or normophagic. The observation that food intake
is regulated by insulin and leptin in "normal" but not obese individuals, leads
to the question of whether typical obesity represents resistance to the action of
adiposity signals as a result of pathological dysregulation of neuronal signaling, or is an appropriate biological phenomenon that primarily generates a
rigorous defense against body weight loss? In the context of a discussion on the
role of insulin and leptin as adiposity signals, this is a fundamentally
important question.

19. What is the difference between "experimental obesity" and common human obesity or rodent diet-induced obesity?

A prediction of the model that insulin and leptin function as adiposity
signals is that resistance to the negative feedback effect of these hormones
would lead to relative hyperphagia, decreased energy expenditure and obesity.
The "Experimental Obesity in Man," Guru Walla, other human studies
(Tremblay *et al.*, 1992) and animal studies (Bernstein *et al.*, 1975; Rothwell &
Stock, 1979; Rolls *et al.*, 1980; Rogers, 1985; Harris *et al.*, 1986; Hill *et al.*, 1989)
all support the existence of a physiological system that potently defends
against body weight gain in "normal" individuals. Common human obesity
and the best animal model thereof, diet-induced obesity, are fundamentally
different because hyperphagia and weight gain occurs not with external
motivation or manipulation but with ad libitum feeding. Further, "experimental" subjects achieving weight gain with overfeeding have no appetite and

require far more calories than typical obese subjects to maintain similar degrees of adiposity, indicating activation of catabolic circuits, whereas obese individuals are known to have reduced metabolic rates and obviously are feeding ad lib. Thus, the analysis and interpretation of an array of experimental approaches supports the concept of adiposity negative feedback that becomes disrupted in the setting of obesity.

20.   Typical obesity and CNS adiposity signal resistance

From a molecular perspective, these examples lead to the hypothesis that whereas leptin and insulin normally act within the CNS to suppress appetite, increase energy expenditure, and ultimately reduce feeding and adiposity in "experimental obesity," exposure to ad libitum consumed obesity-inducing diets generates resistance to adiposity signals by blunting their normal signaling mechanisms. It is clear that leptin and insulin levels rise in direct proportion with increased adipose mass (Bagdade et al., 1967; Considine et al., 1996). In the context of involuntary feeding and obesity, the action of these markedly elevated hormones in the ARC (and elsewhere) to potently inhibit food intake is readily observed when ad libitum feeding resumes and food intake drops precipitously. In rodent diet-induced obesity and common human obesity, insulin and leptin levels are likewise dramatically elevated and yet food intake remains elevated or normal (Considine et al., 1996). Because the ARC is one of the major sites of action of insulin and leptin, this finding defines hypothalamic insulin and leptin resistance from a behavioral perspective, analogous to peripheral insulin resistance in type II diabetes. In this case, instead of resistance to the glucose-lowering effects of insulin typical of diabetes, resistance to the food intake-lowering effects of insulin and leptin is observed. A currently accepted hypothesis is that brain insulin and leptin resistance represents a primary acquired "pathological" defect in adiposity regulation.

21.   Concordance of diabetes and obesity: a common mechanism for the development of adiposity signal resistance?

While obesity is often referred to as a distinct entity, obesity per se is strongly associated with insulin resistance and diabetes (Mokdad et al., 2000; Anderson et al., 2003). Epidemiological and interventional studies of human populations (Houmard et al., 2002; Knowler et al., 2002; Anderson et al., 2003) and animal models of obesity support this relationship (Woods et al., 2003). The converse is likewise true, weight loss results in dramatic improvements in peripheral insulin sensitivity (Houmard *et al.*, 2002; Uusitupa *et al.*, 2003). These observations have led to the term "diabesity" in describing the concordance of these pathological states (Astrup & Finer, 2000). Peripheral insulin resistance associated with obesity has similarities with hypothalamic insulin and leptin resistance, and leads to the question of whether similar mechanisms may contribute to the observed resistance in both the periphery and the CNS.

The IRS-PI3K pathway that is at least partially responsible for insulin and leptin's feeding effects is also responsible for the majority of insulin action in peripheral tissues (Kido *et al.*, 2001; Saltiel & Pessin, 2002). The major effect of insulin signaling to recruit and activate the intracellular pool of glucose transporter molecules (Saltiel & Pessin, 2002), for example, is a requisite action of insulin in the periphery and is PI3K-dependent. Recent work implicates defects in IRS-PI3K signaling as a significant contributor to insulin insensitivity. Thus, in the setting of obesity and type II diabetes (Cusi *et al.*, 2000; Houmard *et al.*, 2002; Vollenweider *et al.*, 2002) and intravenous fat infusion models (Dresner *et al.*, 1999; Griffin *et al.*, 1999; Kim *et al.*, 2001; Yu *et al.*, 2002), the ability of insulin to activate PI3K, and thus glucose transport, is impaired.

The molecular mechanism for this impairment appears to involve the intracellular accumulation of long chain fatty acyl CoA (LCFA) molecules (Griffin *et al.*, 1999). LCFAs appear to activate "pathological" signal transduction systems when chronically elevated, including PKC (Griffin *et al.*, 1999) and/ or a pathway initiated by IκB kinase-β (IKK-β) (Kim *et al.*, 2001). These pathways are "pathological" in the setting of insulin action because they act to dampen insulin signal transduction by serine/threonine phosphorylation of targets such as the insulin receptor and IRS proteins, molecules normally activated by tyrosine phosphorylation (Saltiel & Pessin, 2002). Thus, muscle cell insulin resistance is a common effect of exposure to high fat or obesity, and the molecular mechanism for this defect results in an inability to activate IRS-PI3K signaling (Griffin *et al.*, 1999; Kim *et al.*, 2001; Houmard *et al.*, 2002). Because IRS-PI3K appears to be an important target for CNS insulin and leptin signaling, the hypothesis that hypothalamic resistance at the level of PI3K may at least partially account for CNS insulin and leptin resistance is intriguing.

While IRS-PI3K signaling appears to be critical for the food intake-lowering response to insulin and leptin, JAK-STAT signaling in response to leptin is similarly fundamental to energy balance (Bates *et al.*, 2003), and is also an attractive candidate as a target of resistance (Bjorbaek *et al.*, 1999; El-Haschimi *et al.*, 2000; Bates & Myers, 2003; Bates *et al.*, 2003; Niswender & Schwartz, 2003). In the model of diet-induced obesity published by El-Haschimi *et al.*, however, leptin resistance to STAT3 activation was not observed until well after the animals had become obese (El-Haschimi *et al.*, 2000). An impaired ability of peripherally administered leptin to activate STAT3 was observed at 4 weeks, implicating a defect of leptin access to the CNS; however, high-fat fed animals were significantly heavier even at this time-point (El-Haschimi *et al.*, 2000). If a defect in hypothalamic adiposity signal transduction is proposed to cause obesity it should occur prior to or concomitant with the onset of obesity. Recently, regional hypothalamic resistance to leptin has been described that adds compelling support to a causal role of leptin resistance in obesity. Munzberg *et al.* (2004) have reported decreased STAT3 activation specifically in ARC of mice fed a high-fat diet in as early as 6 days whereas other hypothalamic and extrahypothalamic sites maintained sensitivity to leptin in terms of STAT3 activation at 14 weeks of high-fat feeding. In the context of the current discussion on the role of insulin and leptin as adiposity signals, these data are consistent both with an important role of the ARC in energy balance and of the concept that pathophysiological changes proposed to result in obesity should precede its development (Schwartz & Niswender, 2004). The observation of increased SOCS3 expression in ARC in these studies (Munzberg *et al.*, 2004) further supports the concept presented earlier that the presence of mechanisms to terminate insulin and leptin signaling are yet another "target" or potential mechanism for dysfunction in obesity (Munzberg & Myers, 2005). Despite recent gains in our understanding of the pathophysiology of obesity, clearly a number of unresolved questions remain regarding potential interactions of leptin-JAK-STAT signaling and IRS-PI3K signaling in the pathological transition to frank obesity (Niswender & Schwartz, 2003).

22.   Dietary induction of adiposity signal resistance and propensity to weight gain

The "Western lifestyle" is hypothesized to be a major predisposing factor to the rapid development of obesity within human populations. The Western lifestyle typically consists of the consumption of calorically dense, high fat, high carbohydrate foods (Tseng & DeVillis, 2000) coupled with the absolute absence of a requirement for physical exertion for survival. A frequently cited example of the metabolic effects of this lifestyle are the Pima Indians of Northern Mexico and Arizona (Lillioja & Bogardus, 1988a). While maintaining a traditional lifestyle in Mexico, Pima remain relatively lean (Valencia *et al.*, 1999), however on exposure to a "Western" lifestyle in the southwestern USA, the rates of obesity and diabetes increase dramatically (Lillioja & Bogardus, 1988b; Pratley, 1998). This dramatic phenotype may represent the ultimate manifestation of thrifty genes; however, available evidence suggests that Mexican Pima exhibit intact energy homeostasis (i.e. match caloric intake with expenditure) without true caloric restriction (Valencia *et al.*, 1999) and rapidly acquire hypothalamic defects in response to energy dense diets and relative inactivity. According to this hypothesis, a dosage of leptin would likely reduce food intake in Mexican Pima, but would have little or no effect in obese US Pima given acquired "resistance." Pima may be an example where inherited "thrifty" genes potently predispose to pathological changes in insulin and leptin signal transduction resulting in diabetes and obesity but only under certain environmental conditions. Thus, Pima appear to demonstrate a genetic–environment interaction. Likewise, a similar "Western" lifestyle has been developed by rodent obesity researchers, who have determined that in many rodent strains the most efficient mechanism to generate obesity is to feed a diet high in both fat and simple carbohydrate (Surwit *et al.*, 1988). Because of these observations, it is worthwhile to examine the effects of dietary fat and carbohydrate on body adiposity.

While a detailed review of macronutrient composition and weight gain is well beyond the scope of this chapter, a molecular model that may yield insight into "diabesity" is related to cellular intermediary metabolism (Niswender *et al.*, 2004b). As discussed, insulin resistance in tissues such as muscle (Shulman, 2000) appears to involve the intracellular accumulation of LCFA (long chain fatty acyl) molecules. Both insulin resistance and relative pancreatic beta cell secretory failure must occur to develop overt diabetes (De-Fronzo, 1988). It is increasingly recognized that a similar mechanism involving LCFA accumulation and toxicity may be responsible for beta cell failure (Prentki *et al.*, 2002; El-Assaad *et al.*, 2003). This concept has been referred to as "glucolipotoxicity" (Unger, 1995; Prentki *et al.*, 2002; El-Assaad *et al.*, 2003; Robertson *et al.*, 2003), given that glucose metabolism and/or toxicity is closely linked to lipotoxicity mediated by LCFA (Poitout *et al.*, 2001).

Muscle and pancreatic beta cells are both susceptible to functional toxicity mediated by LCFA. Furthermore, hypothalamic neurons share both intracellular signal transduction mechanisms (IRS-PI3K) with muscle and a number of secretion-coupling mechanisms with pancreatic beta cells. It is compelling to hypothesize, therefore, that since the CNS would also be exposed to the same metabolic milieu, neurons could be susceptible to the same "glucolipotoxic" mechanisms that would function to generate CNS adiposity signal resistance.

In brief, LCFAs can be synthesized both *de novo* via citrate efflux from the TCA cycle, malonyl CoA and the fatty acid synthase complex and by the assimilation of exogenous free fatty acids into LCFA (Semenkovich, 1997). In a general sense, cellular metabolism under normal physiological conditions tends to be either glucose predominant, such as in the fed state, or fatty acid predominant, such as in fasting and starvation (Sugden *et al.*, 2001). In the fed state, glucose fuels glycolysis and the TCA cycle and citrate efflux generates malonyl CoA via acetyl CoA carboxylase (Sugden *et al.*, 2001). Malonyl CoA is thought to function as a cellular fuel sensor by virtue of its ability to inhibit the mitochondrial LCFA transporter carnitine palmitoyl transferase 1 (CPT-1) (Ruderman *et al.*, 1999; McGarry, 2001), thereby inhibiting LCFA oxidation, while also being a substrate for the *de novo* synthesis of LCFA, in total favoring the accumulation of LCFA. Low malonyl CoA levels, such as in the fasted state when cellular glucose metabolism is decreased via several mechanisms (Semenkovich, 1997), leads to disinhibition of CPT-1 and the oxidation of LCFA for energy. Therefore, in this simple model, LCFA is stored in times of glucose plenty and burned in times of relative glucose deficit based upon cellular malonyl CoA levels. A variety of data exists to suggest that physiological equilibrium between LCFA production and consumption is critical for normal cellular function and the avoidance of "toxicity," particularly in metabolic sensing cell types (Corkey *et al.*, 2000).

In obesity and diabetes, both glucose levels and circulating free fatty acids are elevated due to insulin resistance at various levels (Hawkins *et al.*, 2003). The target tissues include muscle, liver, pancreatic beta cells, and hypothalamic neurons, an expansion of the "triumvirate" of diabetes (Defronzo, 1988). According to this model, susceptible tissues are exposed to both substrates leading to inhibition of CPT-1 and accumulation of LCFA via *de novo* synthesis and exposure to free fatty acids. The model proposes that the obesity metabolic milieu disrupts the physiological equilibrium between LCFA production and consumption leading to pathological accumulation in susceptible tissues and finally to cellular dysfunction. While this model is clearly oversimplified, it can also be utilized in a discussion about the effect of macronutrient diets on weight loss and adiposity signal sensitivity.

23.   Macronutrient composition and weight loss

The number of diets proposing a macronutrient preference for the induction of weight loss has increased dramatically over the years and several have now been studied in randomized clinical trials (Bravata *et al.*, 2003). Two of these diets are worthy of comment in comparison to the obesity-producing Western diet in the context of LCFA toxicity. One diet, originally developed for the prevention of coronary artery disease, is vegetarian based, and could be characterized as ultra-low fat. "Experimentally" the "Ornish" diet could be considered a "Western diet" minus fat. The second diet, the ketotic or "Atkin's" diet consists of very little or no carbohydrate with the objective of minimizing prandial insulin secretion and of reaching a mild ketotic state.

By virtue of being low in carbohydrate content, this diet is necessarily high in fat (and protein), and "experimentally" represents our "Western diet" minus carbohydrate.

In controlled trials, patients randomized to the Ornish diet lost on average 10 kg and > 10% of their body weight at one year (Ornish, 1998; Ornish et al., 1998). The subjects achieved a decrease in dietary fat from 30% to 8.5% and went from 53% to 76.5% dietary carbohydrate content (all as a percentage of calories). Thus, low fat intake in the context of high carbohydrate intake results in significant short-term weight loss in this and in other low fat clinical trials (Pirozzo et al., 2003).

Surprisingly to many investigators, the "Atkins" diet also demonstrated efficacy for weight loss in randomized controlled trials. Foster et al. (2003) observed a significant weight loss of approximately 7% and greater than that of "standard" low-fat diet approaches at 3 and 6 months although these differences were no longer statistically significant at one year. Likewise, Samaha et al. (2003) and Brehm et al. (2003) demonstrated an approximately 5% and 10% weight loss in patients following the Atkins diet in these trials respectively, but these patients were only studied for 6 months. With the molecular model described above in mind, it is interesting to note that in short-term trials, both very low-fat and very low-carbohydrate consumption have similar efficacy in leading to loss of body weight, loosely supporting the hypothesis that fat and carbohydrate combined increases susceptibility to obesity in humans, and by inference results in adiposity signal resistance.

It is important to note that caloric restriction was not necessarily the goal of these dietary interventions. For weight loss to occur, fewer calories must be consumed than expended. Under normal conditions and especially in obesity, compensatory changes in energy homeostasis result in hunger, decreased energy expenditure and, most often, the reaccumulation of lost body weight (Schwartz et al., 2000). In these studies patients ate the diets essentially ad libitum, implying that they became sated with fewer calories consumed (i.e. became sensitive to insulin and leptin) (Brehm et al., 2003), although significant limitations of self-reporting of food intake and appetite are recognized. Such observations do raise the interesting possibility that hypothalamic insulin and leptin resistance induced by high-fat and high-carbohydrate consumption may be reversible by consuming either very low fat or very low carbohydrate diets, at least in the short term. This is clearly a controversial issue and a difficult point to prove experimentally in human studies. Data concerning long-term weight loss certainly suggest that re-establishing the sensitivity of the CNS to insulin and leptin is not common, given the very small percentage of individuals maintaining weight loss. Nonetheless, the integration of recent work regarding the molecular biochemistry of insulin resistance, data from human macronutrient diet trials and the model of insulin and leptin as adiposity signals leads to potentially testable new hypotheses.

24.   "Reward" and potentiation of obesity; role of insulin and leptin

The proposed roles of insulin and leptin as long-term, day to day, week to week, and year to year regulators of energy homeostasis, described thus far as the "homeostatic" feeding system, need to potentially be expanded. It is clear that animals and humans consume food for reasons other than these "homeostatic" cues related to hunger and satiety. Certainly, most individuals reading this chapter can likely personally relate to the "dessert" phenomenon, having divulged in a "rewarding" rich dessert despite being quite full from the prior meal. For those that treat obese patients, it is clear that for a significant proportion of patients seen in this setting, food is used as a rewarding and soothing adaptation to life stress (Dallman et al., 2003). Thus, it is also clear that certain food traits have rewarding or "hedonistic" qualities to both animals and humans (Levine et al., 2003a, 2003b; MacDonald et al., 2003).

Rewarding and motivational aspects of feeding have been localized to important CNS structures such as the limbic system, cortical areas, hippocampus, amygdala and striatonigral structures (Figlewicz, 2003a). Palatability (defined here as an indication of food's hedonic value) is known to influence both the amount and type (Levine et al., 2003a, 2003b; MacDonald et al., 2003) of food that is ingested (Berridge & Grill, 1983; Berridge, 1991, 1996). For example, it is well known that even non-caloric solutions will elicit drinking behavior in sated rats if they are made to taste sweet (Capaldi et al., 1997). Thus, palatability can be a major factor driving ingestion and an intriguing hypothesis is that reward- or palatability-mediated food intake accounts for the hyperphagia observed in some models of diet-induced obesity. Upon presentation with a palatable and obesity-inducing diet, rodents initially exhibit a marked hyperphagia for several days that precedes obesity and that may be mediated by the reward aspects of the diet itself. This is followed by a subsequent, lower magnitude hyperphagia that is hypothesized to be mediated by relative hypothalamic adiposity signal resistance (Ricci & Levin, 2003; Woods et al., 2003).

Collectively, these observations question whether the leptin/insulin feedback loop is able to adequately regulate food intake that is controlled by non-regulatory factors such as reward, motivation, hedonics or learning (Figlewicz, 2003a, 2003b). If the answer to this question is, at least in some circumstances, "no," then it would be important to understand the role that such non-regulatory factors play in the development of diet-induced obesity.

In fact, "hypothalamic feeding" circuits and "reward feeding" circuits are not structurally and functionally distinct; it is likely that central regulators of food intake also influence palatability mechanisms and vice versa (Figlewicz, 2003a, 2003b). Intriguingly, Figlewicz et al. have recently demonstrated that both central insulin and leptin reduce the reinforcement potency of palatable foods (Figlewicz et al., 2001, 2003). The doses of leptin and insulin used in these studies were insufficient to reduce daily food intake or body weight, suggesting that CNS reward centers are more sensitive to these hormones than are hypothalamic centers. Thus, adiposity signals per se, presumably based upon their action in reward brain areas, appear to also negatively regulate the reward aspects of certain foods.

As mentioned above, it is hypothesized that acquired defects in the ability of key hypothalamic neurons to sense and respond to adipostatic signals is one potential mechanism for the maintenance of excess body fat. A related, but slightly different, question is what drives the initial hyperphagia necessary to generate the metabolic milieu proposed to lead to both peripheral and central insulin and leptin resistance. The clear possibility that arises from an under-standing of the role of reward systems addressed here is that under certain circumstances, ingestive behavior is the result of systems that operate inde-pendently of the hypothalamically based regulatory systems. This leads to the hypothesis that consumption of high-calorie, high-fat, high-carbohydrate foods, which appear to be the perfect substrate to generate the insulin and leptin resistant milieu, are highly rewarding to consume, and may in fact, based upon the work of Figlewicz, also generate resistance to the reward dampening effects of insulin and leptin signaling (Figlewicz, 2003a, 2003b; Figlewicz et al., 2003b).

One consideration for this hypothesis is that the rate of development of leptin or insulin insensitivity in brain areas that control these motivated behaviors may be different than systems (e.g., hypothalamus) that regulate body weight. If, for example, these reward centers were even more susceptible to the development of insulin and leptin resistance leading to uncontrolled, reward-based feeding, powerful potentiation of the development of resistance in hypothalamic centers could ensue. Such a model for the rapid potentiation of obesity is attractive, given the rapid pace of the development of obesity in human populations. This hypothesis, importantly, allows for the possibility that defects in insulin and leptin action in CNS structures *other* than the hypothalamus participate in the pathological transition to frank obesity. The efficacy of agents targeting this system in animals (Ravinet Trillou et al., 2003), and currently in clinical trials (Despres *et al.*, 2005; Van Gaal *et al.*, 2005; Pi-Sunyer *et al.*, 2006), lend credence to this hypothesis.

25.   Conclusions

A compelling body of work, both historical and more recent, utilizing a variety of model systems and experimental approaches strongly supports the idea that insulin and leptin play a fundamentally important role as adiposity signals in the hypothalamic control of energy homeostasis. Given the current prevalence and societal cost of obesity and diabetes, an improved understanding of homeostatic mechanisms involving insulin and leptin may yield new therapeutic targets and ultimately new treatments.

References

Air, E. L., Benoit, S. C., Blake Smith, K. A., Clegg, D. J. & Woods, S. C. (2002). Acute third ventricular administration of insulin decreases food intake in two paradigms. *Pharmacol. Biochem. Behav.* **72**, 423-9.

Anderson, J. W., Kendall, C. W. & Jenkins, D. J. (2003). Importance of weight management in type 2 diabetes: review with meta-analysis of clinical studies. *J. Am. Coll. Nutr.* **22**, 331-9.

Anderwald, C., Muller, G., Koca, G., Furnsinn, C., Waldhausl, W. & Roden, M. (2002). Short-term leptin-dependent inhibition of hepatic gluconeogenesis is mediated by insulin receptor substrate-2. *Mol. Endocrinol.* **16**, 1612-28.

Association, A. D. (2000). National Diabetes Fact Sheet. http://www.diabetes.org/info/facts/facts_natl.jsp.

Astrup, A. & Finer, N. (2000). Redefining type 2 diabetes: 'diabesity' or 'obesity dependent diabetes mellitus'? *Obes. Rev.* **1**, 57-9.

Bagdade, J. D., Bierman, E. L. & Porte, D., Jr. (1967). The significance of basal insulin levels in the evaluation of the insulin response to glucose in diabetic and nondiabetic subjects. *J. Clin. Invest.* **46**, 1549-57.

Banks, A. S., Davies, S. M., Bates, S. H. & Myers, M. G., Jr. (2000). Activation of downstream signals by the long form of the leptin receptor. *J. Biol. Chem.* **275**, 14563-72.

Banks, W. A. & Farrell, C. L. (2003). Impaired transport of leptin across the blood-brain barrier in obesity is acquired and reversible. *Am. J. Physiol. Endocrinol. Metab.* **285**, E10-15.

Banks, W. A., Kastin, A. J., Huang, W., Jaspan, J. B. & Maness, L. M. (1996). Leptin enters the brain by a saturable system independent of insulin. *Peptides* **17**, 305-11.

Bates, S. H. & Myers, M. G. (2003). The role of leptin->STAT3 signaling in neuroendocrine function: an integrative perspective. *J. Mol. Med.* Epub 2003. Published 2004, *J. Mol. Med.* **82**, 12-20.

Bates, S. H., Stearns, W. H., Dundon, T. A. *et al.* (2003). STAT3 signalling is required for leptin regulation of energy balance but not reproduction. *Nature* **421**, 856–9.

Baura, G. D., Foster, D. M., Porte, D., Jr. *et al.* (1993). Saturable transport of insulin from plasma into the central nervous system of dogs in vivo. A mechanism for regulated insulin delivery to the brain. *J. Clin. Invest.* **92**, 1824–30.

Beck, B., Burlet, A., Nicolas, J. P. & Burlet, C. (1990). Hypothalamic neuropeptide Y (NPY) in obese Zucker rats: implications in feeding and sexual behaviors. *Physiol. Behav.* **47**, 449–53.

Benoit, S. C., Air, E. L., Coolen, L. M. *et al.* (2002). The catabolic action of insulin in the brain is mediated by melanocortins. *J. Neurosci.* **22**, 9048–52.

Bernstein, I. L., Lotter, E. C., Kulkosky, P. J., Porte, D., Jr. & Woods, S. C. (1975). Effect of force-feeding upon basal insulin levels of rats. *Proc. Soc. Exp. Biol. Med.* **150**, 546–8.

Berridge, K. C. (1991). Modulation of taste affect by hunger, caloric satiety, and sensory specific satiety in the rat. *Appetite* **16**, 103–20.

Berridge, K. C. (1996). Food reward: brain substrates of wanting and liking. *Neurosci. Biobehav. Rev.* **20**, 1–25.

Berridge, K. C. & Grill, H. J. (1983). Alternating ingestive and aversive consummatory responses suggest a two-dimensional analysis of palatability in rats. *Behav. Neurosci.* **97**, 563–73.

Berthoud, H. R. (2002). Multiple neural systems controlling food intake and body weight. *Neurosci. Biobehav. Rev.* **26**, 393–428.

Berthoud, H. R. (2004). Mind versus metabolism in the control of food intake and energy balance. *Physiol. Behav.* **81**, 781–93.

Bjorbaek, C., Elmquist, J. K., Frantz, J. D., Shoelson, S. E. & Flier, J. S. (1998). Identification of SOCS-3 as a potential mediator of central leptin resistance. *Mol. Cell.* **1**, 619–25.

Bjorbaek, C., El-Haschimi, K., Frantz, J. D. & Flier, J. S. (1999). The role of SOCS-3 in leptin signaling and leptin resistance. *J. Biol. Chem.* **274**, 30 059–65.

Bravata, D. M., Sanders, L., Huang, J., Krumholz, H. M., Olkin, I. & Gardner, C. D. (2003). Efficacy and safety of low-carbohydrate diets: a systematic review. *J. Am. Med. Assoc.* **289**, 1837–50.

Bray, G. A. (2003). Risks of obesity. *Endocrinol. Metab. Clin. North Am.* **32**, 787–804, viii.

Brehm, B. J., Seeley, R. J., Daniels, S. R. & D'Alessio, D. A. (2003). A randomized trial comparing a very low carbohydrate diet and a calorie-restricted low fat diet on body weight and cardiovascular risk factors in healthy women. *J. Clin. Endocrinol. Metab.* **88**, 1617–23.

Brobeck, J., Tepperman, J. & Long, C. (1943). Experimental hypothalamic hyperphagia in the albino rat. *Yale J. Biol. Med.* **15**, 831.

Bruning, J. C., Gautam, D., Burks, D. J. *et al.* (2000). Role of brain insulin receptor in control of body weight and reproduction. *Science* **289**, 2122–5.

Burks, D. J., De Mora, J. F., Schubert, M. *et al.* (2000). IRS-2 pathways integrate female reproduction and energy homeostasis. *Nature* **407**, 377–82.

Butler, A. A. (2006). The melanocortin system and energy balance. *Peptides* **27**, 281–90.

Campfield, L. A., Smith, F. J., Guisez, Y., Devos, R. & Burn, P. (1995). Recombinant mouse OB protein: evidence for a peripheral signal linking adiposity and central neural networks. *Science* **269**, 546–9.

Capaldi, E. D., Hunter, M. J. & Lyn, S. A. (1997). Conditioning with taste as the CS in conditioned flavor preference learning. *An. Learn. Behav.* **25**, 427–36.

Carlson, M. G. & Campbell, P. J. (1993). Intensive insulin therapy and weight gain in IDDM. *Diabetes* **42**, 1700–7.

Carvalheira, J. B., Ribeiro, E. B., Araujo, E. P. *et al.* (2003). Selective impairment of insulin signalling in the hypothalamus of obese Zucker rats. *Diabetologia* **46**, 1629–40.

Clegg, D. J., Riedy, C. A., Smith, K. A., Benoit, S. C. & Woods, S. C. (2003). Differential sensitivity to central leptin and insulin in male and female rats. *Diabetes* **52**, 682–7.

Cohen, P., Zhao, C., Cai, X. *et al.* (2001). Selective deletion of leptin receptor in neurons leads to obesity. *J. Clin. Invest.* **108**, 1113–21.

Coll, A. P., Farooqi, I. S., Challis, B. G., Yeo, G. S. & O'Rahilly, S. (2004). Proopiomelanocortin and energy balance: insights from human and murine genetics. *J. Clin. Endocrinol. Metab.* **89**, 2557–62.

Cone, R. D., Cowley, M. A., Butler, A. A., Fan, W., Marks, D. L. & Low, M. J. (2001). The arcuate nucleus as a conduit for diverse signals relevant to energy homeostasis. *Int. J. Obes. Relat. Metab. Disord.* **25** Suppl. 5, S63–7.

Considine, R. V., Sinha, M. K., Heiman, M. L. *et al.* (1996). Serum immunoreactive-leptin concentrations in normal-weight and obese humans [see comments]. *N. Engl. J. Med.* **334**, 292–5.

Control, C. F. D. (2003) Overweight and obesity, obesity trends. http://www.cdc.gov/nccdphp/dnpa/obesity/trend/maps/index.htm.

Corkey, B. E., Deeney, J. T., Yaney, G. C., Tornheim, K. & Prentki, M. (2000). The role of long-chain fatty acyl-CoA esters in beta-cell signal transduction. *J. Nutr.* **130**, 299S–304S.

Corp, E. S., Woods, S. C., Porte, D., Jr., Dorsa, D. M., Figlewicz, D. P. & Baskin, D. G. (1986). Localization of 125I-insulin binding sites in the rat hypothalamus by quantitative autoradiography. *Neurosci. Lett.* **70**, 17–22.

Cowley, M. A., Smart, J. L., Rubinstein, M. *et al.* (2001). Leptin activates anorexigenic POMC neurons through a neural network in the arcuate nucleus. *Nature* **411**, 480–4.

Cusi, K., Maezono, K., Osman, A. *et al.* (2000). Insulin resistance differentially affects the PI 3-kinase- and MAP kinase-mediated signaling in human muscle. *J. Clin. Invest.* **105**, 311–20.

Dallman, M. F., Pecoraro, N., Akana, S. F. *et al.* (2003). Chronic stress and obesity: a new view of "comfort food". *Proc. Natl. Acad. Sci. USA* **100**, 11 696–701.

De Luca, C., Kowalski, T. J., Zhang, Y. *et al.* (2005). Complete rescue of obesity, diabetes, and infertility in db/db mice by neuron-specific LEPR-B transgenes. *J. Clin. Invest.* **115**, 3484–93.

Defronzo, R. A. (1988). Lilly lecture 1987. The triumvirate: beta-cell, muscle, liver. A collusion responsible for NIDDM. *Diabetes* **37**, 667–87.

Despres, J. P., Golay, A. & Sjostrm, L. (2005). Effects of rimonabant on metabolic risk factors in overweight patients with dyslipidemia. *N. Engl. J. Med.* **353**, 2121–34.

Dhillon, H., Zigman, J. M., Ye, C. *et al.* (2006). Leptin directly activates SF1 neurons in the VMH, and this action by leptin is required for normal body-weight homeostasis. *Neuron* **49**, 191–203.

Dresner, I., Laurent, D., Marcucci, M. *et al.* (1999). Effects of free fatty acids on glucose transport and IRS-1-associated phosphatidylinositol 3-kinase activity. *J. Clin. Invest.* **103**, 253–9.

Dryden, S., Pickavance, L., Henderson, L. & Williams, G. (1998). Hyperphagia induced by hypoglycemia in rats is independent of leptin and hypothalamic neuropeptide Y (NPY). *Peptides* **19**, 1549–55.

Eckel, R. H., Grundy, S. M. & Zimmet, P. Z. (2005). The metabolic syndrome. *Lancet* **365**, 1415–28.

El-Assaad, W., Buteau, J., Peyot, M. L. *et al.* (2003). Saturated fatty acids synergize with elevated glucose to cause pancreatic beta-cell death. *Endocrinology* **144**, 4154–63.

El-Haschimi, K., Pierroz, D. D., Hileman, S. M., Bjorbaek, C. & Flier, J. S. (2000). Two defects contribute to hypothalamic leptin resistance in mice with diet-induced obesity. *J. Clin. Invest.* **105**, 1827–32.

Elchebly, M., Payette, P., Michaliszyn, E. *et al.* (1999). Increased insulin sensitivity and obesity resistance in mice lacking the protein tyrosine phosphatase-1B gene. *Science* **283**, 1544–8.

Elias, C. F., Aschkenasi, C., Lee, C. *et al.* (1999). Leptin differentially regulates NPY and POMC neurons projecting to the lateral hypothalamic area. *Neuron* **23**, 775–86.

Emanuelli, B., Peraldi, P., Filloux, C., Sawka-Verhelle, D., Hilton, D. & Van Obberghen, E. (2000). SOCS-3 is an insulin-induced negative regulator of insulin signaling. *J. Biol Chem.* **275**, 15 985–91.

Emanuelli, B., Peraldi, P., Filloux, C. *et al.* (2001). SOCS-3 inhibits insulin signaling and is up-regulated in response to tumor necrosis factor-alpha in the adipose tissue of obese mice. *J. Biol. Chem.* **276**, 47 944–9.

Erickson, J. C., Hollopeter, G. & Palmiter, R. D. (1996). Attenuation of the obesity syndrome of ob/ob mice by the loss of neuropeptide Y. *Science* **274**, 1704–7.

Farooqi, I. S., Jebb, S. A., Langmack, G. *et al.* (1999). Effects of recombinant leptin therapy in a child with congenital leptin deficiency. *N. Engl. J. Med.* **341**, 879–84.

Faulconbridge, L. F., Cummings, D. E., Kaplan, J. M. & Grill, H. J. (2003). Hyperphagic effects of brainstem ghrelin administration. *Diabetes* **52**, 2260–5.

Faulconbridge, L. F., Grill, H. J. & Kaplan, J. M. (2005). Distinct forebrain and caudal brainstem contributions to the neuropeptide Y mediation of ghrelin hyperphagia. *Diabetes* **54**, 1985–93.

Figlewicz, D. P. (2003a). Adiposity signals and food reward: expanding the CNS roles of insulin and leptin. *Am. J. Physiol. Regul. Integr. Comp. Physiol.* **284**, R882–92.

Figlewicz, D. P. (2003b). Insulin, food intake, and reward. *Semin. Clin. Neuropsych.* **8**, 82–93.

Figlewicz, D. P., Higgins, M. S., Ng-Evans, S. B. & Havel, P. J. (2001). Leptin reverses sucrose-conditioned place preference in food-restricted rats. *Physiol. Behav.* **73**, 229–34.

Figlewicz, D. P., Evans, S. B., Murphy, J., Hoen, M. & Baskin, D. G. (2003). Expression of receptors for insulin and leptin in the ventral tegmental area/substantia nigra (VTA/SN) of the rat. *Brain Res.* **964**, 107–15.

Figlewicz, D. P., Bennett, J., Evans, S. B., Kaiyala, K., Sipols, A. J. & Benoit, S. C. (2004). Intraventricular insulin and leptin reverse place preference conditioned with high fat diet in rats. *Behav. Neurosci.* **118**, 479–87.

Flier, J. S. (1998). Clinical review 94: What's in a name? In search of leptin's physiologic role. *J. Clin. Endocrinol. Metab.* **83**, 1407–13.

Foster, G. D., Wyatt, H. R., Hill, J. O. *et al.* (2003). A randomized trial of a low carbohydrate diet for obesity. *N. Engl. J. Med.* **348**, 2082–90.

Foster, L. A., Ames, N. K. & Emery, R. S. (1991). Food intake and serum insulin responses to intraventricular infusions of insulin and IGF-I. *Physiol. Behav.* **50**, 745–9.

Garofalo, R. S. (2002). Genetic analysis of insulin signaling in Drosophila. *Trends Endocrinol. Metab.* **13**, 156–62.

Georgescu, D., Sears, R. M., Hommel, J. D. *et al.* (2005). The hypothalamic neuropeptide melanin-concentrating hormone acts in the nucleus accumbens to modulate feeding behavior and forced-swim performance. *J. Neurosci.* **25**, 2933–40.

Griffin, M. E., Marcucci, M. J., Cline, G. W. *et al.* (1999). Free fatty acid-induced insulin resistance is associated with activation of protein kinase C theta and alterations in the insulin signaling cascade. *Diabetes* **48**, 1270–4.

Grill, H. J. & Kaplan, J. M. (2002). The neuroanatomical axis for control of energy balance. *Front. Neuroendocrinol.* **23**, 2–40.

Grill, H. J., Schwartz, M. W., Kaplan, J. M., Foxhall, J. S., Breininger, J. & Baskin, D. G. (2002). Evidence that the caudal brainstem is a target for the inhibitory effect of leptin on food intake. *Endocrinology* **143**, 239–46.

Gulick, A. (1922). A study of weight regulation in the adult human body during over nutrition. *Am. J. Physiol.* **60**, 371–95.

Halaas, J. L., Gajiwala, K. S., Maffei, M. *et al.* (1995). Weight-reducing effects of the plasma protein encoded by the obese gene. *Science* **269**, 543–6.

Harris, R. B., Kasser, T. R. & Martin, R. J. (1986). Dynamics of recovery of body composition after overfeeding, food restriction or starvation of mature female rats. *J. Nutr.* **116**, 2536–46.

Harvey, J., McKay, N. G., Walker, K. S., Van Der Kaay, J., Downes, C. P. & Ashford M. L. (2000). Essential role of phosphoinositide 3-kinase in leptin-induced K(ATP) channel activation in the rat CRI-G1 insulinoma cell line. *J. Biol. Chem.* **275**, 4660–9.

Hawkins, M., Tonelli, J., Kishore, P. *et al.* (2003). Contribution of elevated free fatty acid levels to the lack of glucose effectiveness in type 2 diabetes. *Diabetes* **52**, 2748–58.

He, W., Lam, T. K., Obici, S. & Rossetti, L. (2006). Molecular disruption of hypothalamic nutrient sensing induces obesity. *Nat. Neurosci.* **9**, 227–33.

Hill, J. O., Dorton, J., Sykes, M. N. & Digirolamo, M. (1989). Reversal of dietary obesity is influenced by its duration and severity. *Int. J. Obes.* **13**, 711–22.

Houmard, J. A., Tanner, C. J., Yu, C. *et al.* (2002). Effect of weight loss on insulin sensitivity and intramuscular long-chain fatty acyl-CoAs in morbidly obese subjects. *Diabetes* **51**, 2959–63.

Howard, J. K., Cave, B. J., Oksanen, L. J., Tzameli, I., Bjorbaek, C. & Flier, J. S. (2004). Enhanced leptin sensitivity and attenuation of diet-induced obesity in mice with haploinsufficiency of Socs3. *Nat. Med.* **10**, 734–8.

James, P. (2003). Call for obesity review as overweight numbers reach 1.7 billion. *International Obesity Task Force press release.*

Kaiyala, K. J., Prigeon, R. L., Kahn, S. E., Woods, S. C. & Schwartz, M. W. (2000). Obesity induced by a high-fat diet is associated with reduced brain insulin transport in dogs. *Diabetes* **49**, 1525–33.

Katso, R., Okkenhaug, K., Ahmadi, K., White, S., Timms, J. & Waterfield, W. D. (2001). Cellular function of phosphoinositide 3-kinase: implications for development, homeostasis, and cancer. *Annu. Rev. Cell. Dev. Biol.* **17**, 615–75.

Keen Rhinehart, E., Kalra, S. P. & Kalra, P. S. (2004). Neuropeptidergic characterization of the leptin receptor mutated obese Koletsky rat. *Regul. Pept.* **119**, 3–10.

Kellerer, M., Koch, M., Metzinger, E., Mushack, J., Capp, E. & Haring, H. U. (1997). Leptin activates PI-3 kinase in C2C12 myotubes via janus kinase-2 (JAK- 2) and insulin receptor substrate-2 (IRS-2) dependent pathways. *Diabetologia* **40**, 1358–62.

Kennedy, G. C. (1953). The role of depot fat in the hypothalamic control of food intake in the rat. *Proc. R. Soc. Lond.* **140**, 579–592.

Kido, Y., Nakae, J. & Accili, D. (2001). Clinical review 125: the insulin receptor and its cellular targets. *J. Clin. Endocrinol. Metab.* **86**, 972–9.

Kim, E. M., O'Hare, E., Grace, M. K., Welch, C. C., Billington, C. J. & Levine, A. S. (2000). ARC POMC mRNA and PVN alpha-MSH are lower in obese relative to lean zucker rats. *Brain Res.* **862**, 11–6.

Kim, J. K., Kim, Y. J., Fillmore, J. J. *et al.* (2001). Prevention of fat-induced insulin resistance by salicylate. *J. Clin. Invest.* **108**, 437–46.

Knowler, W. C., Barrett-Connor, E., Fowler, S. E. *et al.* (2002). Reduction in the incidence of type 2 diabetes with lifestyle intervention or metformin. *N. Engl. J. Med.* **346**, 393–403.

Kopelman, P. G. (2000). Obesity as a medical problem. *Nature* **404**, 635–43.

Krisch, B. & Leonhardt, H. (1978). The functional and structural border of the neurohemal region of the median eminence. *Cell Tissue Res.* **192**, 327–39.

Kurrimbux, D., Gaffen, Z., Farrell, C. L., Martin, D. & Thomas, S. A. (2004). The involvement of the blood–brain and the blood–cerebrospinal fluid barriers in the distribution of leptin into and out of the rat brain. *Neurosci.* **123**, 527–36.

Lam, T. K., Schwartz, G. J. & Rossetti, L. (2005). Hypothalamic sensing of fatty acids. *Nat. Neurosci.* **8**, 579–84.

Lee, G. H., Pronca, R., Montez, J. M. *et al.* (1996). Abnormal splicing of the leptin receptor in diabetic mice. *Nature* **379**, 632–5.

Lee, S. S., Kennedy, S., Tolonen, A. C. & Ruvkun, G. (2003). DAF-16 target genes that control *C. elegans* life-span and metabolism. *Science* **300**, 644–7.

Leibel, R. L. (2002). The role of leptin in the control of body weight. *Nutr. Rev.* **60**, S15–19; discussion S68–84, 85–7.

Levine, A. S., Kotz, C. M. & Gosnell, B. A. (2003a). Sugars and fats: the eurobiology of preference. *J. Nutr.* **133**, 831S–4S.

Levine, A. S., Kotz, C. M. & Gosnell, B. A. (2003b). Sugars: hedonic aspects, neuroregulation, and energy balance. *Am. J. Clin. Nutr.* **78**, 834S–42S.

Lillioja, S. & Bogardus, C. (1988a). Insulin resistance in Pima Indians. A combined effect of genetic predisposition and obesity-related skeletal muscle cell hypertrophy. *Acta. Med. Scand. Suppl.* **723**, 103–19.

Lillioja, S. & Bogardus, C. (1988b). Obesity and insulin resistance: lessons learned from the Pima Indians. *Diabetes Metab. Rev.* **4**, 517–40.

Lopez, M., Tovar, S., Vazquez, M. J., Nogueiras, R., Senaris, R. & Dieguez, C. (2005). Sensing the fat: fatty acid metabolism in the hypothalamus and the melanocortin system. *Peptides* **26**, 1753–8.

MacDonald, A. F., Billington, C. J. & Levine, A. S. (2003). Effects of the opioid antagonist naltrexone on feeding induced by DAMGO in the ventral tegmental area and in the nucleus accumbens shell region in the rat. *Am. J. Physiol. Regul. Integr. Comp. Physiol.* **285**, R999–1004.

Marks, J. L., Porte, D., Jr., Stahl, W. L. & Baskin, D. G. (1990). Localization of insulin receptor mRNA in rat brain by in situ hybridization. *Endocrinology* **127**, 3234–6.

Marshall, N. B., Barrnett, R. J. & Mayer, J. (1955). Hypothalamic lesions in goldthioglucose injected mice. *Proc. Soc. Exp. Biol. Med.* **90**, 240–4.

Mayer, J., French, R. G., Zighera, C. F. & Barrnett, R. J. (1955). Hypothalamic obesity in the mouse: production, description and metabolic characteristics. *Am. J. Physiol.* **182**, 75–82.

McGarry, J. D. (2001). Travels with carnitine palmitoyltransferase I: from liver to germ cell with stops in between. *Biochem. Soc. Trans.* **29**, 241–5.

Merchenthaler, I. (1991). Neurons with access to the general circulation in the central nervous system of the rat: a retrograde tracing study with fluoro-gold. *Neuroscience* **44**, 655–62.

Mirshamsi, S., Laidlaw, H. A., Ning, K. *et al.* (2004). Leptin and insulin stimulation of signalling pathways in arcuate nucleus neurones: PI3K dependent actin reorganization and KATP channel activation. *BMC Neurosci.* **5**, 54.

Mizuno, T. M., Kleopoulos, S. P., Bergen, H. T., Roberts, J. L., Priest, C. A. & Mobbs, C. V. (1998). Hypothalamic pro-opiomelanocortin mRNA is reduced by fasting and [corrected] in ob/ob and db/db mice, but is stimulated by leptin. *Diabetes* **47**, 294–7.

Mokdad, A. H., Ford, E. S., Bowman, B. A. *et al.* (2000). Diabetes trends in the U.S.: 1990–1998. *Diabetes Care* **23**, 1278–83.

Mokdad, A. H., Bowman, B. A., Ford, E. S., Vinicor, F., Marks, J. S. & Koplan, J. P. (2001). The continuing epidemics of obesity and diabetes in the United States. *J. Am. Med. Assoc.* **286**, 1195–200.

Montague, C. T., Farooqi, I. S., Whitehead, J. P. *et al.* (1997). Congenital leptin deficiency is associated with severe early-onset obesity in humans. *Nature* **387**, 903–8.

Mori, H., Hanada, R., Hanada, T. *et al.* (2004). Socs3 deficiency in the brain elevates leptin sensitivity and confers resistance to diet-induced obesity. *Nat. Med.* **10**, 739–43.

Munzberg, H. & Myers, M. G., Jr. (2005). Molecular and anatomical determinants of central leptin resistance. *Nat. Neurosci.* **8**, 566–70.

Munzberg, H., Flier, J. S. & Bjorbaek, C. (2004). Region-specific leptin resistance within the hypothalamus of diet-induced obese mice. *Endocrinology* **145**, 4880–9.

Myers, M. G., Jr. (2004). Leptin receptor signaling and the regulation of mammalian physiology. *Rec. Prog. Horm. Res.* **59**, 287–304.

Neel, J. V. (1999). The "thrifty genotype" in 1998. *Nutr. Rev.* **57**, S2–9.

Neel, J. V., Weder, A. B. & Julius, S. (1998). Type II diabetes, essential hypertension, and obesity as "syndromes of impaired genetic homeostasis": the "thrifty genotype" hypothesis enters the 21st century. *Perspect Biol. Med.* **42**, 44–74.

Neumann, R. O. (1902). Experimental contributions to the science of human daily nutritional needs with particular regard to the necessary amount of protein (author's experiments). *Arch. Hyg.* **45**, 69–78.

Niswender, K. D. & Schwartz, M. W. (2003). Insulin and leptin revisited: adiposity signals with overlapping physiological and intracellular signaling capabilities. *Front. Neuroendocrinol.* **24**, 1–10.

Niswender, K. D., Morton, G. J., Stearns, W. H., Rhodes, C. J., Myers, M. G. Jr. & Schwartz, M. W. (2001). Key enzyme in leptin-induced anorexia. *Nature* **413**, 795–6.

Niswender, K. D., Gallis, B., Blevins, J. E., Corson, M. A., Schwartz, M. W. & Baskin, D. G. (2003a). Immunocytochemical detection of phosphatidylinositol 3-kinase activation by insulin and leptin. *J. Histochem. Cytochem.* **51**, 275–83.

Niswender, K. D., Morrison, C. D., Clegg, D. J. *et al.* (2003b). Insulin activation of phosphatidylinositol 3 kinase in the hypothalamic arcuate nucleus: a key mediator of insulin-induced anorexia. *Diabetes* **52**, 227–31.

Niswender, K. D., Baskin, D. G. & Schwartz, M. W. (2004a). Insulin and its evolving partnership with leptin in the hypothalamic control of energy homeostasis. *Trends Endocrinol. Metab.* **15**, 362–9.

Niswender, K. D., Clegg, D. J., Morrison, C. D., Morton, G. J. & Benoit, S. C. (2004b). The human obesity epidemic – a physiological perspective. *Curr. Med. Chem. - Immun. Endoc. Metab. Agents* **4**, 91–104.

Obici, S., Feng, Z., Karkanias, G., Baskin, D. G. & Rossetti, L. (2002a). Decreasing hypothalamic insulin receptors causes hyperphagia and insulin resistance in rats. *Nat. Neurosci.* **5**, 566–72.

Obici, S., Feng, Z., Morgan, K., Stein, D., Karkanias, G. & Rossetti, L. (2002b). Central administration of oleic acid inhibits glucose production and food intake. *Diabetes* **51**, 271–5.

Obici, S., Wang, J., Chowdury, R. *et al.* (2002c). Identification of a biochemical link between energy intake and energy expenditure. *J. Clin. Invest.* **109**, 1599–605.

Ogden, C. L., Flegal, K. M., Carroll, M. D. & Johnson, C. L. (2002). Prevalence and trends in overweight among US children and adolescents, 1999–2000. *J. Am. Med. Assoc.* **288**, 1728–32.

Ollmann, M. M., Wilson, B. D., Yang, Y. K. *et al.* (1997). Antagonism of central melanocortin receptors in vitro and in vivo by agouti- related protein. *Science* **278**, 135–8.

Ornish, D. (1998). Avoiding revascularization with lifestyle changes: The Multicenter Lifestyle Demonstration Project. *Am. J. Cardiol.* **82**, 72T–76T.

Ornish, D., Scherwitz, L. W., Billings, J. H. *et al.* (1998). Intensive lifestyle changes for reversal of coronary heart disease. *J. Am. Med. Assoc.* **280**, 2001–7.

Pasquet, P. & Apfelbaum, M. (1994). Recovery of initial body weight and composition after long-term massive overfeeding in men. *Am. J. Clin. Nutr.* **60**, 861–3.

Pasquet, P., Brigant, L., Froment, A. *et al.* (1992). Massive overfeeding and energy balance in men: the Guru Walla model. *Am. J. Clin. Nutr.* **56**, 483–90.

Peraldi, P., Filloux, C., Emanuelli, B., Hilton, D. J. & Van Obberghen, E. (2001). Insulin induces suppressor of cytokine signaling-3 tyrosine phosphorylation through janus-activated kinase. *J. Biol. Chem.* **276**, 24 614–20.

Pi-Sunyer, F. X., Aronne, L. J., Heshmati, H. M., Devin, J. & Rosenstock, J. (2006). Effect of rimonabant, a cannabinoid-1 receptor blocker, on weight and cardiometabolic risk factors in overweight or obese patients: RIO-North America: a randomized controlled trial. *J. Am. Med. Assoc.* **295**, 761–75.

Pirozzo, S., Summerbell, C., Cameron, C. & Glasziou, P. (2003). Should we recommend low-fat diets for obesity? *Obes. Rev.* **4**, 83–90.

Pocai, A., Muse, E. D. & Rossetti, L. (2006). Did a muscle fuel gauge conquer the brain? *Nat. Med.* **12**, 50–1.

Poitout, V., Tanaka, Y., Reach, G. & Robertson, R. P. (2001). Oxidative stress, insulin secretion, and insulin resistance. *J. Annu. Diabetol. Hotel. Dieu.* 75–86.

Pratley, R. E. (1998). Gene-environment interactions in the pathogenesis of type 2 diabetes mellitus: lessons learned from the Pima Indians. *Proc. Nutr. Soc.* **57**, 175–81.

Prentki, M., Joly, E., El-Assaad, W. & Roduit, R. (2002). Malonyl-CoA signaling, lipid partitioning, and glucolipotoxicity: role in beta-cell adaptation and failure in the etiology of diabetes. *Diabetes* **51** Suppl. 3, S405–13.

Ravinet Trillou, C., Arnone, M., Delgorge, C. *et al.* (2003). Anti-obesity effect of SR141716, a CB1 receptor antagonist, in diet induced obese mice. *Am. J. Physiol. Regul. Integr. Comp. Physiol.* **284**, R345–53.

Ricci, M. R. & Levin, B. E. (2003). Ontogeny of diet-induced obesity in selectively bred Sprague–Dawley rats. *Am. J. Physiol. Regul. Integr. Comp. Physiol.* **285**, R610–18.

Roberts, S. B., Young, V. R., Fuss, P. *et al.* (1990). Energy expenditure and subsequent nutrient intakes in overfed young men. *Am. J. Physiol.* **259**, R461–9.

Robertson, R. P., Harmon, J., Tran, P. O., Tanaka, Y. & Takahashi, H. (2003). Glucose toxicity in beta-cells: type 2 diabetes, good radicals gone bad, and the glutathione connection. *Diabetes* **52**, 581–7.

Rogers, P. J. (1985). Returning 'cafeteria-fed' rats to a chow diet: negative contrast and effects of obesity on feeding behaviour. *Physiol. Behav.* **35**, 493–9.

Rolls, B. J., Rowe, E. A. & Turner, R. C. (1980). Persistent obesity in rats following a period of consumption of a mixed, high energy diet. *J. Physiol.* **298**, 415–27.

Rosenbaum, M., Leibel, R. L. & Hirsch, J. (1997). Obesity. *N. Engl. J. Med.* **337**, 396–407.

Rothwell, N. J. & Stock, M. J. (1979). Regulation of energy balance in two models of reversible obesity in the rat. *J. Comp. Physiol. Psychol.* **93**, 1024–34.

Ruderman, N. B., Saha, A. K., Vavvas, D. & Witters, L. A. (1999). Malonyl-CoA, fuel sensing, and insulin resistance. *Am. J. Physiol.* **276**, E1–E18.

Rui, L., Yuan, M., Frantz, D., Shoelson, S. & White, M. F. (2002). SOCS-1 and SOCS-3 block insulin signaling by ubiquitin-mediated degradation of IRS1 and IRS2. *J. Biol. Chem.* **277**, 42 394–8.

Saad, M. J., Folli, F., Kahn, J. A. & Kahn, C. R. (1993). Modulation of insulin receptor, insulin receptor substrate-1, and phosphatidylinositol 3-kinase in liver and muscle of dexamethasone-treated rats. *J. Clin. Invest.* **92**, 2065–72.

Saltiel, A. R. & Pessin, J. E. (2002). Insulin signaling pathways in time and space. *Trends Cell Biol.* **12**, 65–71.

Samaha, F. F., Iqbal, N., Seshadri, P. *et al.* (2003). A low-carbohydrate as compared with a low-fat diet in severe obesity. *N. Engl. J. Med.* **348**, 2074–81.

Schuit, F. C., Huypens, P., Heimberg, H. & Pipeleers, D. G. (2001). Glucose sensing in pancreatic beta-cells: a model for the study of other glucose-regulated cells in gut, pancreas, and hypothalamus. *Diabetes* **50**, 1–11.

Schwartz, M. W. & Niswender, K. D. (2004). Adiposity signaling and biological defense against weight gain: absence of protection or central hormone resistance? *J. Clin. Endocrinol. Metab.* **89**, 5889–97.

Schwartz, M. W. & Porte, D., Jr. (2005). Diabetes, obesity, and the brain. *Science* **307**, 375–9.

Schwartz, M. W., Marks, J. L., Sipols, A. J. *et al.* (1991). Central insulin administration reduces neuropeptide Y mRNA expression in the arcuate nucleus of food-deprived lean (Fa/Fa) but not obese (fa/fa) Zucker rats. *Endocrinology* **128**, 2645–7.

Schwartz, M. W., Baskin, D. G., Bukowski, T. R. *et al.* (1996a). Specificity of leptin action on elevated blood glucose levels and hypothalamic neuropeptide Y gene expression in ob/ob mice. *Diabetes* **45**, 531–5.

Schwartz, M. W., Seeley, R. J., Campfield, L. A., Burn, P. & Baskin, D. G. (1996b). Identification of targets of leptin action in rat hypothalamus. *J. Clin. Invest.* **98**, 1101–6.

Schwartz, M. W., Woods, S. C., Porte, D., Jr., Seeley, R. J. & Baskin, D. G. (2000). Central nervous system control of food intake. *Nature* **404**, 661–71.

Schwartz, M. W., Woods, S. C., Seeley, R. J., Barsh, G. S., Baskin, D. G. & Leibel, R. L. (2003). Is the energy homeostasis system inherently biased toward weight gain? *Diabetes* **52**, 232–8.

Semenkovich, C. F. (1997). Regulation of fatty acid synthase (FAS). *Prog. Lipid Res.* **36**, 43–53.

Shaver, S. W., Pang, J. J., Wainman, D. S., Wall, K. M. & Gross, P. M. (1992). Morphology and function of capillary networks in subregions of the rat tuber cinereum. *Cell Tissue Res.* **267**, 437–48.

Shulman, G. I. (2000). Cellular mechanisms of insulin resistance. *J. Clin. Invest.* **106**, 171–6.

Sims, E. A., Goldman, R. F., Gluck, C. M., Horton, E. S., Kelleher, P. C. & Rowe, D. W. (1968). Experimental obesity in man. *Trans. Assoc. Am. Physicians*, **81**, 153–70.

Sims, E. A., Danforth, E., Jr., Horton, E. S., Glennon, J. A., Bray, G. A. & Salans, L. B. (1972). Experimental obesity in man. A progress report. *Isr. J. Med. Sci.* **8**, 813–14.

Sims, E. A., Danforth, E., Jr., Horton, E. S., Bray, G. A., Glennon, J. A. & Salans, L. B. (1973). Endocrine and metabolic effects of experimental obesity in man. *Recent Prog. Horm. Res.* **29**, 457–96.

Sindelar, D. K., Havel, P. J., Seeley, R. J., Wilkinson, C. W., Woods, S. C. & Schwartz, M. W. (1999). Low plasma leptin levels contribute to diabetic hyperphagia in rats. *Diabetes* **48**, 1275–80.

Sipols, A. J., Baskin, D. G. & Schwartz, M. W. (1995). Effect of intracerebroventricular insulin infusion on diabetic hyperphagia and hypothalamic neuropeptide gene expression. *Diabetes* **44**, 147–51.

Spanswick, D., Smith, M. A., Groppi, V. E., Logan, S. D. & Ashford, M. L. (1997). Leptin inhibits hypothalamic neurons by activation of ATP-sensitive potassium channels. *Nature* **390**, 521–5.

Spanswick, D., Smith, M. A., Mirshamsi, S., Routh, V. H. & Ashford, M. L. (2000). Insulin activates ATP-sensitive K+ channels in hypothalamic neurons of lean, but not obese rats. *Nat. Neurosci.* **3**, 757–8.

Speakman, J. R., Stubbs, R. J. & Mercer, J. G. (2002). Does body mass play a role in the regulation of food intake? *Proc. Nutr. Soc.* **61**, 473–87.

Spiegelman, B. M. & Flier, J. S. (2001). Obesity and the regulation of energy balance. *Cell* **104**, 531–43.

Stephens, T. W., Basinski, M., Bristow, P. K. *et al.* (1995). The role of neuropeptide Y in the antiobesity action of the obese gene product. *Nature* **377**, 530–2.

Sugden, M. C., Bulmer, K. & Holness, M. J. (2001). Fuel-sensing mechanisms integrating lipid and carbohydrate utilization. *Biochem. Soc. Trans.* **29**, 272–8.

Surwit, R. S., Kuhn, C. M., Cochrane, C., McCubbin, J. A. & Feinglos, M. N. (1988). Diet induced type II diabetes in C57BL/6J mice. *Diabetes* **37**, 1163–7.

Tremblay, A., Despres, J. P., Theriault, G., Fournier, G. & Bouchard, C. (1992). Overfeeding and energy expenditure in humans. *Am. J. Clin. Nutr.* **56**, 857–62.

Tseng, M. & DeVillis, R. (2000). Correlates of the "western" and "prudent" diet patterns in the us. *Ann. Epidemiol.* **10**, 481–2.

Ueki, K., Kondo, T. & Kahn, C. R. (2004a). Suppressor of cytokine signaling 1 (SOCS-1) and SOCS-3 cause insulin resistance through inhibition of tyrosine phosphorylation of insulin receptor substrate proteins by discrete mechanisms. *Mol. Cell Biol.* **24**, 5434–46.

Ueki, K., Kondo, T., Tseng, Y. H. & Kahn, C. R. (2004b). Central role of suppressors of cytokine signaling proteins in hepatic steatosis, insulin resistance, and the metabolic syndrome in the mouse. *Proc. Natl. Acad. Sci. USA*, **101**, 10422–7.

Unger, R. H. (1995). Lipotoxicity in the pathogenesis of obesity-dependent NIDDM. Genetic and clinical implications. *Diabetes* **44**, 863–70.

Uusitupa, M., Lindi, V., Loueranta, A., Salopuro, T., Lindstrom, J. & Tuomilehto, J. (2003). Long-term improvement in insulin sensitivity by changing lifestyles of people with impaired glucose tolerance: 4-year results from the Finnish Diabetes Prevention Study. *Diabetes* **52**, 2532–8.

Valencia, M. E., Bennett, P. H., Ravussin, E., Esparza, J., Fox, C. & Schulz, L. O. (1999). The Pima Indians in Sonora, Mexico. *Nutr. Rev.* **57**, S55–7; discussion S57–8.

Van Gaal, L. F., Rissanen, A. M., Scheen, A. J., Ziegler, O. & Rossner, S. (2005). Effects of the cannabinoid-1 receptor blocker rimonabant on weight reduction and cardiovascular risk factors in overweight patients: 1-year experience from the RIO-Europe study. *Lancet* **365**, 1389–97.

Vanhaesebroeck, B., Ali, K., Bilancio, A., Geering, B. & Foukas, L. C. (2005). Signalling by PI3K isoforms: insights from gene-targeted mice. *Trends Biochem. Sci.* **30**, 194–204.

Vollenweider, P., Menard, B. & Nicod, P. (2002). Insulin resistance, defective insulin receptor substrate 2-associated phosphatidylinositol-3' kinase activation, and impaired atypical protein kinase C (zeta/lambda) activation in myotubes from obese patients with impaired glucose tolerance. *Diabetes* **51**, 1052–9.

Wallum, B. J., Taborsky, G. J., Jr., Porte, D., Jr. *et al.* (1987). Cerebrospinal fluid insulin levels increase during intravenous insulin infusions in man. *J. Clin. Endocrinol. Metab.* **64**, 190–4.

Weigle, D. S. (1994). Appetite and the regulation of body composition. *FASEB J.* **8**, 302–10.

Weigle, D. S., Bukowski, T. R., Foster, D. C. *et al.* (1995). Recombinant ob protein reduces feeding and body weight in the ob/ob mouse. *J. Clin. Invest.* **96**, 2065–70.

Willett, W. C., Dietz, W. H. & Colditz, G. A. (1999). Guidelines for healthy weight. *N. Engl. J. Med.* **341**, 427–34.

Wilson, B. E., Meyer, G. E., Cleveland, J. C., Jr. & Weigle, D. S. (1990). Identification of candidate genes for a factor regulating body weight in primates. *Am. J. Physiol.* **259**, 1148–55.

Wolkow, C. A., Kimura, K. D., Lee, M. S. & Ruvkun, G. (2000). Regulation of *C. elegans* life-span by insulinlike signaling in the nervous system. *Science* **290**, 147–50.

Wolkow, C. A., Munoz, M. J., Riddle, D. L. & Ruvkun, G. (2002). Insulin receptor substrate and p55 orthologous adaptor proteins function in the *Caenorhabditis elegans* daf-2/insulin-like signaling pathway. *J. Biol. Chem.* **277**, 49 591–7.

Woods, S. C. & Porte, D., Jr. (1977). Relationship between plasma and cerebrospinal fluid insulin levels of dogs. *Am. J. Physiol.* **233**, E331–4.

Woods, S. C. & Porte, D., Jr. (1978). The central nervous system, pancreatic hormones, feeding, and obesity. *Adv. Metab. Disord.* **9**, 283–312.

Woods, S. C. & Seeley, R. J. (2001). Insulin as an adiposity signal. *Int. J. Obes. Relat. Metab. Disord.* **25** Suppl. 5, S35–8.

Woods, S. C., Lotter, E. C., McKay, L. D. & Porte, D., Jr. (1979). Chronic intracerebroventricular infusion of insulin reduces food intake and body weight of baboons. *Nature* **282**, 503–5.

Woods, S. C., Seeley, R. J., Rushing, P. A., D'Alessio, D. & Tso, P. (2003). A controlled high-fat diet induces an obese syndrome in rats. *J. Nutr.* **133**, 1081–7.

Xu, A. W., Kaelin, C. B., Takeda, K., Akira, S., Schwartz, M. W. & Barsh, G. S. (2005). Phosphatidylinositol 3-kinase integrates the action of insulin and leptin on hypothalamic neurons. *J. Clin. Invest.* **115**, 951–8.

Yu, C., Chen, Y., Zong, H. *et al.* (2002). Mechanism by which fatty acids inhibit insulin activation of IRS-1 associated phosphatidylinositol 3-kinase activity in muscle. *J. Biol. Chem.* **277**, 50 230–6.

Zabolotny, J. M., Bence-Hanulec, K. K., Stricker-Krongrad, A. *et al.* (2002). PTP1B regulates leptin signal transduction in vivo. *Dev. Cell.* **2**, 489–95.

Zhang, Y., Proenca, R., Maffei, M., Barone, M., Leopold, L. & Friedman, J. M. (1994). Positional cloning of the mouse obese gene and its human homologue. *Nature* **372**, 425–32.

Zhao, A. Z., Shinohara, M. M., Huang, D. *et al.* (2000). Leptin induces insulin-like signaling that antagonizes cAMP elevation by glucagon in hepatocytes. *J. Biol. Chem.* **275**, 11 348–54.

Zhao, A. Z., Huan, J. N., Gupta, S., Pal, R. & Sahu, A. (2002). A phosphatidylinositol 3 kinase phosphodiesterase 3B cyclic AMP pathway in hypothalamic action of leptin on feeding. *Nat. Neurosci.* **5**, 727–8.

5

Convergence of leptin and insulin signaling networks in obesity

CALUM SUTHERLAND AND MIKE ASHFORD

1.   Introduction

Leptin (a 146 residue peptide) and insulin (a 30 amino acid dipeptide) are synthesized in distinct locations in the periphery but share a common function of long-term regulation of body weight and energy balance through direct alterations in hypothalamic arcuate nucleus (ARC) signaling (Sahu, 2004; Cone, 2005). Insulin is synthesized as a prohormone almost exclusively by pancreatic β-cells, and secreted into plasma in response to rising glucose levels. The mRNA for insulin has been found in some brain areas, suggesting that specific neurons may be capable of producing an 'insulin-like' peptide. Meanwhile leptin is synthesized and secreted mainly by adipocytes, and circulating levels are normally related to adiposity (Zhang *et al.*, 1994; Frederich *et al.*, 1995; Considine *et al.*, 1996). There is some evidence that leptin is also produced by cells of the immune system such as T-cells and macrophages, bone, skeletal muscle, placenta, stomach, hypothalamus and by stellate cells of the liver. Direct administration of either hormone to the ARC has significant effects on feeding and body weight, while both hormones can cross the blood-brain barrier, probably via specific and saturable transport systems (Niswender & Schwartz, 2003; Niswender *et al.*, 2004). Leptin and insulin stimulate pro-opiomelanocortin (POMC) expressing neurons in the ARC, resulting in processing of POMC to α-melanocyte-stimulating hormone (α-MSH) and subsequent activation of the melanocortin-3 and -4 receptors, leading to anorexigenic outputs. Leptin and insulin also inhibit neurons in the ARC that

Neurobiology and Obesity, ed. Jenni Harvey and Dominic J. Withers. Published by Cambridge University Press. © Cambridge University Press 2008

express neuropeptide Y (NPY) and agouti-related peptide (AGRP) (Morton & Schwartz, 2001; Niswender & Schwartz, 2003; Niswender et al., 2004). Neuro-peptide Y is a 36 amino acid neuropeptide and the most potent appetite-stimulating agent identified to date (Stanley et al., 1986; Zarjevski et al., 1993), while AGRP, a powerful and long-lasting orexigenic agent directly inhibits melanocortin-3 and -4 receptors (and thus inhibit melanocortin-driven appetite suppression) (Fong et al., 1997; Ollmann et al., 1997). This is a major part of the mechanism by which these hormones repress food intake (for reviews see Niswender & Schwartz, 2003; Niswender et al., 2004; Sahu, 2004; Cone, 2005). These common functions of insulin and leptin suggest overlapping intracel-lular signaling processes and recent work has confirmed a high degree of homology in the major events initiated by these hormones. These will be the focus of this chapter.

In the periphery the primary function of insulin is to regulate glucose homeostasis in response to increasing glucose load (e.g. feeding). Meanwhile, leptin modulates insulin action through control of body fat, since excess adi-posity promotes insulin resistance (Hotamisligil et al., 1993; Ahmad et al., 1997; Bray et al., 2002; Kern et al., 2003). In addition, leptin has a direct effect on glucose homeostasis through hepatic expression of leptin receptors and the CNS-mediated regulation of hepatic glucose production. Indeed leptin and insulin can act directly on the hypothalamus to regulate hepatic glucose pro-duction (Liu et al., 1998; Pocai et al., 2005a, 2005b). The importance of the loss of this latter function on the generation of insulin resistance in obesity (where leptin resistance is present) may not yet be fully appreciated. There is some controversy in the literature over the nature of the cross-talk between leptin and insulin in hepatocytes. Some studies suggest that direct application of leptin to liver cell lines antagonizes insulin signaling (Cohen et al., 1996; Benomar et al., 2005), while others identify insulin sensitizing or insulin mimetic effects of leptin (Szanto & Kahn, 2000; Zhao et al., 2000; Carvalheira et al., 2003).

This chapter will introduce the molecular signaling mechanisms known to mediate at least some of the effects of insulin and leptin both in the periphery and the ARC. Particular attention will be given to common signaling compon-ents that explain the overlapping cellular effects of both hormones. However, we will also highlight the obvious differences in the signaling cascades, as well as the subtle variation in signal kinetics that permit the cells to respond in different ways to each agent. Defects in these signaling processes that contribute to obesity and diabetes will be discussed. Finally, we will review recent attempts to manipulate signaling processes common to both leptin and insulin in order to identify therapeutics for both obesity and diabetes.

2.   Signaling networks

2.1   *Distinct insulin and leptin signaling components*

Receptors

The expression of cell surface insulin or leptin specific receptors is the major determinant on whether the cell will respond to either agent. A specific transmembrane protein for each allows sensing of ligand and initiation of intracellular signaling (Figure 5.1). There is no cross reactivity between the two receptor types, that is, leptin does not bind to the insulin receptor and vice versa, however once activated each receptor can influence the signaling capacity of the other (see later). This specificity of receptor proteins represents a major distinction between the two signaling pathways.

The insulin receptor (IR) is a heterotetrameric membrane glycoprotein composed of two a subunits and two β subunits linked by disulphide bonds. Binding of insulin to the a subunit leads to a conformational change that activates the intrinsic intracellular tyrosine kinase domain of the β subunit. The resultant receptor autophosphorylation on specific tyrosine residues enhances the ability of the IR to recruit and regulate target proteins (Kahn & White, 1988; White & Kahn, 1994; Withers & White, 2000). The liver, muscle and adipose tissue represent the major sites of expression of the IR, however it is found in several other tissues including the CNS. It is expressed in many regions of the brain, but predominantly in the hypothalamus, hippocampus, cerebellum and olfactory bulb (Havrankova *et al.*, 1978; Marks *et al.*, 1990). Neuronal IR expression decreases with age. Interestingly, the glycation of the neuronal IR appears different from that found in peripheral tissues (or glial cells) but the functional outcome of this is not clear. Neuron-specific deletion of the IR renders the animal more sensitive to diet-induced obesity (Bruning *et al.*, 2000), implicating neuronal IR in the satiety response.

The leptin receptor (Ob-R) is a member of the cytokine class 1 type receptor family (Baumann *et al.*, 1996) and is encoded by the diabetes gene (db) (Tartaglia *et al.*, 1995). It contains four fibronectin Type III domains and one Ig-like domain. At least six splice variants of the human receptor have been reported, with the major signaling form thought to be 'the long form' also known as Ob-Rb (120 kDa) (Chen *et al.*, 1996; Lee *et al.*, 1996; Friedman & Halaas, 1998). It is the lack of a functional Ob-Rb isoform that underlies the obese phenotype of the *db/db* mouse and the *fa/fa* rat (Chua *et al.*, 1996; Phillips *et al.*, 1996). Upon binding of leptin the receptor homodimerizes resulting in interaction with various intracellular signaling components (Sweeney, 2002; Hegyi *et al.*, 2004; Sahu, 2004). The main differences between the splice variants lie in the intracellular domain of the receptor. However, all Ob-R proteins

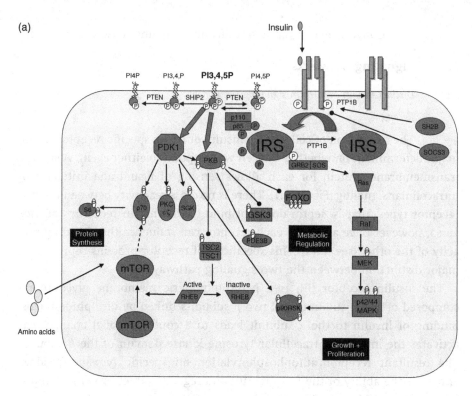

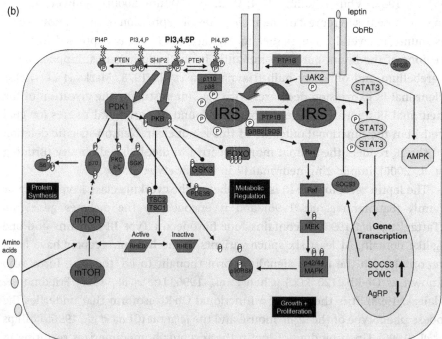

Figure 5.1 Comparison of insulin and leptin signalling pathways. The major signalling pathways for insulin (a) and leptin (b) action are depicted, with common elements colored red, insulin specific molecules in green and leptin specific in yellow. Due to limitations of space the molecules involved in insulin induction of glucose transport have been omitted. Activation →, inhibition –•.

contain a proline rich box1 that mediates association with members of the Jak family of tyrosine kinases, primarily Jak2 (Jiang, *et al.*, 1996). The Ob-Rb isoform has additional proline rich boxes that are required for full Jak-STAT signaling capability. The exact function of the shorter isoforms remains unclear, although ObRa and ObRc may function as leptin transport proteins (Hileman *et al.*, 2002) and the secreted soluble isoform, ObRe may act as a protein buffering system for free circulating leptin (Lammert *et al.*, 2001).

JAK-STAT signaling

The first signaling pathway identified downstream of the leptin receptor was the JAK-STAT pathway (Ihle & Kerr, 1995; Baumann *et al.*, 1996; Bates *et al.*, 2003). The Ob-Rb protein (which unlike insulin does not have intrinsic tyrosine kinase activity) activates an associated tyrosine kinase (JAK2) upon binding of leptin, thereby initiating phosphorylation of a number of tyrosine residues within the Ob-Rb sequence (see (Hekerman *et al.*, 2005; Munzberg *et al.*, 2005 for review). These phosphotyrosines act as docking sites for the phosphotyrosine phosphatase SHP2 (at Y985) and the transcription factor STAT3 (at Y1138). The coordinated recruitment of JAK2 and STAT3 results in phosphorylation of STAT3 by JAK2, promoting STAT3 dimerization, nuclear translocation and activation. Numerous genes have been identified as STAT3 targets, including the neuropeptide POMC and the Ob-Rb antagonist SOCS3 (Bates *et al.*, 2003; and see later). Other STAT family members may also be regulated by Ob-Rb (e.g. STAT5 through interaction with phosphoY1077), however STAT3 activation is the best characterized to date.

Athough insulin increases STAT3 phosphorylation in liver (Carvalheira *et al.*, 2003; Benomar *et al.*, 2005), SH-SY5Y cells (Benomar *et al.*, 2005) and rat hypothalamus (Mirshamsi *et al.*, 2004) the mechanism by which this is mediated is uncertain. Although some studies have implicated JAK2 in insulin-induced STAT3 activation (Carvalheira *et al.*, 2003; Benomar *et al.*, 2005), work on myoblasts and cell lines indicate the possible involvement of other signaling proteins (such as the tyrosine kinase Fer and the adaptor RACK1) as effectors of insulin-stimulated STAT3 activation (Taler *et al.*, 2003; Zhang *et al.*, 2006). It has also been reported that insulin-mediated activation of STAT5 requires JAK family kinases and IRS1 phosphorylation (Le *et al.*, 2002).

2.2   *Signalling molecules common to insulin and leptin action*

The receptor substrates

Proximal substrates of the insulin receptor include members of the insulin receptor substrate family (IRS). There are four closely related IRSs, namely IRS1, IRS2, IRS3 and IRS4 (White, 1998; Uchida *et al.*, 2000), as well as the functionally related Shc (Pelicci *et al.*, 1992), and p62dok (Yamanashi & Baltimore, 1997; Wick *et al.*, 2001), that all act as molecular adapters to relay the insulin signal (see Pawson, 1995, 2004 for reviews). IRS1 and IRS2 are widely expressed while IRS4 is expressed in brain, kidney and thymus. Rodents express IRS3 predominantly within the adipose tissue, however this isoform does not appear in human tissue. Although originally identified as substrates of the insulin receptor, the IRS1 and IRS2 proteins are now known to be important in leptin signaling (Burks *et al.*, 2000; Suzuki *et al.*, 2004), however IRS2 is not required for the CNS actions of leptin (Kubota *et al.*, 2004; Choudhury *et al.*, 2005). Indeed, deletion of IRS2 in the hypothalamus promotes increased food intake and obesity (Kubota *et al.*, 2004; Lin *et al.*, 2004; Choudhury *et al.*, 2005). The leptin receptor does not contain an intrinsic tyrosine kinase activity therefore the mechanism that links this receptor to IRSs is not identical to the IR. The non-covalent interaction between the tyrosine kinase Jak2 and the leptin receptor, and the ligand-induced recruitment of the adaptor protein SH2-B probably facilitates the phosphorylation of IRSs.

All IRSs possess an N-terminal pleckstrin homology (PH) domain that is necessary for protein–lipid interaction and is involved in targeting the IRS to the membrane in proximity to the receptor. Adjacent to this domain lies a phospho-tyrosine binding domain (PTB) followed by a variable length C-terminal tail (White, 1998). The IRSs are phosphorylated by the insulin receptor tyrosine kinase on a number of tyrosine residues that lie in YMXM or YXXM motifs within the C-terminal tail. Activated IRS proteins subsequently interact with various effector proteins that contain src homology (SH) 2 domains (White, 1998; Kaburagi *et al.*, 1999; Cantley, 2002). These include Grb-2 (growth receptor bound protein-2), the regulatory subunit of PI 3-kinase (see later), the tyrosine kinases fyn and csk and the tyrosine phosphatase SHP2 (see later). These interactions initiate further downstream signaling events. In addition to phosphorylation, IRS1 protein levels in the periphery are induced acutely by insulin, thereby increasing the capacity of the signaling network (Ruiz-Alcaraz *et al.*, 2005). It is not known if this occurs in the brain or if leptin promotes the same induction. Conversely, chronic insulin exposure, or obesity, promotes degradation of IRS1, and this has been hypothesized to be a potential mechanism for the generation of insulin and leptin resistance (Greene *et al.*, 2003; Harrington *et al.*, 2004; Kim *et al.*, 2004; Um *et al.*, 2004; Hers & Tavare, 2005; Morino *et al.*, 2005; Ueno *et al.*, 2005).

Inositol lipid signaling

Phosphoinositide 3-kinase (PI 3-kinase) is activated by insulin and leptin, as well as many growth factors and cytokines (Kapeller & Cantley, 1994;

Vanhaesebroeck *et al.*, 1997; Shepherd *et al.*, 1998; Cantley, 2002; Foukas *et al.*, 2006). The PI 3-kinase family consists of three classes of enzymes with related but distinct structural features and substrate specificities (Vanhaesebroeck *et al.*, 1997, 2001). The Class Ia subgroup of the PI 3-kinases represent the major form of this enzyme activated by insulin (Vanhaesebroeck *et al.*, 2001). The Class Ib PI 3-kinase subgroup contains only one member, p110γ, that trans-duces signals that originate from G-protein coupled receptors (GPCRs). Mean-while, the Class II PI 3-kinase family can also be activated by insulin, and although less well defined, may therefore play a role in insulin signaling (Domin *et al.*, 1997; Brown & Shepherd, 2001; Katso *et al.*, 2001) and leptin can activate the Class IIa PI3K isoform (Ktori *et al.*, 2003). The Class III PI 3-kinases are the homologues of the yeast vesicular sorting protein and are widely expressed. However there is currently little evidence that they are involved in insulin or leptin signaling with respect to physiological outputs. Indeed little work has been performed to assess the PI 3-kinase family that is regulated by leptin.

PI 3-kinase catalyses the phosphorylation of the 3' hydroxyl of the phos-phatidylinositols. In vitro, phosphatidylinositols (PtdIns), PtdIns(4)P and PtdIns$(4,5)P_2$ can all serve as substrates for the Class I PI 3-kinases. Upon PI 3-kinase stimulation, cellular levels of PtdIns$(3,4)P_2$ and PtdIns$(3,4,5)P_3$ but not PtdIns(3)P are elevated (Stephens *et al.*, 1991; Hawkins *et al.*, 1992; Cantley, 2002). Although PtdIns$(3,4)P_2$ can be produced from PtdIns(4)P via the activation of PI 3-kinase, the bulk of this product is actually generated from the dephos-phorylation of PtdIns$(3,4,5)P_3$ by a Type II 5'phosphatase, termed SHIP2. Thus, PtdIns$(3,4,5)P_3$ is the major phosphatidylinositol that is generated directly upon activation of PI 3-kinase, and PtdIns$(3,4)P_2$ levels are dictated by the combined activity of PI 3-kinase and SHIP2.

Wortmannin (Ui *et al.*, 1995) and LY294002 (Vlahos *et al.*, 1994) are two cell permeable compounds that are widely used to elucidate the cellular actions of PI 3-kinase. Wortmannin is a fungal metabolite that potently inhibits PI 3-kinase with an IC50 of around 5 nM. LY294002 (2–4(-Morpholinyl)8-phenyl-4H-1benzopyran-4-one) inhibits Class I family with an IC50 of 1 μM, however Class II PI 3-kinases are relatively resistant to this compound (Domin *et al.*, 1997). The employment of these inhibitors has established a role for PI 3-kinase in almost all the major actions of insulin such as glycogen synthesis, protein synthesis, lipolysis, glucose uptake, membrane trafficking, cytoskeletal arrangement and apoptosis (Shepherd *et al.*, 1998; Vanhaesebroeck *et al.*, 2001; Fisher & White, 2004). Interestingly, the regulation of transcription of genes involved in metabolism by insulin also appears predominantly dependent on PI 3-kinase activation (Sutherland *et al.*, 1995; Gabbay *et al.*, 1996; Dickens *et al.*, 1998; Patel *et al.*, 2003). Leptin activates PI 3-kinase in a wide variety of cells, and this pathway is key for the leptin activation of ATP-sensitive K^+ (K_{ATP}) channels present in insulin-secreting cells (Harvey *et al.*, 2000) and hypothalamic neurons (Mirshamsi *et al.*, 2004), activation of BK channels (Shanley *et al.*, 2002), hippo-campal synaptic plasticity (Shanley *et al.*, 2001; Durakoglugil *et al.*, 2005) and inhibition of glucagon signaling (Zhao *et al.*, 2000). Furthermore, icv adminis-tration of PI3K inhibitors has been reported to inhibit the actions of leptin and insulin to suppress food intake in rats (Niswender *et al.*, 2001, 2003), and to reduce some leptin- and insulin-mediated sympathoactivation processes (Rahmouni & Haynes, 2004). Importantly in diet-induced obesity leptin induc-tion of hepatic PI 3-kinase is impaired (Huang *et al.*, 2004), suggesting a block in the pathway upstream of PI 3-kinase activation. Such a defect would simultan-eously reduce leptin and insulin signaling (see later).

The products of the PI 3-kinase reaction, PtdIns $(3,4,5)P_3$ and PtdIns $(3,4)P_2$, regulate cellular processes through interactions with proteins that contain PH domains. The best-characterized targets for these lipids are members of the AGC subfamily of protein kinases (Alessi & Downes, 1998; Williams *et al.*, 2000). These include PDK1 (3'-phosphoinositide-dependent kinase 1) and PKB (protein kinase B). The activation of other members of this family, such as SGK (Serum and glucocorticoid-induced kinase), S6K (S6 kinase), p90rsk and MSK (mitogen and stress activated protein kinase), requires phosphorylation by PDK1 (Williams *et al.*, 2000), therefore they are indirectly regulated by the binding of PtdIns$(3,4,5)P_3$ to PDK1. However, each of these protein kinases also receives signaling inputs from other insulin-regulated pathways (Lizcano & Alessi, 2002). For example, S6K requires mTOR activity (see below and Chung *et al.*, 1992), while p90rsk requires p42/p44 MAPK activity (see below and Sturgill *et al.*, 1988). Thus, inhibitors of mTOR (rapamycin) and the p42/p44 MAPK pathway (e.g. PD98059, U0126) block activation of S6K and p90rsk, respectively. Both of these inhibitors are known to antagonize some aspects of insulin and leptin action.

The p42/p44 MAPK cascade

The adaptor molecules Shc and Grb2 bind to the IRSs via their SH2 domain or their PTB domains either singly or in combination (Pawson & Scott, 1997). Grb2 is complexed to the Ras guanine exchange factor mSOS (son of sevenless). Recruitment of mSOS from the cytosol to the plasma membrane activates Ras (a 21 kDa GTPase). In its active GTP bound form Ras associates with the N-terminal region of the serine/threonine kinase Raf, bringing it to the plasma membrane to become activated (Moodie *et al.*, 1993; Stokoe *et al.*, 1994). Activated Raf forms a stable complex with another protein kinase termed MKK1 (Mitogen activated protein kinase kinase1, also known as MEK1). Phosphorylation of MKK1 by Raf increases MKK1 activity (Dent *et al.*, 1992; Kyriakis *et al.*, 1992; Zheng & Guan, 1994). MKK1, in turn, phosphorylates and activates p42/p44 mitogen activated protein kinase (MAPK). This pathway can be activated by insulin and leptin, however these are relatively weak activators in comparison to the growth factors (e.g. BDNF, NGF, PDGF, EGF etc.). Interestingly, leptin can activate this pathway independently of the IRSs, through the phosphotyrosine phosphatase SHP2, which binds directly to phospho-Y985 of the activated LRb and to phosphotyrosine sites in JAK2 (Banks *et al.*, 2000; Bjorbaek *et al.*, 2001). Interestingly, mice lacking the gene for p44 MAPK (namely ERK1) demonstrate decreased adiposity, fewer adipocytes, resistance to diet-induced obesity and protection from insulin resistance (Bost *et al.*, 2005).

p42/p44 MAPKs are members of the MAPK superfamily that also include the p38 MAPK and jun N-terminal protein kinase (JNK) isoforms (Chang & Karin, 2001). These latter MAPKs are activated predominantly by cellular stresses such as osmotic stress, oxidative stress, UV irradiation, heat stress and cytokines. There are reports that leptin increases phosphorylation and activation of p38 MAPK in human mononuclear cells (van den Brink *et al.*, 2000) and muscle cells, which in smooth muscle and heart induces hypertrophy (Maroni *et al.*, 2003; Shin *et al.*, 2005). Leptin has also been reported to increase JNK activity in human smooth muscle cells (Bouloumie *et al.*, 1999) and in prostate cancer cells (Onuma *et al.*, 2003). In some cells insulin is a very weak activator of p38 MAPK and JNK, but their role in insulin action is unclear as strong activation of either of these molecules can promote insulin and leptin resistance (Hirosumi *et al.*, 2002; Lee *et al.*, 2003; Hers & Tavare, 2005). Indeed genetic deletion of JNK1 protects animals from diet-induced obesity and associated leptin and insulin resistance (see Bost *et al.*, 2005 for review).

Once activated, p42/p44 MAPK phosphorylates many downstream substrates that are involved in numerous cellular processes such as proliferation, differentiation, cell survival and gene transcription. Indeed, MAPK can translocate to the nucleus upon activation (Whitehurst *et al.*, 2002) suggesting that it has important nuclear substrates. In addition, MAPK is involved in the activation of several downstream serine/threonine protein kinases, such as the p90rsk isoforms (RSKs 1-3), MSK1/MSK2 (mitogen and stress activated protein kinases) and MNK1/MNK2 (MAPK interacting kinases) (Pearson *et al.*, 2001). The three p90rsk isoforms also require PDK1 in order to become activated (Frodin & Gammeltoft, 1999; Williams *et al.*, 2000). Once activated p90rsk phosphorylates downstream targets that are involved in gene transcription, cell cycle regulation and cellular metabolism. The p42/p44 MAPK is linked to the regulation of many immediate early genes, and as its name suggests, is key in the mitogenic actions of many hormones and growth factors. Indeed, this molecule appears crucial in the regulation of immediate early genes by insulin, in a variety of tissues. It also mediates regulation of NPY gene expression by growth factors (Williams *et al.*, 1998). Shc, Grb2, and the SH2 containing protein tyrosine phosphatase (SHP2) bind directly to the leptin receptor following its phosphorylation by Jak2 at Y985. Receptors that lack Y985 have a greatly reduced ability to activate p42/p44 MAPK (Bjorbaek *et al.*, 2001). Therefore there are potentially two mechanisms that link the leptin receptor to this pathway, one requiring IRS phosphorylation and one mediated by Shc, Grb2 and SHP2 binding to Y985. Leptin activates p42/p44 MAPK in the hypothalamus, pancreatic β-cells, adipose, skeletal muscle and liver (Bjorbaek *et al.*, 2001; Machinal-Quelin *et al.*, 2002; Benomar *et al.*, 2005; Maroni *et al.*, 2005; Cao *et al.*, 2006), and in the β-cells at least this induces proliferation (Tanabe *et al.*, 1997). Insulin has been shown to activate p42/p44 MAPK in the hypothalamus (Mirshamsi *et al.*, 2004; Carvalheira *et al.*, 2005), although it is presently unclear what the underlying functional role of this may be. However, recent work does indicate that p42/p44 MAPK plays a significant role in insulin and leptin regulation of brain ion channel and receptor functions. For example, insulin activation of recombinant and native hippocampal neuron BK channels is dependent on MAPK activation (O'Malley & Harvey, 2004), which contrasts to the PI3K dependent action of leptin on this channel type (Shanley *et al.*, 2002). Furthermore, leptin has been reported to enhance N-methyl-D-aspartate receptor mediated calcium influx in cerebellar granule cells via a MAPK dependent signaling process (Irving *et al.*, 2006). Leptin can also inhibit voltage-gated calcium channels in lateral hypothalamic neurons by activation of JAK2 and p42/44 MAPK (Jo *et al.*, 2005). Consequently, both leptin and insulin appear capable of coupling to a variety of ion channel proteins utilizing either PI3K or MAPK pathways.

SH2-B

The cytoplasmic adaptor protein SH2-B is ubiquitously expressed, multiply phosphorylated and contains both an SH2 domain and a PH domain (Rui *et al.*, 1997). It interacts with many tyrosine kinase receptors including the IGF-1, NGF and PDGF receptors (Wang & Riedel, 1998; Rui *et al.*, 1999; Kong *et al.*, 2002). Most interestingly this protein binds to the insulin receptor, IRS2 and to JAK2 via the SH2 domain of SH2-B (Wang & Riedel, 1998; O'Brien *et al.*, 2002; Duan *et al.*, 2004). It plays a pivotal role in leptin activation of PI 3-kinase following IRS2 phosphorylation by JAK2 (Duan *et al.*, 2004), and can sensitize cells to insulin (Ahmed & Pillay, 2003). Mice deficient in SH2-B develop insulin and leptin resistance, hyperphagia, obesity, diabetes and reproductive defects (Ohtsuka *et al.*, 2002; Duan *et al.*, 2004; Ren *et al.*, 2005). In particular, leptin activation of hypothalamic Jak-STAT is defective, while expression of hypothalamic NPY and AGRP is increased (Ren *et al.*, 2005). Therefore this protein clearly plays an important part in both insulin and leptin signaling, although it remains to be seen if both the glucose homeostasis and hyperphagic defects are due to central and/or peripheral loss of this protein.

Suppressor of cytokine signaling (SOCS)-3

SOCS-3 is a protein that can bind to the activated leptin receptor at both of the major signaling phosphotyrosines (Y1138 and Y985), as well as to phosphorylated JAK2 (Bjorbaek *et al.*, 1999; Eyckerman *et al.*, 2000; Dunn *et al.*, 2005). This antagonizes the binding (and therefore activation) of STAT3, SHP2 and the IRSs both to LRb and to JAK2 (Bjorbaek *et al.*, 2001; Dunn *et al.*, 2005; Fruhbeck, 2005; Munzberg & Myers, 2005). STAT3 activation actually induces SOCS3 expression (Dunn *et al.*, 2005) providing a negative feedback mechanism to regulate leptin signaling, by ultimately reducing tyrosine phosphorylation of ObRb. Consistent with this model, overexpression of SOCS3 in cultured cells blocks leptin action, while RNAi knockdown of SOCS3 enhances leptin signaling (Dunn *et al.*, 2005). In addition, heterozygous deletion of SOCS3 in mouse CNS increases leptin sensitivity, reduces body weight and confers resistance to diet-induced obesity (Howard *et al.*, 2004; Mori *et al.*, 2004). This role for SOCS3 in the antagonism of leptin action suggests that abnormal SOCS3 expression could promote leptin resistance and obesity. Indeed, SOCS3 expression is high in several animal models of obesity, however the interpretation of this observation is complicated by the fact that leptin regulates SOCS3 expression. Whether increased SOCS3 expression predates the hyperleptinemia and/or leptin resistance in these models or in obese humans is not known. Interestingly, inflammatory mediators such as IL6 and TNFa (Starr *et al.*, 1997; Fasshauer *et al.*, 2004; Rieusset *et al.*, 2004), or fatty acids themselves (Gual *et al.*, 2005), can induce SOCS3 expression, and this may suggest that increased SOCS3 expression is a consequence of obesity or inflammation. Increased SOCS3 expression is also found in muscle after exercise, and this is also likely to be linked to increased IL-6 production (Spangenburg *et al.*, 2006). Importantly, SOCS3 over-expression antagonizes insulin as well as leptin signaling, possibly through direct binding to the phosphorylated IR (Emanuelli *et al.*, 2000), and reduction in IRS-1 levels and subsequent signals (Shi *et al.*, 2006), and the heterozygotic deletion of SOCS3 increases insulin sensitivity in the CNS (Howard *et al.*, 2004). Therefore, the abnormal SOCS3 expression in obesity or inflammation represents a potential molecular link between leptin and insulin resistance (Rieusset *et al.*, 2004; Dunn *et al.*, 2005; Fruhbeck, 2005; Gual *et al.*, 2005; Munzberg & Myers, 2005).

The mTOR pathway

The mammalian Target of Rapamycin (mTOR) lies downstream of PI 3-kinase signaling (for review see Fisher & White, 2004; Martin & Hall, 2005). Activation of PKB promotes phosphorylation and inhibition of the TSC1-TSC2 complex (Figure 5.1). The result is activation of the small G-protein Rheb and stimulation of mTOR. Interestingly this pathway receives additional information from a nutrient sensing pathway (Gingras *et al.*, 2001; Beugnet *et al.*, 2003), as well as the AMP-activated protein kinase (AMPK), which acts as a cellular energy status monitor (see later). Hence mTOR can be regulated by a number of environmental cues, and is key to coordinating responses to the overall nutritional status of the cell (Fisher & White, 2004).

The immunosuppressant rapamycin is a highly specific inhibitor of mTOR, indeed it was fundamental in the original identification of the protein (Heitman *et al.*, 1991). Rapamycin blocks insulin activation of p70S6 kinase and subsequent phosphorylation of the S6 ribosomal protein (Chung *et al.*, 1992; Jefferies *et al.*, 1994; von Manteuffel *et al.*, 1997) thereby demonstrating a requirement for mTOR in their regulation. This pathway controls the rate of translation of specific mRNA species (Jefferies *et al.*, 1997). Interestingly, a recent report (Cota *et al.*, 2006) demonstrates that icv administration of rapamycin inhibits icv leptin-induced inhibition of food intake and body weight gain. These authors show that phosphorylated forms of mTOR, S6 and S6K are present in the ARC, particularly NPY neurons, and that their levels are modulated by fasting (decreased) and by icv leucine (increased), corresponding to orexigenic and anorexigenic outputs, respectively. The leucine-induced anorexia was also inhibited by rapamycin indicating that mTOR signaling may be an important component of the ARC sensing and integration system for nutrients and hormones. It has also been suggested that the mTOR pathway connects leptin regulation of AMPK (see below) to appetite control (Flier, 2006).

Interestingly, hyperactivation of the mTOR pathway can promote serine/threonine phosphorylation of the IRSs (Potashnik *et al.*, 2003; Harrington *et al.*, 2004; Khamzina *et al.*, 2005; Ueno *et al.*, 2005). Prolonged stimulation of cells with activators of mTOR (3-24h) results in increased ser/thr phosphorylation of IRS1 and IRS2, which antagonizes tyrosine phosphorylation by the insulin receptor, as well as inducing ubiquitin-mediated degradation (see Shulman, 2000; Withers & White, 2000; White, 2002; Gual *et al.*, 2005 for reviews). The obesity-induced degradation of IRSs has been proposed as a potential site of insulin and leptin resistance, and could also be a point of cross-talk between the two pathways. For example, long-term exposure to insulin would reduce the ability of leptin to promote IRS-dependent signaling, and vice versa. Rather paradoxically, inhibitors of mTOR are thus potential sensitizers of some actions of insulin and leptin.

AMP kinase

The AMP-activated protein kinase (AMPK) is a ubiquitously expressed protein kinase that was first identified as a regulator of acetyl CoA carboxylase (ACC) in response to changing energy status of the cell (for review see Hardie et al., 1999; Kahn et al., 2005). AMPK activity is increased by 5'-AMP and antagonized by ATP hence it is a molecular sensor of the chemical energy of a cell. Its major cellular roles appear to be to reduce ATP utilizing processes and increase ATP repletion. Leptin activates AMPK in skeletal muscle thereby inducing fatty acid oxidation (Merrill et al., 1997; Minokoshi et al., 2002), mitochondrial biogenesis (Zong et al., 2002) and glucose uptake (Merrill et al., 1997). Meanwhile supraphysiological concentrations of leptin promote an oxidative phenotype in adipocytes, and this correlates with alterations in AMPK activity (Orci et al., 2004). Therefore leptin signaling through AMPK may contribute to induction of fat utilization and removal in the periphery.

Interestingly, activation of AMPK in the hypothalamus (either pharmacologically or by overexpression) induces food intake (Andersson et al., 2004; Minokoshi et al., 2004). Since leptin injection into the 3rd ventricle inhibits AMPK activity in the ARC (Andersson et al., 2004; Minokoshi et al., 2004), it seems reasonable to hypothesize that leptin regulation of AMPK contributes to its inhibitory effects on food intake. The mechanisms underlying this divergent tissue specific regulation of AMPK by leptin (activation in muscle, inhibition in ARC) remain undefined. There is also evidence to link leptin, AMPK and the control of blood glucose levels. Chemical activation of AMPK during hypoglycemia, by intra-VMH injection of AICAR, stimulated hepatic glucose production (McCrimmon et al., 2004). In addition, inhibition of hypothalamic AMPK by icv administration of compound C or by intrahypothalamic injection of dominant negative AMPK results in impaired counter-regulatory responses to hypoglycemia (Han et al., 2005). As AMPK activity is reported to be reduced by leptin in the hypothalamus (Andersson et al., 2004; Minokoshi et al., 2004) it might be expected that this hormone would therefore act to depress hepatic glucose output and suppress the counter-regulatory responses to hypoglycemia (and so exacerbate the hypoglycemic condition). These CNS actions appear counter-intuitive as defective compensatory response to systemic hypoglycemia is associated with type I diabetes, an insulin-deficient state. Furthermore, central activity of leptin is important for maintaining peripheral glucose homeostasis (Liu et al., 1998; Pocai et al., 2005a, b). However, recent studies complicate the picture further, as deletion of liver AMPKα2 subunit indicates that this AMPK isoform is required for maintenance of regulation of hepatic glucose fluxes by leptin (Andreelli et al., 2006).

Insulin inhibition of AMPK activity has been reported in muscle cells (Witters & Kemp, 1992; Gamble & Lopaschuk, 1998). Meanwhile, pharmacological AMPK activation antagonizes insulin up-regulation of glucose transport in adipocytes (Salt et al., 2000) but mimics the effect of insulin on hepatic gene transcription (although insulin did not activate AMPK in this system) (Lochhead et al., 2000). Furthermore, loss of hepatic AMPKα2 did not alter insulin sensitivity of this tissue with respect to glucose production or transcriptional regulation of enzymes (Andreelli et al., 2006). Therefore AMPK does not appear to be required for normal insulin action. This enzyme clearly influences both leptin and insulin action, however it appears to be a mediator of leptin action and a modulator of insulin action.

The most commonly prescribed treatment for T2DM is metformin, an insulin-sensitizing agent that also activates AMPK in cells and in vivo (Fryer et al., 2002; Hawley et al., 2003). Indeed the glucose-lowering effects of metformin appear to require AMPK activation, at least in rodents (Shaw et al., 2005). Therefore AMPK has attracted attention as a therapeutic target for diabetes and obesity (see later).

PDE3B

Cyclic nucleotide phosphodiesterases (PDE) are a large group of enzymes, derived from 11 different gene families (Francis et al., 2001). PDE3B is localized to several tissues involved in metabolic homeostasis, including adipocytes, liver, pancreatic β-cells and the hypothalamus. Studies on pancreatic β-cells have shown that leptin causes a PI3K-dependent increase in PDE3B activity, which results in reduced levels of cAMP and suppression of glucagon-like peptide 1 induced insulin secretion (Zhao et al., 1998). PDE3B activation in the hypothalamus may also play a role in leptin signaling, as icv injection of cilostamide, a selective PDE3B inhibitor, is reported to reverse the actions of leptin on food intake and body weight and to inhibit leptin-mediated increased STAT3 phosphorylation and DNA binding (Zhao et al., 2002). Furthermore, leptin increases the activity of hypothalamic PDE3B in a PI3K-dependent manner and chronic central leptin infusion in rats, which induces central leptin resistance, uncoupled the leptin and cAMP signals, in contrast to that of the STAT3 pathway (Sahu & Metlakunta, 2005). At present, it is unclear which hypothalamic neurons are responsible for transducing these signals, or whether PDE3B is also involved in other aspects of leptin function such as glucose homeostasis.

Insulin also activates PDE3B and the mechanism is more clearly established. Tyrosine phosphorylation of IRS1 promotes activation of PI 3-kinase and a PKB-mediated phosphorylation of S273 of PDE3B (Kitamura et al., 1999). Since leptin also increases PKB activity it is plausible that the same mechanism links leptin and PDE3B activation. Although an insulin-induced increase in PDE3B activity inhibits lipolysis and hepatocyte glycogenolysis (Manganiello & Vaughan, 1973; Beebe et al., 1985), it has not yet been demonstrated whether PDE3B is also associated with any hypothalamic-mediated insulin action.

Other signaling molecules

There are multiple protein kinase C (PKC) isoforms, all of which require phosphorylation by PDK1 for activity (see Parekh et al., 2000 for review). There is increasing evidence that PKC's have an important role in some aspects of insulin action (Messina & Weinstock, 1994; Toker et al., 1994; Bandyopadhay et al., 1997; Le Good et al., 1998; Parekh et al., 1999). In particular, the activation of the atypical class of PKC isoforms in adipocytes may involve interaction with PtdIns(3,4,5)P$_3$ (the product of the PI 3-kinase reaction) (Standaert et al., 1997). In addition, many of the actions of insulin can be observed when cells are incubated with phorbol esters (which activate classical and novel PKCs). Leptin can induce PKC activity in muscle and this promotes phosphorylation of S318 of IRS1 resulting in reduced insulin signaling (Hennige et al., 2006). Therefore it is possible that PKC activation due to hyperleptinemia contributes to both leptin and insulin resistance.

Meanwhile, insulin treatment of cells can lead to the generation of hydrogen peroxide (H$_2$O$_2$) (Krieger-Brauer & Kather, 1992; Prasad & Ismail-Beigi, 1999; Mahadev et al., 2001a, 2001b). Treatment of cells with this agent can mimic many of the effects of insulin (Sutherland et al., 1997). The mechanism of H$_2$O$_2$ generation is not fully understood, however this molecule is one of many reactive oxygen species known to influence the activity of the transcription factor NFkB (for review see Morel & Barouki, 1999) and the phosphatase PTP1B. Recent studies have also indicated that leptin can drive the increased production of reactive oxygen species in heart (Hu et al., 2006) and endothelial cells (Bouloumie et al., 1999; Yamagishi et al., 2001). In human cultured hepatic stellar cells, leptin increases production of H$_2$O$_2$ in a JAK2 dependent manner and this acts as a signal to cause p42/p44 and p38 MAPK activation (Cao et al., 2006). Studies like these have led to suggestions that high levels of circulating leptin observed in obesity may be increasing oxidative stress in certain tissues leading to adverse cardiovascular effects. It is not clear whether leptin or insulin induced production of ROS occurs centrally and is involved in energy and glucose homeostatic mechanisms. However, mice that over-express glutathione peroxidase 1, an enzyme responsible for reducing H_2O_2 in vivo, develop elevated leptin levels, hyperglycemia, hyperinsulinemia coupled with increased body weight and adiposity (McClung et al., 2004). This insulin resistance was demonstrated to be associated with reduced liver IR and PKB phosphorylation. Thus, leptin and insulin induction of H_2O_2 as a second messenger may play a role in the maintenance of cellular leptin and insulin sensitivity.

Common gene targets

An important aspect of insulin and leptin action in the ARC is the regulation of expression of the neuropeptides NPY, POMC, AGRP and CART. Insulin and leptin inhibit NPY and AGRP expression, while inducing POMC and CART production (Niswender et al., 2004; Sahu, 2004; Wynne et al., 2005). Little is known about the mechanisms of repression of NPY other than that PI 3-kinase activation is required (Niswender et al., 2003). However there is strong evidence that leptin (and possibly insulin) induction of POMC is mediated by activation of the JAK2-STAT3 pathway (Bates et al., 2003; Munzberg et al., 2003) and possibly by SHP2 (Zhang et al., 2004). A recent study indicates a role for the forkhead protein, Foxo1 in the leptin-mediated control of AGRP (and possibly POMC) mRNA expression (Kitamura et al., 2006). Glucose injection (ip) can alter the expression of NPY and AGRP within 30 min, independently of changes in leptin or insulin (Chang et al., 2005). The effects of leptin and insulin on NPY and POMC expression are less rapid, peaking between 6 and 12 h, and are independent of glucose. Meanwhile, NPY mRNA levels are abnormally high in the hypothalamic neurons of the obese Zucker rats, presumably reflecting the leptin and insulin resistance of these animals (Bogacka et al., 2004). Therefore, there appears to be a complex interplay between food intake, body adiposity and ARC neuropeptide expression.

2.3   Negative regulation of the pathways

SHP2

As discussed above, the protein tyrosine phosphatase, SHP2, physically associates with LRb by docking to Y985 and acts as a positive regulator of p42/p44 MAPK (Bjorbaek et al., 2001). Brain-specific knock-out of SHP2 results in early-onset obesity and an accelerated body weight increase, an action that was linked to deficient leptin regulation of NPY expression (Zhang et al., 2004). Consequently, although this phosphatase has been suggested to negatively regulate JAK2/STAT3 signaling, it may enhance leptin signaling through the MAPK pathway.

PTP1B

The phosphotyrosine phosphatases PTP1B and TCP1a are key modulators of insulin and leptin action, as they dephosphorylate the phosphotyrosine residues targeted by the insulin receptor as well as leptin receptor associated kinases. PTP1B knockout mice display an overt metabolic phenotype, characterized by resistance to diet-induced obesity and insulin resistance, with higher energy expenditure and enhanced whole body glucose disposal (Elchebly *et al.*, 1999; Klaman *et al.*, 2000). Studies of these mice coupled with use of antisense oligonucleotide knock-down of PTP1B in rodents demonstrated increased insulin sensitivity, with prolonged phosphorylation of the insulin receptor and enhanced signaling through the IRS–PI3K–PKB pathway (Zinker *et al.*, 2002; Gum *et al.*, 2003). There is also evidence to suggest that PTP1B affects leptin signaling. PTP1B knockout mice display increased sensitivity to leptin and an increase in leptin driven hypothalamic STAT3 phosphorylation (Zabolotny *et al.*, 2002). In vitro studies indicate that PTP1B negatively regulates leptin signaling by targeting JAK2 and STAT3 causing their dephosphorylation (Myers *et al.*, 2001; Kaszubska *et al.*, 2002; Lund *et al.*, 2005). Thus the levels, activity and cellular location of PTP1B may well play crucial roles in tissue sensitivity to leptin and insulin levels, as well as resistance to these hormones. The mechanisms that control these aspects of PTP1B function are presently unclear, with conflicting data present in the literature. Indeed, insulin has been reported to cause inactivation of PTP1B activity in three distinct ways; via H_2O_2 production (Mahadev *et al.*, 2001a), by phosphorylation of Ser-50 of PTP1B by the insulin (and leptin) induced kinase PKB (Ravichandran *et al.*, 2001) and by direct phosphorylation of PTP1B by the insulin receptor (Tao *et al.*, 2001). Conversely, direct phosphorylation of PTP1B by the insulin receptor has also been reported to cause activation of this enzyme (Dadke *et al.*, 2001). Complete elucidation of these mechanisms is vital if we are to understand whether insulin regulation of PTP1B enhances signaling or is a negative feedback mechanism. The results of the PTP1B depletion studies do suggest that PTP1B inhibitors would be potential anti-obesity and anti-diabetic therapeutics.

PTEN

The generation of PIP3 by the action of PI 3-kinase is opposed by the lipid phosphatase PTEN (phosphatase and tensin homologue deleted on chromosome 10; for review see Leslie & Downes, 2004). The amount of PIP3 present in the cell is a measure of the relative activity of these two enzymes. Insulin and leptin both activate PI 3-kinase, however it is becoming clear that

PTEN activity is also regulated. Leptin, but not insulin, stimulation of the hypothalamic cell lines GT1-7 and N29/4 promotes phosphorylation of PTEN at C-terminal residues, and this reduces the activity of PTEN towards PIP3 (Ning et al., 2006). This partially explains differences in signal strength and duration following insulin or leptin stimulation of cells (Ning et al., 2006). In addition, the leptin signal in these cells also appears to require inhibition of PTEN protein phosphatase activity, to induce further downstream effector outputs such as cytoskeletal rearrangement and opening of K_{ATP} channels in pancreatic β-cells (Ning et al., 2006). Thus, the detection of leptin-induced co-incident signals may differ from that of insulin in certain cells and allow differential coupling to cellular effectors and hence separate outputs. Inhibition or deletion of PTEN in liver (Stiles et al., 2004), adipose (Butler et al., 2002; Kurlawalla-Martinez et al., 2005) or muscle (Wijesekara et al., 2005) improves insulin sensitivity and glucose disposal leading to suggestions that PTEN may be a useful target for treatment or prevention of insulin resistance and diabetes. Amazingly, improved insulin sensitivity in any single tissue (muscle, liver or adipose) appears sufficient to protect against the development of diabetes. It remains to be seen whether reduction of PTEN in the hypothalamus also provides improved whole body insulin and leptin sensitivity. As increased expression of PTEN is associated with muscle insulin resistance in rats (Lo et al., 2004) and a specific polymorphism in the PTEN gene that results in higher PTEN expression is linked with type 2 diabetes in a Japanese cohort (Ishihara et al., 2003), dysregulated PTEN activity due to leptin resistance would be predicted to reduce insulin sensitivity.

SHIP2

There is a second lipid phosphatase capable of limiting insulin signaling by hydrolysing the PI 3-kinase product, $PI(3,4,5)P_3$. This protein, SH-2 containing inositol phosphatase 2 (SHIP2), displays 5' phosphatase activity to $PI(3,4,5)P_3$ resulting in the formation of $PI(3,4)P_2$, an important regulator of PKB. Overexpression of wild-type SHIP2 in 3T3-L1 adipocytes reduces insulin-induced metabolic signaling, whereas the 5'-phosphatase defective SHIP2 causes increased insulin sensitivity (Murakami et al., 2004; Sasaoka et al., 2004). An initial attempt to produce a SHIP2 knockout mouse resulted in an animal with severe postnatal hypoglycemia (Clement et al., 2001), which appeared to fit well with the idea of SHIP2 acting as a negative regulator of insulin action. However, the targeting construct for this study actually caused the loss of two proteins, the second, PHOX2A is a transcription factor, which confused the outcome considerably. A more specific SHIP2 knockout mouse has since been generated and rather surprisingly displayed normal fasted glucose and insulin levels with no evidence of impaired glucose or insulin tolerance (Sleeman *et al.*, 2005). However, these mice were highly resistant to weight gain on a high-fat diet and did not display the insulin resistance observed in the wild-type littermates. Thus, SHIP2-deficient mice show normal glucose homeostasis, despite enhanced insulin signaling. The lean phenotype, which appears to be due to enhanced energy expenditure, is intriguing and it should be instructive to determine the effects of SHIP2 deletion on insulin and leptin signaling in the hypothalamus. Recent studies have shown that polymorphisms in the SHIP2 gene are associated with increased incidence of metabolic dysregulation, including diabetes and obesity (Kaisaki *et al.*, 2004; Kagawa *et al.*, 2005).

3.   Signaling mechanisms as therapeutic targets

3.1   *Interplay between insulin and leptin signaling*

As discussed in detail above there are numerous signaling molecules that are key for *both* insulin and leptin action (Figure 5.1). Of course in many cases it is not yet known whether the strength or duration of regulation of all of these molecules by each agent is identical or indeed whether the regulation by each agent occurs in the same cell type in all cases. Initial studies in hypothalamic and pancreatic cells suggest important kinetic differences in the regulation of the PI 3-kinase pathway by insulin and leptin (Ning *et al.*, 2006). Although insulin and leptin both induce PIP3 production in these cells the mechanisms by which this is achieved by each are subtly different. For example leptin controls PTEN activity, while insulin relies on a large induction of PI 3-kinase activity. The result is differences in the duration of downstream signaling events, with a prolonged activation of PKB by insulin and a much more transient activation by leptin (Ning *et al.*, 2006).

However, there is clear evidence that insulin and leptin stimulation of cells has a distinct outcome to incubation of cells with either agent in isolation. For example prolonged stimulation by leptin induces SOCS3 expression (Dunn *et al.*, 2005), and activates PKC (Hennige *et al.*, 2006) to promote IRS1 serine-318 phosphorylation, a mechanism considered to underlie impaired insulin signaling (Hennige *et al.*, 2006). All of this negatively regulates both insulin and leptin signaling. Hence prior exposure to leptin would result in an insulin resistant phenotype and it is clearly possible that one or more of these processes contributes to insulin resistance found in hyperleptinemic obese individuals (Shulman, 2000; Kim *et al.*, 2004). Similarly, prolonged exposure to insulin can promote IRS degradation (Ueno *et al.*, 2005), and this would also compromise leptin action. Meanwhile, leptin can regulate AMPK, and activation of this protein kinase modulates insulin sensitivity and can promote "insulin-like" beneficial effects on glucose homeostasis. Therefore, in leptin resistance there would be loss of a potential modulation of insulin action that could contribute to the co-existence of insulin and leptin resistance.

Finally, the fact that there are so many common mediators of leptin and insulin action provides multiple potential molecular links between insulin and leptin resistance. For example a single molecular defect (either genetic or environmental) could reduce both insulin and leptin signaling (e.g. reduced IRS1 expression). In such a case the leptin resistance would result in obesity and the same defect would result in insulin resistance, and ultimately T2DM. The obesity would occur simultaneously with the insulin resistance (which is asymptomatic), and only when increased insulin secretion could not overcome the insulin resistance would the T2DM become apparent. This may provide an explanation for the close association between obesity and T2DM. It is not yet clear what percentage of the clinically obese are already insulin resistant.

3.2   Novel therapeutic strategies for the treatment of obesity and T2DM

There is a major effort to identify novel therapeutics to combat the obesity epidemic in order to address the major health implications of this condition. The development of leptin and insulin "sensitisers" has focused on the signaling pathways discussed in this chapter. For example, depletion of PTP1B by antisense or genetic ablation produces an animal that is resistant to weight gain and exhibits high sensitivity to insulin and leptin (Elchebly et al., 1999; Klaman et al., 2000; Zinker et al., 2002; Gum et al., 2003). Indeed reduction of PTP1B in animal models of obesity and insulin resistance has dramatic benefits both to BMI and glucose homeostasis. However, the development of potent, selective inhibitors for this enzyme has proven difficult (Pei et al., 2004; Taylor & Hill, 2004). This is primarily due to the high homology between PTP1B and other members of the phosphotyrosine phosphatase family, and the relatively large size and hydrophilicity of the PTP1B active site. However, although highly selective small molecules with drug-like physiochemical properties remain elusive, antisense oligonucleotide therapeutics for PTP1B have progressed to the clinic (Liu, 2004). Similarly, inhibition of PTEN would clearly improve both leptin and insulin sensitivity of cells, however as this enzyme was initially identified as a tumour suppressor protein it may prove a risky strategy for long-term therapy. Additionally, targeting PTEN generally is likely to lead to an increased risk of hepatic steatosis and hepatomegaly (Horie et al., 2004; Stiles et al., 2004). Inhibition of SHIP2 may prove to be a better prospect for development of small molecule inhibitors as this lipid phosphatase demonstrates higher substrate specificity and regulates stimulated rather than basal PtdIns(3,4,5)P_3 levels and does not appear to be linked to cancer in humans (Lazar & Saltiel, 2006).

Possibly the most exciting breakthrough in recent years is the identification of AMPK as the target of the insulin-sensitizing drug metformin (Fryer et al., 2002; Hawley et al., 2003). This has validated AMPK activators for the treatment of T2DM and as this enzyme is activated by leptin (in non-neuronal tissues) these activators would presumably also have beneficial effects on leptin resistant individuals. Metformin is a relatively weak activator of AMPK and therefore the search is on for more potent AMPK activators. However, such compounds may have potential deleterious effects on weight gain, mediated by AMPK action in the hypothalamus (Andersson et al., 2004; Minokoshi et al., 2004), so tissue specific AMPK activation may be required. This highlights the need to understand the variable signaling that results in opposite actions of leptin on central and peripheral AMPK.

Finally, there is a strong body of evidence linking obesity to reduced signaling through the IRS proteins (see earlier). Protein kinases induced by fatty acids (e.g. PKC), inflammation (e.g. p38MAPK, JNK, IKK, PKC) or hyper-insulinemia (e.g. p70S6K) are known to phosphorylate IRS on serine residues, resulting in ubiquitination and degradation. Therefore inhibitors of these protein kinases are being investigated as agents that could reverse leptin and insulin resistance through the stabilization of IRS molecules. However, there is still much debate as to the contribution of each of these protein kinases to resistance in humans. It will require more detailed molecular analysis of human tissues at different stages of the development of obesity and insulin resistance to establish how effective such inhibitors would be for the treatment of T2DM. If it became possible to diagnose individuals as having hyper-activation of one or more of these IRS kinases, then there would be more confidence to move inhibitor programs forward to clinical trials.

Conclusions

Much remains to be learned regarding the mechanisms by which leptin and insulin coordinate mammalian energy balance. However the identification of numerous signaling molecules regulated at least at some level by both agents suggests that single defects could promote both leptin and insulin resistance. It remains to be seen if such defects account for more than a small percentage of T2DM in the human population, or are fundamental to altered body mass. In the meantime, those molecules with key roles in both leptin and insulin action will be the focus of heightened attention for the immediate future.

References

Ahmad, F., Considine, R. V., Bauer, T. L., Ohannesian, J. P., Marco, C. C. & Goldstein, B. J. (1997). Improved sensitivity to insulin in obese subjects following weight loss is accompanied by reduced protein-tyrosine phosphatases in adipose tissue. *Metabolism* **46**, 1140–5.

Ahmed, Z. & Pillay, T. S. (2003). Adapter protein with a pleckstrin homology (PH) and an Src homology 2 (SH2) domain (APS) and SH2-B enhance insulin-receptor autophosphorylation, extracellular-signal-regulated kinase and phosphoinositide 3 kinase-dependent signaling. *Biochem. J.* **371**, 405–12.

Alessi, D. R. & Downes, C. P. (1998). The role of PI 3-kinase in insulin action. *Biochim. Biophys. Acta* **1436**, 151–64.

Andersson, U., Filipsson, K., Abbott, C. R. et al. (2004). AMPK plays a role in the control of food intake. *J. Biol. Chem.* **279**, 12 005– 8.

Andreelli, F., Foretz, M., Knauf, C. et al. (2006). Liver adenosine monophosphate-activated kinase alpha2 catalytic subunit is a key target for the control of hepatic glucose production by adiponectin and leptin but not insulin. *Endocrinology* **147**, 2432–41.

Bandyopadhay, G., Standaert, M. L., Zhao, L. et al. (1997). Activation of protein kinase C (*a*, *β* and *ζ*) by insulin in 3T3/L1 cells. *J. Biol. Chem.* **272**, 2551–8.

Banks, A. S., Davis, S. M., Bates, S. H. & Myers, M. G. Jr. (2000). Activation of downstream signals by the long form of the leptin receptor. *J. Biol. Chem.* **275**, 14 563–72.

Bates, S. H., Stearns, W. H., Dundon, T. A. et al. (2003). STAT3 signaling is required for leptin regulation of energy balance but not reproduction. *Nature* **421**, 856–9.

Baumann, H., Morella, K. K., White, D. W. et al. (1996). The full-length leptin receptor has signaling capabilities of interleukin 6-type cytokine receptors. *Proc. Natl. Acad. Sci. USA* **93**, 8374–8.

Beebe, S. J., Redmon, J. B., Blackmore, P. F. & Corbin, J. D. (1985). Discriminative insulin antagonism of stimulatory effects of various cAMP analogs on adipocyte lipolysis and hepatocyte glycogenolysis. *J. Biol. Chem.* **260**, 15 781–8.

Benomar, Y., Roy, A. F., Aubourg, A., Djiane, J. & Taouis, M. (2005). Cross down regulation of leptin and insulin receptor expression and signaling in a human neuronal cell line. *Biochem. J.* **388**, 929–39.

Benomar, Y., Wetzler, S., Larue-Achagiotis, C., Djiane, J., Tome, D. & Taouis, M. (2005). In vivo leptin infusion impairs insulin and leptin signaling in liver and hypothalamus. *Mol. Cell. Endocrinol.* **242**, 59–66.

Beugnet, A., Tee, A. R., Taylor, P. M. & Proud, C. G. (2003). Regulation of targets of mTOR (mammalian target of rapamycin) signaling by intracellular amino acid availability. *Biochem. J.* **372**, 555–66.

Bjorbaek, C., El-Haschimi, K., Frantz, J. D. & Flier, J. S. (1999). The role of SOCS-3 in leptin signaling and leptin resistance. *J. Biol. Chem.* **274**, 30059–65.

Bjorbaek, C., Buchholz, R. M., Davis, S. M. et al. (2001). Divergent roles of SHP-2 in ERK activation by leptin receptors. *J. Biol. Chem.* **276**, 4747–55.

Bogacka, I., Roane, D. S., Xi, X. et al. (2004).Expression levels of genes likely involved in glucose-sensing in the obese Zucker rat brain. *Nutr. Neurosci.* **7**, 67–74.

Bost, F., Aouadi, M., Caron, L. & Binetruy, B. (2005). The role of MAPKs in adipocyte differentiation and obesity. *Biochimie* **87**, 51–6.

Bost, F., Aouadi, M., Caron, L. et al. (2005). The extracellular signal-regulated kinase isoform ERK1 is specifically required for in vitro and in vivo adipogenesis. *Diabetes* **54**, 402–411.

Bouloumie, A., Marumo, T., Lafontan, M. & Busse, R. (1999). Leptin induces oxidative stress in human endothelial cells. *FASEB J.* **13**, 1231–8.

Bray, G. A., Lovejoy, J. C., Smith, S. R. et al. (2002). The influence of different fats and fatty acids on obesity, insulin resistance and inflammation. *J. Nutr.* **132**, 2488–91.

Brown, R. A. & Shepherd, P. R. (2001). Growth factor regulation of the novel class II phosphoinositide 3-kinases. *Biochem. Soc. Trans.* **29**, 535–7.

Bruning, J. C., Gautam, D., Burks, D. J. et al. (2000). Role of brain insulin receptor in control of body weight and reproduction. *Science* **289**, 2122–5.

Burks, D. J., Font de Mora, J., Schubert, M. et al. (2000). IRS2 pathways integrate female reproduction and energy homeostasis. *Nature* **407**, 377–82.

Butler, M., McKay, R. A., Popoff, I. J. et al. (2002). Specific inhibition of PTEN expression reverses hyperglycemia in diabetic mice. *Diabetes* **51**, 1028–34.

Cantley, L. C. (2002). The PI 3-kinase pathway. *Science* **296**, 1655–7.

Cao, Q., Mak, K. M. & Lieber, C. S. (2006). Leptin enhances alpha1(I) collagen gene expression in LX-2 human hepatic stellate cells through JAK-mediated H2O2-dependent MAPK pathways. *J. Cell. Biochem.* **97**, 188–97.

Carvalheira, J. B., Ribeiro, E. B., Folli, F., Velloso, L. A. & Saad, M. J. (2003). Interaction between leptin and insulin signaling pathways differentially affects JAK-STAT and PI 3 kinase-mediated signaling in rat liver. *Biol. Chem.* **384**, 151–9.

Carvalheira, J. B., Torsoni, M. A., Ueno, M. et al. (2005). Cross-talk between the insulin and leptin signaling systems in rat hypothalamus. *Obes. Res.* **13**, 48–57.

Chang, G. Q., Karatayev, O., Davydova, Z., Wortley, K. & Leibowitz, S. F. (2005). Glucose injection reduces neuropeptide Y and agouti-related protein expression in the arcuate nucleus: a possible physiological role in eating behavior. *Mol. Brain Res.* **135**, 69–80.

Chang, L. & Karin M. (2001). Mammalian MAP kinase signaling cascades. *Nature* **410**, 37–40.

Chen, H., Charlat, O., Tartaglia, L. A. et al. (1996). Evidence that the diabetes gene encodes the leptin receptor: identification of a mutation in the leptin receptor gene in db/db mice. *Cell* **84**, 491–5.

Choudhury, A. I., Heffron, H., Smith, M. A. et al. (2005). The role of insulin receptor substrate 2 in hypothalamic and beta cell function. *J. Clin. Invest.* **115**, 940–50.

Chua, S. C. J., Chung, W. K., Wu-Peng, X. S. et al. (1996). Phenotypes of mouse diabetes and rat fatty due to mutations in the OB (leptin) receptor. *Science* **271**, 994–6.

Chung, J., Kuo, C. J., Crabtree, G. R. & Blenis, J. (1992). Rapamycin-FKBP specifically blocks growth dependent activation of and signaling by the 70kDa S6 protein kinases. *Cell* **69**, 1227–36.

Clément, S., Krause, U., Desmedt, F. *et al.* (2001). The lipid phosphatase SHIP2 controls insulin sensitivity. *Nature* **409**, 92–7.

Cohen, B., Novick, D. & Rubinstein, M. (1996). Modulation of insulin activities by leptin. *Science* **274**, 1185–8.

Cone, R. D. (2005). Anatomy and regulation of the central melanocortin system. *Nat. Neurosci.* **8**, 571–8.

Considine, R. V., Sinha, M. K., Heiman, M. L. *et al.* (1996). Serum immunoreactive-leptin concentrations in normal-weight and obese humans. *N. Engl. J. Med.* **334**, 292–5.

Cota, D., Proulx, K., Smith, K. A. *et al.* (2006). Hypothalamic mTOR signaling regulates food intake. *Science* **312**, 927–30.

Dadke, S., Kusari, A. & Kusari, J. (2001). Phosphorylation and activation of proteintyrosine phosphatase (PTP) 1B by insulin receptor. *Mol. Cell. Biochem.* **221**, 147–54.

Dent, P., Haser, W., Haystead, T. A., Vincent, L. A., Roberts, T. M. & Sturgill, T. W. (1992). Activation of mitogen-activated protein kinase kinase by v-Raf in NIH 3T3 cells and in vitro. *Science* **257**, 1404–7.

Dickens, M., Svitek, C. A., Culbert, A. A., O'Brien, R. M. & Tavare, J. M. (1998). Central role for PI 3-kinase in the repression of glucose-6-phosphatase gene transcription by insulin. *J. Biol. Chem.* **273**, 20 144–9.

Domin, J., Pages, F., Volinia, S. *et al.* (1997). Cloning of a human phosphoinositide 3-kinase with a C2 domain that displays reduced sensitivity to the inhibitor wortmannin. *Biochem. J.* **326**, 139–47.

Duan, C., Li, M. & Rui, L. (2004). SH2-B promotes IRS1- and IRS2-mediated activation of the PI 3-kinase pathway in response to leptin. *J. Biol. Chem.* **279**, 43 684–91.

Duan, C., Yang, H., White, M. F. & Rui, L. (2004). Disruption of the SH2-B gene causes age-dependent insulin resistance and glucose intolerance. *Mol. Cell. Biol.* **24**, 7435–43.

Dunn, S. L., Bjornholm, M., Bates, S. H., Chen, Z., Seifert, M. & Myers, M. G. Jr. (2005). Feedback inhibition of leptin receptor/Jak2 signaling via Tyr1138 of the leptin receptor and suppressor of cytokine signaling 3. *Mol. Endocrinol.* **19**, 925–38.

Durakoglugil, M., Irving, A. J. & Harvey, J. (2005). Leptin induces a novel form of NMDA receptor-dependent long-term depression. *J. Neurochem.* **95**, 396–405.

Elchebly, M., Payette, P., Michaliszyn, E. *et al.* (1999). Increased insulin sensitivity and obesity resistance in mice lacking the protein tyrosine phosphatase-1B gene. *Science* **283**, 1423–5.

Emanuelli, B., Peraldi, P., Filloux, C., Sawka-Verhelle, D., Hilton, D. & Van Obberghen, E. (2000). SOCS-3 is an insulin-induced negative regulator of insulin signaling. *J. Biol. Chem.* **275**, 15 985–91.

Eyckerman, S., Broekaert, D., Verhee, A., Vandekerckhove, J. & Tavernier, J. (2000). Identification of the Y985 and Y1077 motifs as SOCS3 recruitment sites in the murine leptin receptor. *FEBS Lett.* **486**, 33–7.

Fasshauer, M., Kralisch, S., Klier, M. *et al.* (2004). Insulin resistance-inducing cytokines differentially regulate SOCS mRNA expression via growth factor- and Jak/Stat-signaling pathways in 3T3-L1 adipocytes. *J. Endocrinol.* **181**, 129–38.

Fisher, T. L. & White, M. F. (2004). Signaling pathways: the benefits of good communication. *Curr. Biol.* **14**, R1005–7.

Flier, J. S. (2006). Neuroscience. Regulating energy balance: the substrate strikes back. *Science* **312**, 861–4.

Fong, T. M., Mao, C., MacNeil, T. *et al.* (1997). ART (protein product of agouti-related transcript) as an antagonist of MC-3 and MC-4 receptors. *Biochem. Biophys. Res. Commun.* **237**, 629–31.

Foukas, L. C., Claret, M., Pearce, W. *et al.* (2006). Critical role for the p110alpha phosphoinositide-3 OH kinase in growth and metabolic regulation. *Nature* **441**, 366–70.

Francis, S. H., Turko, I. V. & Corbin, J. D. (2001). Cyclic nucleotide phosphodiesterases: relating structure and function. *Prog. Nucleic Acid Res. Mol. Biol.* **65**, 1–52.

Frederich, R. C., Hamann, A., Anderson, S., Lollmann, B., Lowell, B. B. & Flier, J. S. (1995). Leptin levels reflect body lipid content in mice: evidence for diet-induced resistance to leptin action. *Nat. Med.* **1**, 1211–14.

Friedman, J. M. & Halaas, J. L. (1998). Leptin and the regulation of body weight in mammals. *Nat. Med.* **395**, 763–70.

Frodin, M. & Gammeltoft, S. (1999). Role and regulation of 90 kDa ribosomal S6 kinase (RSK) in signal transduction. *Mol. Cell. Endocrinol.* **151**, 65–77.

Fruhbeck, G. (2005). Intracellular signaling pathways activated by leptin. *Biochem. J.* **393**, 7–20.

Fryer, L. G., Parbu-Patel, A. & Carling, D. (2002). The anti-diabetic drugs rosiglitazone and metformin stimulate AMP-activated protein kinase through distinct pathways. *J. Biol. Chem.* **277**, 25 226–32.

Gabbay, R. A., Sutherland, C., Gnudi, L. *et al.* (1996). Insulin regulation of PEPCK gene expression does not require activation of the Ras/MAP kinase signaling pathway. *J. Biol. Chem.* **271**, 1890–7.

Gamble, J. & Lopaschuk, G. D. (1998). Insulin inhibition of 5' adenosine monophosphate activated protein kinase in the heart results in activation of acetyl coenzyme A carboxylase and inhibition of fatty acid oxidation. *Metabolism* **46**, 1270–4.

Gingras, A.-C., Raught, B. & Sonenberg, N. (2001). Regulation of translational initiation by FRAP/mTOR. *Genes Dev.* **15**, 807–26.

Greene, M. W., Sakaue, H., Wang, L., Alessi, D. R. & Roth, R. A. (2003). Modulation of insulin-stimulated degradation of human insulin receptor substrate-1 by Serine 312 phosphorylation. *J. Biol. Chem.* **278**, 8199–211.

Gual, P., Le Marchand-Brustel, Y. & Tanti, J. F. (2005). Positive and negative regulation of insulin signaling through IRS-1 phosphorylation. *Biochimie* **87**, 99–109.

Gum, R. J., Gaede, L. L., Koterski, S. L. *et al.* (2003). Reduction of protein tyrosine phosphatase 1B increases insulin-dependent signaling in ob/ob mice. *Diabetes* **52**, 21–8.

Han, S. M., Namkoong, C., Jang, P. G. *et al.* (2005). Hypothalamic AMP-activated protein kinase mediates counter-regulatory responses to hypoglycaemia in rats. *Diabetologia* **48**, 2170–8.

Hardie, D. G., Salt, I. P., Hawley, S. A. & Davies, S. P. (1999). AMP-activated protein kinase: an ultrasensitive system for monitoring cellular energy charge. *Biochem. J.* **338**, 717–22.

Harrington, L. S., Findlay, G. M., Gray, A. *et al.* (2004). The TSC1-2 tumor suppressor controls insulin-PI3K signaling via regulation of IRS proteins. *J. Cell Biol.* **166**, 213–23.

Harvey, J., McKay, N. G., Walker, K. S., Downes, C. P. & Ashford, M. L. J. (2000). Essential role of phosphoinositide 3-kinase in leptin-induced KATP channel activation in the rat CRI-G1 insulinoma cell line. *J. Biol. Chem.* **275**, 4660–9.

Havrankova, J., Roth, J. & Brownstein, M. (1978). Insulin receptors are widely distributed in the central nervous system of the rat. *Nature* **272**, 827–9.

Hawkins, P. T., Jackson, T. R. & Stephens, L. R. (1992). Platelet-derived growth factor stimulates synthesis of PtdIns(3,4,5)P3 by activating a PtdIns(4,5)P2 3-OH kinase. *Nature* **358**, 157–9.

Hawley, S. A., Gadalla, A. E., Olsen, G. S. & Hardie, D. G. (2003). The antidiabetic drug metformin activates the AMP-activated protein kinase cascade via an adenine nucleotide independent mechanism. *Diabetes* **51**, 2420–5.

Hegyi, K., Fulop, K., Kovacs, K., Toth, S. & Falus, A. (2004). Leptin-induced signal transduction pathways. *Cell Biol. Int.* **28**, 159–69.

Heitman, J., Movva, N. R. & Hall, M. N. (1991). Targets for cell cycle arrest by the immunosuppressant rapamycin in yeast. *Science* **253**, 905–9.

Hekerman, P., Zeidler, J., Bamberg-Lemper, S. *et al.* (2005). Pleiotropy of leptin receptor signaling is defined by distinct roles of the intracellular tyrosines. *FEBS J.* **272**, 109–19.

Hennige, A. M., Stefan, N., Kapp, K. *et al.* (2006). Leptin down-regulates insulin action through phosphorylation of serine-318 in insulin receptor substrate 1. *FASEB J* Epub.

Hers, I. & Tavare, J. M. (2005). Mechanism of feedback regulation of IRS1 phosphorylation in primary adipocytes. *Biochem. J.* **388**, 713–20.

Hileman, S. M., Pierroz, D. D., Masuzaki, H. *et al.* (2002). Characterizaton of short isoforms of the leptin receptor in rat cerebral microvessels and of brain uptake of leptin in mouse models of obesity. *Endocrinology* **143**, 775–83.

Hirosumi, J., Tuncman, G., Chang, L. *et al.* (2002). A central role for JNK in obesity and insulin resistance. *Nature* **420**, 333–6.

Horie, Y., Suzuki, A., Kataoka, E. *et al.* (2004). Hepatocyte-specific Pten deficiency results in steatohepatitis and hepatocellular carcinomas. *J. Clin. Invest.* **113**, 1774–83.

Hotamisligil, G. S., Shargill, N. S. & Spiegelman, B. M. (1993). Adipose expression of TNF-a: direct role in obesity-linked insulin resistance. *Science* **259**, 87–91.

Howard, J. K., Cave, B. J., Oksanen, L. J., Tzameli, I., Bjorbaek, C. & Flier, J. S. (2004). Enhanced leptin sensitivity and attenuation of diet induced obesity in mice with haploinsufficiency of Socs3. *Nat. Med.* **10**, 734–8.

Hu, T. P., Xu, F. P., Li, Y. J. & Luo, J. D. (2006). Simvastatin inhibits leptin-induced hypertrophy in cultured neonatal rat cardiomyocytes. *Acta Pharmacol. Sin.* **27**, 419–22.

Huang, W., Dedousis, N., Bhatt, B. A. & O'Doherty, R. M. (2004). Impaired activation of PI 3-kinase by leptin is a novel mechanism of hepatic leptin resistance in diet-induced obesity. *J. Biol. Chem.* **279**, 21 695–700.

Ihle, J. N. & Kerr, I. M. (1995). Jaks and Stats in signaling by the cytokine receptor superfamily. *Trends Genet.* **11**, 69–74.

Irving, A. J., Wallace, L., Durakoglugil, D. & Harvey, J. (2006). Leptin enhances NR2B mediated N-methyl-D-aspartate responses via a mitogen-activated protein kinase dependent process in cerebellar granule cells. *Neuroscience* **138**, 1137–48.

Ishihara, H., Sasaoka, T., Kagawa, S. *et al.* (2003). Association of the polymorphisms in the 5' untranslated region of PTEN gene with type 2 diabetes in a Japanese population. *FEBS Lett.* **554**, 450–4.

Jefferies, H. B. J., Reinhard, C., Kozma, S. C. & Thomas, G. (1994). Rapamycin selectively represses translation of the 'polypyrimidine tract ' mRNA family. *Proc. Natl. Acad. Sci.* **91**, 4441–5.

Jefferies, H. B. J., Fumagalli, S., Dennis, P. B., Reinhard, C., Pearson, R. B. & Thomas, G. (1997). Rapamycin suppresses 5'TOP mRNA translation through inhibition of p70S6K. *EMBO J.* **16**, 3693–704.

Jiang, N., He, T. C., Miyajima, A. & Wojchowski, D. M. (1996). The box1 domain of the erythropoietin receptor specifies Janus kinase 2 activation and functions mitogenically within an interleukin 2 beta receptor chimera. *J. Biol. Chem.* **271**, 16 472–6.

Jo, Y. H., Chen, Y. J., Chua, S. C. Jr., Talmage, D. A. & Role, L. W. (2005). Integration of endocannabinoid and leptin signaling in an appetite-related neural circuit. *Neuron* **48**, 1055–66.

Kaburagi, Y., Yamauchi, T., Yamamoto-Honda, R. *et al.* (1999). The mechanism of insulin-induced signal transduction mediated by the insulin receptor substrate family. *Endocr. J.* **46**, S25–34.

Kagawa, S., Sasaoka, T., Yaguchi, S. *et al.* (2005). Impact of SRC homology 2-containing inositol 5' phosphatase 2 gene polymorphisms detected in a Japanese population on insulin signaling. *J. Clin. Endocrinol. Metab.* **90**, 2911–19.

Kahn, B. B., Alquier, T., Carling, D. & Hardie, D. G. (2005). AMP-activated protein kinase: ancient energy gauge provides clues to modern understanding of metabolism. *Cell Metab.* **1**, 15–25.

Kahn, C. R. & White, M. F. (1988). The insulin receptor and the molecular mechanism of insulin action. *J. Clin. Invest.* **82**, 1151–6.

Kaisaki, P. J., Delepine, M., Woon, P. Y. *et al.* (2004). Polymorphisms in type II SH2 domain containing inositol 5-phosphatase (INPPL1, SHIP2) are associated with physiological abnormalities of the metabolic syndrome. *Diabetes* **53**, 1900–4.

Kapeller, R. & Cantley, L. C. (1994). PI 3-kinase. *Bioessays* **16**, 565–76.

Kaszubska, W., Falls, H. D., Schaefer, V. G. *et al.* (2002). Protein tyrosine phosphatase 1B negatively regulates leptin signaling in a hypothalamic cell line. *Mol. Cell. Endocrinol.* **195**, 109–18.

Katso, R., Okkenhaug, K., Ahmadi, K., White, S., Timms, J. & Waterfield, M. D. (2001). Cellular function of phosphoinositide 3-kinases: implications for development, homeostasis, and cancer. *Annu. Rev. Cell Dev. Biol.* **17**, 615–75.

Kern, P. A., Di Gregorio, G. B., Lu, T., Rassouli, N. & Ranganathan, G. (2003). Adiponectin expression from human adipose tissue: relation to obesity, insulin resistance, and tumor necrosis factor-alpha expression. *Diabetes* **52**, 1779–85.

Khamzina, L., Veilleux, A., Bergeron, S. & Marette, A. (2005). Increased activation of the mammalian target of rapamycin pathway in liver and skeletal muscle of obese rats: possible involvement in obesity-linked insulin resistance. *Endocrinology* **146**, 1473–81.

Kim, J. K., Fillmore, J. J., Sunshine, M. J. *et al.* (2004). PKC-theta knockout mice are protected from fat induced insulin resistance. *J. Clin. Invest.* **114**, 823–7.

Kitamura, T., Kitamura, Y., Kuroda, S. *et al.* (1999). Insulin-induced phosphorylation and activation of cyclic nucleotide phosphodiesterase 3B by the serine threonine kinase Akt Mol. *Cell. Biol.* **19**, 6286–96.

Kitamura, T., Feng, Y., Ido, X. *et al.* (2006). Forkhead protein FoxO1 mediates Agrp-dependent effects of leptin on food intake. *Nat. Med.* **12**, 534–40.

Klaman, L. D., Boss, O., Peroni, O. D. *et al.* (2000). Increased energy expenditure, decreased adiposity, and tissue-specific insulin sensitivity in protein-tyrosine phosphatase 1B-deficient mice. *Mol.Cell. Biol.* **20**, 5479–89.

Kong, M., Wang, C. S. & Donohue, D. G. (2002). Interaction of fibroblast growth factor receptor 3 and the adapter protein SH2-B. A role in STAT5 activation. *J. Biol. Chem.* **277**, 15 962–70.

Krieger-Brauer, H. I. & Kather, H. (1992). Human fat cells possess a plasma membrane bound H_2O_2-generating system that is activated by insulin via a mechanism bypassing the receptor kinase. *J. Clin. Invest.* **89**, 1006–13.

Ktori, C., Shepherd, P. R. & O'Rourke, L. (2003). TNF-alpha and leptin activate the alpha-isoform of class II phosphoinositide 3-kinase. *Biochem. Biophys. Res. Commun.* **306**, 139–43.

Kubota, N., Terauchi, Y., Tobe, K. *et al.* (2004). Insulin receptor substrate 2 plays a crucial role in beta cells and the hypothalamus. *J. Clin. Invest.* **114**, 917–27.

Kurlawalla-Martinez, C., Stiles, B., Wang, Y., Devaskar, S. U., Kahn, B. B. & Wu, H. (2005). Insulin hypersensitivity and resistance to streptozotocin-induced diabetes in mice lacking PTEN in adipose tissue. *Mol. Cell. Biol.* **25**, 2498–510.

Kyriakis, J. M., App, H., Zhang, X. F. *et al.* (1992). Raf-1 activates MAP kinase-kinase. *Nature* **358**, 417–21.

Lammert, A., Kiess, W., Bottner, A., Glasow, A. & Kratzsch, J. (2001). Soluble leptin receptor represents the main leptin binding activity in human blood. *Biochem. Biophys. Res. Commun.* **283**, 982–8.

Lazar, D. F. & Saltiel, A. R. (2006). Lipid phosphatases as drug discovery targets for type 2 diabetes. *Nat. Rev. Drug Discov.* **5**, 333–42.

Le Good, J. A., Ziegler, W. H., Parekh, D. B., Alessi, D. R., Cohen, P. & Parker, P. J. (1998). PKC isotypes controlled by PI 3-kinase through the protein kinase PDK1. *Science* **281**, 2042–5.

Le, M. N., Kohanski, R. A., Wang, L. H. & Sadowski, H. B. (2002). Dual mechanism of signal transducer and activator of transcription 5 activation by the insulin receptor. *Mol. Endocrinol.* **16**, 2764–79.

Lee, G. H., Proenca, R., Montez, J. M. *et al.* (1996). Abnormal splicing of the leptin receptor in diabetic mice. *Nature* **379**, 632–5.

Lee, Y. H., Giraud, J., Davis, R. J. & White, M. F. (2003). c-Jun N-terminal kinase (JNK) mediates feedback inhibition of the insulin signaling cascade. *J. Biol. Chem.* **278**, 2896–902.

Leslie, N. R. & Downes, C. P. (2004). PTEN function: how normal cells control it and tumour cells lose it. *Biochem. J.* **382**, 1–11.

Lin, X., Taguchi, A., Park, S. *et al.* (2004). Dysregulation of insulin receptor substrate 2 in beta cells and brain causes obesity and diabetes. *J. Clin. Invest.* **114**, 908–16.

Liu, G. (2004). Technology evaluation: ISIS-113715, Isis. *Curr. Opin. Mol. Ther.* **6**, 331–6.

Liu, L., Karkanias, G. B., Morales, J. C. *et al.* (1998). Intracerebroventricular leptin regulates hepatic but not peripheral glucose fluxes. *J. Biol. Chem.* **273**, 31 160–7.

Lizcano, J. M. & Alessi, D. R. (2002). The insulin signaling pathway. *Curr. Biol.* **12**, R236–8.

Lo, Y. T., Tsao, C. J., Liu, I. M., Liou, S. S. & Cheng, J. T. (2004). Increase of PTEN gene expression in insulin resistance. *Horm. Metab. Res.* **36**, 662–6.

Lochhead, P. A., Salt, I. P., Walker, K. S., Hardie, D. G. & Sutherland, C. (2000). AICAR mimics the effects of insulin on the expression of 2 key gluconeogenic genes PEPCK and G6Pase. *Diabetes* **49**, 896–903.

Lund, I. K., Hansen, J. A., Andersen, H. S., Moller, N. P. & Billestrup, N. (2005). Mechanism of protein tyrosine phosphatase 1B mediated inhibition of leptin signaling. *J. Mol. Endocrinol.* **34**, 339–51.

Machinal-Quelin, F., Dieudonne, M. N., Leneveu, M. C., Pecquery, R. & Giudicelli, Y. (2002). Proadipogenic effect of leptin on rat preadipocytes in vitro: activation of MAPK and STAT3 signaling pathways. *Am. J. Physiol. Cell Physiol.* **282**, C853–63.

Mahadev, K., Wu, X., Zilbering, A., Zhu, L., Lawrence, J. T. & Goldstein, B. J. (2001a). Hydrogen peroxide generated during cellular insulin stimulation is integral to activation of the distal insulin signaling cascade in 3T3-L1 adipocytes. *J. Biol. Chem.* **276**, 48 662–9.

Mahadev, K., Zilbering, A., Zhu, L. & Goldstein, B. J. (2001b). Insulin-stimulated hydrogen peroxide reversibly inhibits protein-tyrosine phosphatase 1b in vivo and enhances the early insulin action cascade. *J. Biol. Chem.* **276**, 21 938–42.

Manganiello, V. & Vaughan, M. (1973). An effect of insulin on cyclic adenosine
3':5'monophosphate phosphodiesterase activity in fat cells. *J. Biol. Chem.* **248**,
7164–70.

Marks, J. L., Porte, D., Stahl, W. L. & Baskin, D. G. (1990). Localization of
insulin receptor mRNA in rat brain by in situ hybridization. *Endocrinology* **127**,
3234–6.

Maroni, P., Bendinelli, P. & Piccoletti, R. (2003). Early intracellular events induced
by in vivo leptin treatment in mouse skeletal muscle. *Mol. Cell. Endocrinol.* **201**,
109–21.

Maroni, P., Bendinelli, P. & Piccoletti, R. (2005). Intracellular signal transduction
pathways induced by leptin in C2C12 cells. *Cell Biol. Int.* **29**, 542–50.

Martin, D. E. & Hall, M. N. (2005). The expanding TOR signaling network. *Curr. Opin.
Cell Biol.* **17**, 158–66.

McClung, J. P., Roneker, C. A., Mu, W. *et al.* (2004). Development of insulin resistance
and obesity in mice overexpressing cellular glutathione peroxidase. *Proc. Natl.
Acad. Sci. USA* **101**, 8852–7.

McCrimmon, R. J., Fan, X., Ding, Y., Zhu, W., Jacob, R. J. & Sherwin, R. S. (2004).
Potential role for AMP-activated protein kinase in hypoglycemia sensing in the
ventromedial hypothalamus. *Diabetes* **53**, 1953–8.

Merrill, G. M., Kurth, E. J., Hardie, D. G. & Winder, W. W. (1997). AICA riboside
increases AMP-activated kinase, fatty acid oxidation and glucose uptake in rat
muscle. *Am. J. Physiol.* **273**, E1107–12.

Messina, J. L. & Weinstock, R. S. (1994). Evidence for diverse roles of PKC in the
inhibition of gene expression by insulin. *Endocrinology* **135**, 2327–34.

Minokoshi, Y., Kim, Y. B., Peroni, O. D., Fryer, L. G., Muller, C., Carling, D. & Kahn,
B. B. (2002). Lepin stimulates fatty-acid oxidation by activating AMPK. *Nature*
415, 339–43.

Minokoshi, Y., Alquier, T., Furukawa, N. *et al.* (2004). AMP-kinase regulates food
intake by responding to hormonal and nutrient signals in the hypothalamus.
Nature **428**, 569–74.

Mirshamsi, S., Laidlaw, H. A., Ning, K. *et al.* (2004). Leptin and insulin stimulation of
signaling pathways in arcuate nucleus neurones: PI3K dependent actin
reorganization and KATP channel activation. *BMC Neurosci.* **5**, 54.

Moodie, S. A., Willumsen, B. M., Weber, M. J. & Wolfman, A. (1993). Complexes of
Ras.GTP with Raf-1 and mitogen-activated protein kinase kinase. *Science* **260**,
1658–61.

Morel, Y. & Barouki, R. (1999). Repression of gene expression by oxidative stress.
Biochem. J. **342**, 481–96.

Mori, H., Hanada, R., Hanada, T. *et al.* (2004). Socs3 deficiency in the brain elevates
leptin sensitivity and confers resistance to diet-induced obesity. *Nat. Med.* **10**,
739–43.

Morino, K., Petersen, K. F., Dufour, S. *et al.* (2005). Reduced mitochondrial density
and increased IRS-1 serine phosphorylation in muscle of insulin resistant
offspring of type 2 diabetic parents. *J. Clin. Invest.* **115**, 3587–93.

Morton, G. J. & Schwartz, M. W. (2001). The NPY/AgRP neuron and energy homeostasis. *Int. J. Obes. Relat. Metab. Disord.* **25**, S56–62.

Munzberg, H. & Myers, M. G. Jr. (2005). Molecular and anatomical determinants of central leptin resistance. *Nat. Neurosci.* **5**, 566–70.

Munzberg, H., Huo, L., Nillni, E. A., Hollenberg, A. N. & Bjorbaek, C. (2003). Role of signal transducer and activator of transcription 3 in regulation of hypothalamic proopiomelanocortin gene expression by leptin. *Endocrinology* **144**, 2121–31.

Munzberg, H., Bjornholm, M., Bates, S. H. & Myers, M. G. Jr. (2005). Leptin receptor action and mechanisms of leptin resistance. *Cell. Mol. Life Sci.* **62**, 642–52.

Murakami, S., Sasaoka, T., Wada, T. *et al.* (2004). Impact of Src homology 2-containing inositol 5' phosphatase 2 on the regulation of insulin signaling leading to protein synthesis in 3T3 L1 adipocytes cultured with excess amino acids. *Endocrinology* **145**, 3215–23.

Myers, M. P., Andersen, J. N., Cheng, A. *et al.* (2001). TYK2 and JAK2 are substrates of protein tyrosine phosphatase 1B. *J. Biol. Chem.* **276**, 47771–4.

Ning, K., Miller, L. C., Laidlaw, H. A. *et al.* (2006). A novel leptin signaling pathway via PTEN inhibition in hypothalamic cell lines and pancreatic beta-cells. *EMBO J.* doi:10.1038/sj.embboj.7601118.

Niswender, K. D. & Schwartz, M. W. (2003). Insulin and leptin revisited: adiposity signals with overlapping physiological and intracellular signaling capabilities. *Front. Neuroendocrinol.* **24**, 1–10.

Niswender, K. D., Morton, G. J., Stearns, W. H., Rhodes, C. J., Myers, M. G. Jr. & Schwartz, M. W. (2001). Intracellular signaling. Key enzyme in leptin-induced anorexia. *Nature* **413**, 794–5.

Niswender, K. D., Morrison, C. D., Clegg, D. J. *et al.* (2003). Insulin activation of phosphatidylinositol 3 kinase in the hypothalamic arcuate nucleus: a key mediator of insulin-induced anorexia. *Diabetes* **52**, 227–31.

Niswender, K. D., Baskin, D. G. & Schwartz, M. W. (2004). Insulin and its evolving partnership with leptin in the hypothalamic control of energy homeostasis. *Trends Endocrinol. Metab.* **15**, 362–9.

O'Brien, K. B., O'Shea, J. J. & Carter-Su, C. (2002). SH2-B family members differentially regulate JAK family tyrosine kinases. *J. Biol. Chem.* **277**, 8673–81.

Ohtsuka, S., Takaki, S., Iseki, M. *et al.* (2002). SH2-B is required for both male and female reproduction. *Mol. Cell. Biol.* **22**, 3066–77.

Ollmann, M. M., Wilson, B. D., Yang, Y. K. *et al.* (1997). Antagonism of central melanocortin receptors in vitro and in vivo by agouti related protein. *Science* **278**, 135–8.

O'Malley, D. & Harvey, J. (2004). Insulin activates native and recombinant large conductance Ca^{2+}-activated potassium channels via a mitogen-activated protein kinase-dependent process. *Mol. Pharmacol.* **65**, 1352–63.

Onuma, M., Bub, J. D., Rummel, T. L. & Iwamoto, Y. (2003). Prostate cancer cell adipocyte interaction: leptin mediates androgen-independent prostate cancer cell proliferation through c-Jun NH2 terminal kinase. *J. Biol. Chem.* **278**, 42660–7.

Orci, L., Cook, W. S., Ravazzola, M. et al. (2004). Rapid transformation of white adipocytes into fat oxidising machines. Proc. Natl. Acad. Sci. USA **101**, 2058–63.

Parekh, D., Ziegler, W., Yonezawa, K., Hara, K. & Parker, P. J. (1999). Mammalian TOR controls one of two kinase pathways acting upon nPKCd and nPKCe. J. Biol. Chem. **274**, 34 758–64.

Parekh, D. B., Ziegler, W., Yonezawa, K., Hara, K. & Parker, P. J. (2000). Multiple pathways control PKC phosphorylation. EMBO J. **19**, 496–503.

Patel, S., Lipina, C. & Sutherland, C. (2003). Different mechanisms are used by insulin to repress three genes that contain a homologous thymine-rich insulin response element. FEBS Lett **549**, 72–6.

Pawson, T. (1995). Protein modules and insulin signaling networks. Nature **373**, 573–80.

Pawson, T. (2004). Specificity in signal transduction: from phosphotyrosine-SH2 domain interactions to complex cellular systems. Cell **116**, 191–203.

Pawson, T. & Scott, J. D. (1997). Signaling through scaffold, anchoring, and adaptor proteins. Science **278**, 2075–80.

Pearson, G., Robinson, F., Beers, M. et al. (2001). Mitogen-activated protein (MAP) kinase pathways: regulation and physiological functions. Endocrin. Rev. **22**, 153–83.

Pei, Z., Liu, G., Lubben, T. H. & Szczepankiewicz, B. G. (2004). Inhibition of protein tyrosine phosphatase 1B as a potential treatment of diabetes and obesity. Curr. Pharm. Des. **10**, 3481–504.

Pelicci, G., Lanfrancone, L., Grignani, F. et al. (1992). A novel transforming protein (SHC)with an SH2 domain is implicated in mitogenic signal transduction. Cell **70**, 93–104.

Phillips, M. S., Liu, Q., Hammond, H. A. et al. (1996). Leptin receptor missense mutation in the fatty Zucker rat. Nat. Genet. **13**, 18–19.

Pocai, A., Lam, T. K. T., Gutierrez-Juarez, R. et al. (2005a). Hypothalamic KATP channels control hepatic glucose production. Nature **434**, 1026–31.

Pocai, A., Morgan, K., Buettner, C., Gutierrez-Juarez, R., Obici, S. & Rossetti, L. (2005b). Central leptin acutely reverses diet-induced hepatic insulin resistance. Diabetes **54**, 3182–9.

Potashnik, R., Bloch-Damti, A., Bashan, N. & Rudich, A. (2003). IRS1 degradation and increased serine phosphorylation cannot predict the degree of metabolic insulin resistance induced by oxidative stress. Diabetologia **46**, 639–48.

Prasad, R. K. & Ismail-Beigi, F. (1999). Mechanism of stimulation of glucose transport by H2O2: role of PLC. Arch. Biochem. Biophys. **362**, 113–22.

Rahmouni, K. & Haynes, W. G. (2004). Leptin and the cardiovascular system. Rec. Prog. Horm. Res. **59**, 225–44.

Ravichandran, L. V., Chen, H., Li, Y. & Quon, M. J. (2001). Phosphorylation of PTP1B at Ser(50) by Akt impairs its ability to dephosphorylate the insulin receptor. Mol. Endocrinol. **15**, 1768–80.

Ren, D., Li, M., Duan, C. & Rui, L. (2005). Identification of SH2-B as a key regulator of leptin sensitivity, energy balance, and body weight in mice. Cell Metab. **2**, 95–104.

Rieusset, J., Bouzakri, K., Chevillotte, E. et al. (2004). Suppressor of cytokine signaling 3 expression and insulin resistance in skeletal muscle of obese and type 2 diabetic patients. Diabetes **53**, 2232–41.

Rui, L., Mathews, L. S., Hotta, K., Gustafson, T. A. & Carter-Su, C. M. (1997). Identification of SH2-Bbeta as a substrate of the tyrosine kinase JAK2 involved in growth hormone signaling. Mol. Cell. Biol. **17**, 6633–44.

Rui, L., Herrington, J. & Carter-Su, C. (1999). SH2-B is required for nerve growth factor induced neuronal differentiation. J. Biol. Chem. **274**, 10 590–4.

Ruiz-Alcaraz, A. J., Liu, H. K., Cuthbertson, D. J. et al. (2005). A novel regulation of IRS1 (insulin receptor substrate-1) expression following short term insulin administration. Biochem. J. **392**, 345–52.

Sahu, A. (2004). Leptin signaling in the hypothalamus: emphasis on energy homeostasis and leptin resistance. Front. Neuroendocrinol. **24**, 225–53.

Sahu, A. & Metlakunta, A. S. (2005). Hypothalamic phosphatidylinositol 3-kinase phosphodiesterase 3B-cyclic AMP pathway of leptin signaling is impaired following chronic central leptin infusion. J. Neuroendocrinol. **17**, 720–6.

Salt, I. P., Connell, J. M. & Gould, G. W. (2000). 5-aminoimidazole-4-carboxamide ribonucleoside (AICAR) inhibits insulin-stimulated glucose transport in 3T3-L1 adipocytes. Diabetes **49**, 1649–56.

Sasaoka, T., Wada, T., Fukui, K. et al. (2004). SH2-containing inositol phosphatase 2 predominantly regulates Akt2, and not Akt1, phosphorylation at the plasma membrane in response to insulin in 3T3-L1 adipocytes. J. Biol. Chem. **279**, 14 835–43.

Shanley, L. J., Irving, A. J. & Harvey, J. (2001). Leptin enhances NMDA receptor function and modulates hippocampal synaptic plasticity. J. Neurosci. **21**, RC186.

Shanley, L. J., O'Malley, D., Irving, A. J., Ashford, M. L. J. & Harvey, J. (2002). Leptin inhibits epileptiform-like activity in rat hippocampal neurones via PI 3-kinase-driven activation of BK channels. J. Physiol. **545**, 933–44.

Shaw, R. J., Lamia, K. A., Vasquez, D. et al. (2005). The kinase LKB1 mediates glucose homeostasis in liver and therapeutic effects of metformin. Science **310**, 1642–6.

Shepherd, P. R., Withers, D. J. & Siddle, K. (1998). Phosphoinositide 3-kinase: the key switch mechanism in insulin signaling. Biochem. J. **333**, 471–90.

Shi, H., Cave, B., Inouye, K., Bjorbaek, C. & Flier, J. S. (2006). Overexpression of suppressor of cytokine signaling 3 in adipose tissue causes local but not systemic insulin resistance. Diabetes **55**, 699–707.

Shin, H. J., Oh, J., Kang, S. M. et al. (2005). Leptin induces hypertrophy via p38 mitogen-activated protein kinase in rat vascular smooth muscle cells. Biochem. Biophys. Res. Commun. **329**, 18–24.

Shulman, G. I. (2000). Cellular mechanisms of insulin resistance. J. Clin. Invest. **106**, 171–6.

Sleeman, M. W., Wortley, K. E., Lai, K. M. et al. (2005). Absence of the lipid phosphatase SHIP2 confers resistance to dietary obesity. Nat. Med. **11**, 199–205.

Spangenburg, E. E., Brown, D. A., Johnson, M. S. & Moore, R. L. (2006). Exercise increases SOCS-3 expression in skeletal muscle: potential relationship to IL-6 expression. J. Physiol. Epub.

Standaert, M. L., Galloway, L., Karnam, P., Bandyopadhyay, G., Moscat, J. & Farese, R. V. (1997). Protein kinase C-z as a downstream effector of phosphatidylinositol 3 kinase during insulin stimulation in rat adipocytes. *J. Biol. Chem.* **272**, 30 075–82.

Stanley, B. G., Kyrkouli, S. E., Lampert, S. & Leibowitz, S. F. (1986). Neuropeptide Y chronically injected into the hypothalamus: a powerful neurochemical inducer of hyperphagia and obesity. *Peptides* **7**, 1189–92.

Starr, R., Willson, T. A., Viney, E. M. *et al.* (1997). A family of cytokine-inducible inhibitors of signaling. *Nature* **387**, 917–21.

Stephens, L. R., Hughes, K. T. & Irvine, R. F. (1991). Pathway of phosphatidylinositol (3,4,5)-trisphosphate synthesis in activated neutrophils. *Nature* **351**, 33–9.

Stiles, B., Wang, Y., Stahl, A. *et al.* (2004). Liver-specific deletion of negative regulator Pten results in fatty liver and insulin hypersensitivity. *Proc. Natl. Acad. Sci. USA* **101**, 2082–7.

Stokoe, D., Macdonald, S. G., Cadwallader, K., Symons, M. & Hancock, J. F. (1994). Activation of Raf as a result of recruitment to the plasma membrane. *Science* **264**, 1463–7.

Sturgill, T. W., Ray, L. B., Erikson, E. & Maller, J. L. (1988). Insulin-stimulated MAP-2 kinase phosphorylates and activates ribosomal protein S6 kinase II. *Nature* **334**, 715–18.

Sutherland, C., O'Brien, R. M. & Granner, D. K. (1995). Phosphatidylinositol 3-kinase, but not p70/p85 ribosomal S6 protein kinase, is required for the regulation of phosphoenolpyruvate carboxykinase gene expression by insulin. *J. Biol. Chem.* **270**, 15 501–6.

Sutherland, C., Tebbey, P. W. & Granner, D. K. (1997). Oxidative and chemical stress mimic insulin by selectively inhibiting the expression of phosphoenolpyruvate carboxykinase in hepatoma cells. *Diabetes* **46**, 17–22.

Suzuki, R., Tobe, K., Aoyama, M. *et al.* (2004). Both insulin signaling defects in the liver and obesity contribute to insulin resistance and cause diabetes in Irs2(-/-) mice. *J. Biol. Chem.* **279**, 25 039–49.

Sweeney, G. (2002). Leptin signaling. *Cell Signal.* **14**, 655–63.

Szanto, J. & Kahn, C. R. (2000). Selective interaction between leptin and insulin signaling pathways in a hepatic cell line. *Proc. Natl. Acad. Sci. USA* **97**, 2355–60.

Taler, M., Shpungin, S., Salem, Y., Malovani, H., Pasder, O. & Nir, U. (2003). Fer is a downstream effector of insulin and mediates the activation of signal transducer and activator of transcription 3 in myogenic cells. *Mol. Endocrinol.* **17**, 1580–92.

Tanabe, K., Okuya, O., Tanizawa, Y., Matsutani, A. & Oka, Y. (1997). Leptin induces proliferation of pancreatic beta cell line MIN6 through activation of mitogen-activated protein kinase. *Biochem. Biophys. Res. Commun.* **241**, 765–8.

Tao, J., Malbon, C. C. & Wang, H. Y. (2001). Insulin stimulates tyrosine phosphorylation and inactivation of protein-tyrosine phosphatase 1B in vivo. *J. Biol. Chem.* **276**, 29 520–5.

Tartaglia, L. A., Dembski, M., Weng, X. *et al.* (1995). Identification and expression cloning of a leptin receptor, OB-R. *Cell* **83**, 1263–71.

Taylor, S. D. & Hill, B. (2004). Recent advances in protein tyrosine phosphatase 1B inhibitors. *Expert Opin. Investig. Drugs* **13**, 199–214.

Toker, A., Meyer, M., Reddy, K. K. *et al.* (1994). Activation of PKC family members by the novel polyphosphoinositides PI-3,4-P2 and PI-3,4,5-P3. *J. Biol. Chem.* **269**, 32 358–67.

Uchida, T., Myers Jr, M. G. & White, M. F. (2000). IRS-4 mediates protein kinase B signaling during insulin stimulation without promoting antiapoptosis. *Mol. Cell. Biol.* **20**, 126–38.

Ueno, M., Carvalheira, J. B., Tambascia, R. C. *et al.* (2005). Regulation of insulin signaling by hyperinsulinaemia: role of IRS-1/2 serine phosphorylation and the mTOR/p70 S6K pathway. *Diabetologia* **48**, 506–18.

Ui, M., Okada, T., Hazeki, K. & Hazeki, O. (1995). Wortmannin as a unique probe for an intracellular signaling protein, phosphoinositide 3-kinase. *Trends Biochem. Sci.* **20**, 303–7.

Um, S. H., Frigerio, M., Watanabe, M. *et al.* (2004). Absence of S6K1 protects against age- and diet-induced obesity while enhancing insulin sensitivity. *Nature* **431**, 200–5.

van den Brink, G. R., O'Toole, T., Hardwick, J. C. *et al.* (2000). Leptin signaling in human peripheral blood mononuclear cells, activation of p38 and p42/44 mitogen-activated protein (MAP) kinase and p70 S6 kinase. *Mol. Cell. Biol. Res. Commun.* **4**, 144–50.

Vanhaesebroeck, B., Leevers, S. J., Panayotou, G. & Waterfield, M. D. (1997). Phosphoinositide 3-kinases: a conserved family of signal transducers. *Trends Biochem. Sci.* **22**, 267–72.

Vanhaesebroeck, B., Leevers, S. J., Ahmadi, K. *et al.* (2001). Synthesis and function of 3 phosphorylated inositol lipids. *Annu. Rev. Biochem.* **70**, 535–602.

Vlahos, C. J., Matter, W. F., Hui, K. Y. & Brown, R. F. (1994). A specific inhibitor of phosphatidylinositol 3-kinase, 2-(4-morpholinyl)-8-phenyl-4H-1-benzopyran-4-one (LY294002). *J. Biol. Chem.* **269**, 5241–8.

von Manteuffel, S. R., Dennis, P. B., Pullen, N., Gingras, A. C., Sonenberg, N. & Thomas, G. (1997). The insulin-induced signaling pathway leading to S6 and initiation factor 4E binding protein 1 phosphorylation bifurcates at a rapamycin-sensitive point immediately upstream of p70s6k. *Mol. Cell. Biol.* **17**, 5426–36.

Wang, J. & Riedel, H. (1998). Insulin-like growth factor-I receptor and insulin receptor association with a Src homology-2 domain-containing putative adapter. *J. Biol. Chem.* **273**, 3136–9.

White, M. F. (1998). The IRS-signaling system: a network of docking proteins that mediate insulin action. *Mol. Cell. Biochem.* **182**, 3–11.

White, M. F. (2002). IRS proteins and the common path to diabetes. *Am. J. Physiol. Endocrinol. Metab.* **283**, E413–22.

White, M. F. & Kahn, C. R. (1994). The insulin signaling system. *J. Biol. Chem.* **269**, 1–4.

Whitehurst, A. W., Wilsbacher, J. L., You, Y., Luby-Phelps, K., Moore, M. S. & Cobb, M. H. (2002). ERK2 enters the nucleus by a carrier independent mechanism. *Proc. Natl. Acad. Sci. USA* **99**, 7496–501.

Wick, M. J., Dong, L. Q., Hu, D., Langlais, P. & Liu, F. (2001). Insulin-receptor-mediated p62dok tyrosine phosphorylation at residues 362 and 398 plays distinct roles for binding GAP and Nck and is essential for inhibiting insulin-stimulated activation of Ras and Akt. *J. Biol. Chem.* **278**, 42 843–50.

Wijesekara, N., Konrad, D., Eweida, M. *et al.* (2005). Muscle specific Pten deletion protects against insulin resistance and diabetes. *Mol. Cell. Biol.* **25**, 1135–45.

Williams, A. G., Hargreaves, A. C., Gunn-Moore, F. J. & Tavare, J. M. (1998). Stimulation of NPY gene expression by BDNF requires both the PLCg and shc binding sites on its receptor, TrkB. *Biochem. J.* **333**, 505–9.

Williams, M. R., Arthur, J. S., Balendran, A. *et al.* (2000). The role of 3-phosphoinositide-dependent protein kinase 1 in activating AGC kinases defined in embryonic stem cells. *Curr. Biol.* **10**, 439–48.

Withers, D. J. & White, M. (2000). Perspective: the insulin signaling system – a common link in the pathogenesis of type 2 diabetes. *Endocrinology* **141**, 1917–21.

Witters, L. A. & Kemp, B. E. (1992). Insulin activation of acetyl-CoA carboxylase accompanied by inhibition of the 5′-AMP-activated protein kinase. *J. Biol. Chem.* **267**, 2864–7.

Wynne, K., Stanley, S., McGowan, B. & Bloom, S. (2005). Appetite control. *J. Endocrinol.* **184**, 291–318.

Yamagishi, S. I., Edelstein, D., Du, X. L., Kaneda, Y., Guzman, M. & Brownlee, M. (2001). Leptin induces mitochondrial superoxide production and monocyte chemoattractant protein-1 expression in aortic endothelial cells by increasing fatty acid oxidation via protein kinase A. *J. Biol. Chem.* **276**, 25096–100.

Yamanashi, Y. & Baltimore, D. (1997). Identification of the Abl- and rasGAP-associated 62 kDa protein as a docking protein, Dok. *Cell* **88**, 205–11.

Zabolotny, J. M., Bence-Hanulec, K. K., Stricker-Krongrad, A. *et al.* (2002). PTP1B regulates leptin signal transduction in vivo. *Dev. Cell* **2**, 489–95.

Zarjevski, N., Cusin, I., Vettor, R., Rohner-Jeanrenaud, F. & Jeanrenaud, B. (1993). Chronic intracerebroventricular neuropeptide-Y administration to normal rats mimics hormonal and metabolic changes of obesity. *Endocrinology* **133**, 1753–8.

Zhang, E. E., Chapeau, E., Hagihara, K. & Feng, G. S. (2004). Neuronal Shp2 tyrosine phosphatase controls energy balance and metabolism. *Proc. Natl. Acad. Sci. USA* **101**, 16064–9.

Zhang, W., Zong, C. S., Hermanto, U., Lopez-Bergami, P., Ronai, Z. & Wang, L. H. (2006). RACK1 recruits STAT3 specifically to insulin and insulin-like growth factor 1 receptors for activation, which is important for regulating anchorage-independent growth. *Mol. Cell. Biol.* **26**, 413–24.

Zhang, Y., Proenca, R., Maffei, M., Barone, M., Leopold, L. & Friedman, J. M. (1994). Positional cloning of the mouse obese gene and its human homologue. *Nature* **372**, 425–32.

Zhao, A. Z., Bornfeldt, K. E. & Beavo, J. A. (1998). Leptin inhibits insulin secretion by activation of PDE 3B. *J. Clin. Invest.* **102**, 869–73.

Zhao, A. Z., Shinohara, M. M., Huang, D. *et al.* (2000). Leptin induces insulin-like signaling that antagonises cAMP elevation by glucagon in hepatocytes. *J. Biol. Chem.* **275**, 11 348–54.

Zhao, A. Z., Huan, J. N., Gupta, S., Pal, R. & Sahu, A. (2002). A phosphatidylinositol 3 kinase phosphodiesterase 3B-cyclic AMP pathway in hypothalamic action of leptin on feeding. *Nat. Neurosci.* **5**, 727–8.

Zheng, C. F. & Guan, K. L. (1994). Activation of MEK family kinases requires phosphorylation of two conserved Ser/Thr residues. *Embo. J.* **13**, 1123–31.

Zinker, B. A., Rondinone, C. M., Trevillyan, J. M. *et al.* (2002). PTP1B antisense oligonucleotide lowers PTP1B protein, normalizes blood glucose, and improves insulin sensitivity in diabetic mice. *Proc. Natl. Acad. Sci. USA* **99**, 11 357–62.

Zong, H., Ren, J. M., Young, L. H. *et al.* (2002). AMP kinase is required for mitochondrial biogenesis in skeletal muscle in response to chronic energy deprivation. *Proc. Natl. Acad. Sci. USA* **99**, 15 983–7.

6

Diet-induced obesity in animal models and what they tell us about human obesity

BARRY E. LEVIN AND ALISON M. STRACK

1.   Introduction

Animals have been used extensively as surrogates for the study of factors that contribute to the development and persistence of obesity in human beings. Each model has its own set of advantages and disadvantages in relation to its similarities and differences from humans. In fact, obesity rarely occurs in feral animals outside of the pre-hibernating period. For the majority of individuals obesity is a relatively recent event in human history because food availability was generally limited and a relatively high degree of physical activity was required to procure sufficient food to maintain survival. The switch from hunter-gatherer to agricultural societies has allowed increasing numbers of individuals to obtain food with reduced expenditure of energy. In the developed world, the prevalence of obesity has increased precipitously in the last 20–30 years as the availability of cheap, highly palatable, energy-dense food has become more widely available and physical activity has declined (Popkin & Doak, 1999). Clearly, the gene pool has not changed substantially over such a short period of time to explain the rapid increase in obesity prevalence. Thus, environmental factors must be the critical variable which has promoted the current epidemic of human obesity. Animal models of obesity have become a useful tool in our quest to understand the factors contributing to the recent obesity epidemic in humans. Although other animals differ from humans in many ways, they share many common physiological properties that assure their survival during periods of

Neurobiology and Obesity, ed. Jenni Harvey and Dominic J. Withers. Published by Cambridge University Press. © Cambridge University Press 2008

famine. It is these similarities that make animal models valuable for understanding the basic mechanisms underlying the regulation of energy homeostasis and its physiological, metabolic and neuroendocrine underpinnings. Because of their relatively low cost and ease of use, rodents have gained wide acceptance as models of human obesity. For this reason, this review will focus primarily on rodent models of diet-induced obesity (DIO). However, we will also provide an overview of some of the other animal models of DIO which have been used for this purpose although the data in such models are much more limited. We will not include genetically modified rodent models since those will be covered in other chapters.

1.1   Survival, the "thrifty phenotype" and obesity

Survival of the species depends upon the ability of an organism to ingest and store as much energy as possible during times of plenty against times of scarcity. Even more important is the ability to preserve existing energy stores when little food is available. Those individuals who are most efficient at both of these tasks are the most likely to survive cycles of feast and famine. Such individuals have been said to have a "thrifty genotype" (Neel, 1962) or "thrifty phenotype" (Hales & Barker, 1992). Virtually all mammals share the common ability to reduce energy expenditure when food is scarce by utilizing a series of physiological and metabolic processes. However, the ability to ingest more calories than one needs to meet ongoing metabolic demands is unique to those individuals with the thrifty phenotype. Lean individuals monitor their caloric intake, make appropriate corrections in subsequent intake and energy expenditure and maintain their defended body weights within relatively narrow limits over long periods of time (Levin et al., 1985, 2003; Weinsier et al., 1995). However, such tight regulation of adipose stores is not necessarily the best survival strategy in times of intermittent famine. The most efficient survivors are able to eat beyond their metabolic needs to store as much energy as fat as possible when food is abundant to act as a buffer against times when the food supplies become scarce. One way of accomplishing this is to have an elevated threshold for sensing and responding to hormonal and metabolic cues from the periphery which normally limit food intake (Levin & Dunn-Meynell, 2002c; Levin et al., 2003; Ricci & Levin, 2003; Levin, 2004). On the other hand, when food is scarce, virtually all individuals are able to minimize catabolic processes and maximize the anabolic drive to eat and conserve stored calories by reducing their metabolic rate (Levin & Dunn-Meynell, 1997a; Levin, 1999; MacLean et al., 2004).

1.2   Neural plasticity and the defended body weight

Energy homeostasis is the balance between intake and expenditure where adipose stores represent the major buffer in which energy is stored when intake exceeds expenditure and which supplies energy during periods of negative energy balance. In obesity-prone individuals the "set-point" or "set-tling-point" (Davis & Wirtshafter, 1978; Stunkard, 1982) about which energy homeostasis is regulated tends to rise throughout life. At each successively higher level, the defended body weight can be permanently lowered by caloric restriction or pharmacotherapy in only ~10% of individuals (Kramer et al., 1989). This unidirectional movement of the defended body weight suggests that some permanent change occurs in the pathways involved in the regulation of energy homeostasis. The brain is the major controller of energy homeostasis through its interactions with the periphery and is a likely location for such permanent change since it is capable of forming new neural pathways throughout life as occurs during the formation of long-term memories (Levin & Keesey, 1998; Levin, 2000). In fact, long-term changes in dietary composition and body weight do lead to permanent changes in neural circuits involved in energy homeostasis (Wilmot et al., 1988; Levin, 1990a, 1990b, 1994; Levin & Hamm, 1994). Also, a variety of lesions within some of these same circuits can markedly and permanently alter the level about which body weight is defended (Keesey et al., 1979; King et al., 1993; Bellinger & Bernardis, 2002). Thus, there is good evidence that certain alterations in the connectivity and function of pathways regulating energy homeostasis, whether naturally occurring or experimentally imposed, can lead to major changes in the level of defended body weight and adiposity.

1.3   Metabolic sensing neurons and the regulation of energy homeostasis

The brain requires neural, hormonal and metabolic signals from the body and external environment to enable it to regulate energy homeostasis. Animal models provide a convenient and accessible means to study these interactions. From such models we have learned that mammals have evolved a unique set of "metabolic-sensing" neurons which receive these multiple inputs from the periphery (Levin, 2002a; Levin et al., 2004). Metabolic sensing neurons are arrayed in a distributed network of multiple interconnected sites throughout the brain (Levin, 2001, 2002a, 2002b). Originally described as "glucose-sensing" because they alter their firing rate when ambient glucose levels change (Anand et al., 1964; Oomura et al., 1964), it is now clear that many of these same neurons can also utilize metabolites such as lactate (Yang et al., 1999; Yang et al., 2004; Song & Routh, 2005), ketone bodies (Minami et al., 1990) and fatty acids (Oomura et al., 1975; Wang et al., 2005) as signaling molecules. They also have receptors for and respond to hormones such as leptin and insulin (Spanswick et al., 1997; Kang et al., 2004; Wang et al., 2004). Collectively, these signals inform the brain of the status of adipose and glucose stores and visceral function. Hindbrain areas such as the nucleus tractus solitarius, area postrema, raphe pallidus and obscurus and A1/C1 and C3 areas contain such metabolic-sensing neurons (Adachi et al., 1984; Dallaporta et al., 1999; Ritter et al., 2000; Levin et al., 2004; Sanders et al., 2004). These neurons express the monoamines norepinephrine (NE), epinephrine (Epi) and serotonin (5HT) (Ritter et al., 2000) and neuropeptides such as the neuropeptide Y (NPY), proopiomelanocortin (POMC; Li & Ritter, 2004) and glucagon-like peptide-2 (Tang-Christensen et al., 2000). Some receive direct neural inputs from sensors in peripheral organs such as the gastrointestinal tract and hepatic portal vein (Niijima, 1969; Adachi et al., 1984) but also have receptors for and respond to leptin (Grill et al., 2002). These hindbrain sensing neurons relay information from the periphery to hypothalamic and other forebrain areas which mediate feeding behavior and metabolic processes involved in the control of energy homeostasis (Tang-Christensen et al., 2000; Ritter et al., 2001). They also project to limbic and forebrain structures involved in the affective and rewarding properties of food (Ricardo & Koh, 1978). Metabolic-sensing NPY and POMC neurons in the hypothalamic arcuate nucleus (ARC) receive some of these hindbrain inputs as do several neuropeptide and neurotransmitter expressing neurons within the paraventricular nucleus (PVN) and lateral hypothalamus (LH). The PVN and LH are major effector areas involved in neuroendocrine function, food intake, energy assimilation and expenditure (Ritter et al., 2001; Dunn-Meynell et al., 2002).

2.   Animal models of diet-induced obesity

While there is good evidence that metabolic-sensing neurons do exist and that they play an important role in energy homeostasis in rodents, there are no comparable sets of data showing that similar neurons exist within the human brain. Certainly there are comparable sets of neurons such as the NPY and POMC neurons in the ARC which are likely to represent metabolic sensors (Bai et al., 2005). Also, in vivo imaging studies suggest that there are areas within the hypothalamus that respond to alterations in plasma glucose (Matsuda et al., 1999) comparably to those in the rodent brain (Mahankali et al., 2000). But our ability to study the function of the human brain either in vivo or in vitro at the cellular level is severely limited, leading us to rely on animal models as useful surrogates. We do so with the full realization that these animal models are similar to but not identical to human beings in terms of their neural, hormonal, physiologic and metabolic functions.

2.1   Diet-induced obesity in rodents

While there are many differences between rodents and humans, there are also many important similarities with regard to the mechanisms which underlie the development of obesity. A few major differences include the complexity and the ontogeny of brain development, the dependence of adult rodents on brown adipose tissue for some aspects of thermogenesis (Foster & Frydman, 1978) and most importantly, the fact that obesity in rodents rarely has the pathological consequences that it does in humans. However, there are many similarities depending upon the specific strain and species of rodent used. The development of DIO in rodents resembles the majority of human obesity in being of polygenic origin (Stunkard et al., 1990; Bouchard & Perusse, 1993; Levin et al., 1997, 2003) and being associated with the development of the metabolic syndrome (Levin et al., 1997, 2003; Ricci & Levin, 2003), hyperleptinemia and with leptin resistance (Caro et al., 1996; Van Heek et al., 1997; El-Haschimi et al., 2000; Levin & Dunn-Meynell, 2002a) and reduced ghrelin levels (Tschop et al., 2001; Levin et al., 2003). Some obese humans and rodents also have reduced growth hormone secretion (Williams et al., 1984; Lauterio & Perez, 1997), abnormalities of brain glucosensing (Levin & Sullivan, 1989a, 1989b; Levin, 1992; Levin & Planas, 1993; Levin et al., 1996; Levin & Dunn-Meynell, 1997b; Song et al., 2001; Dunn-Meynell et al., 2002) and reduced oxidation of fatty acids when the fat content of the diet is increased (Chang et al., 1990; Zurlo et al., 1990). Perhaps the most important similarity is the shared ability to avidly defend their elevated levels of carcass adiposity against most attempts to reduce them by caloric restriction (Rolls et al., 1980; Leibel & Hirsch, 1984; Levin & Keesey, 1998; Levin & Dunn-Meynell, 2000, 2002b; MacLean et al., 2004). Also, both obese humans and rodents respond to several drugs which reduce food intake and/or increase thermogenesis but such drugs have no lasting effect beyond the period over which they are administered (Stunkard, 1982; Rowland & Carlton, 1986; Levin & Dunn-Meynell, 2000).

The idea of producing DIO in rodents to study human obesity goes back at least as far as 1949 (Ingle, 1949). Since that time there have been a number of seminal studies which have guided our use of rodents in this field. Gordon Kennedy (Kennedy, 1953) utilized rat models to test his "lipostatic hypothesis" which stated that there was an adipose-derived signal that allowed the brain to regulate adipose stores. Cohn et al. (1957) demonstrated the often overlooked point that rats could be made obese without necessarily increasing their body weight, and Hollifield & Parson (1962) showed that restricting the amount of time that food was available could induce rats to become obese. In two landmark studies, Schemmel et al. established that the propensity to become obese varied as a function of dietary composition, gender, age and starting body weight (Schemmel et al., 1969). They also demonstrated the important genetic component of obesity by showing that there was huge variability in the degree of obesity that developed among different rats strains when they were fed the same high fat diet (Schemmel et al., 1970). These inter-strain differences have been widely exploited in both rats (Lin et al., 1998; Helies et al., 2005) and mice (West et al., 1994) to examine traits which predispose animals to become obese. Sclafani and co-workers were the first to employ a "supermarket" (later called "cafeteria diet"; Rolls et al., 1980) composed of different highly palatable foods to produce obesity (Sclafani & Springer, 1976). Most importantly, they were the first to recognize that there was considerable variability of weight gain among individuals of the same outbred strain. Hill et al. (1983) took advantage of these differences by separating high and low weight gainers on high fat diets into two groups for the purposes of studying those who were prone and those who were resistant to the development of DIO. Finally, Berthoud (1985) noticed that there were large differences among various members of the same rat strain in their cephalic phase insulin responses to food-related cues and that these responses were predictive of future weight gain on a high fat diet. By selectively breeding for high and low weight gainers from an outbred Sprague–Dawley strain and then backcrossing those which expressed the DIO trait we were able to establish a polygenic mode of obesity inheritance in rats (Levin et al., 1997, 2003) similar to that found in the majority of human obesity (Stunkard et al., 1990; Bouchard & Perusse, 1993). Other studies showed that that there can be major differences in the organization and function of the nervous system (Clark et al., 1991) and the propensity to develop DIO on a high fat diet (Levin et al., 1983; Archer et al., 2003) in the same strains of outbred rats derived by different commercial breeders. Even genetically identical, inbred strains of mice can show enormous variability in the amount of adiposity they gain when fed energy-dense diets (Burcelin et al., 2002). Such studies establish a role for environmental factors during the perinatal periods as critical determinants of the development of obesity. These have been supported by others using high fat diets (Guo & Jen, 1995), maternal undernutrition (Jones et al., 1984), diabetes (Reifsnyder et al., 2000), obesity (Levin & Govek, 1998; Levin & Dunn-Meynell, 2002c) or hormonal exposure (Plagemann et al., 1992; Levin et al., 2005) during gestation and lactation to emphasize the role of the perinatal environment and its interaction with genetic predisposition in the development of obesity.

The major problem in the treatment of obesity in both humans and rodents is that it becomes irreversible as long as the individual has an underlying obesity-prone predisposition. Early studies of reversibility in rodents produced variable results, most likely because of the variability of metabolic responses to high fat diet among members of the same strains and because of inter-strain differences. In Wistar rats, switching from a high to low fat diet caused most rats to lose the weight they had gained after 17 weeks, while none lost weight when switched to low fat diet after 30 weeks on a high fat diet (Hill *et al.*, 1989). In hooded Lister rats, 90 days on a cafeteria diet was sufficient to prevent them from losing weight when switched to a low fat diet (Rolls *et al.*, 1980). Furthermore, when their caloric intake was restricted for 27 days to produce weight loss, they regained all of their lost weight when allowed to eat ad libitum. Gender also plays an important role in weight loss strategies. Females are more sensitive to the anorectic effects of leptin while males are more sensitive to the anorectic effects of centrally administered insulin (Clegg *et al.*, 2003). While exercise can reduce obesity in rodents, this effect is more marked in obese males. Lean animals in general and females in particular rarely lose as much adiposity with exercise as obese males (Mayer *et al.*, 1954; Rolls & Rowe, 1979; Levin & Dunn-Meynell, 2005).

In summary, the seminal studies cited above demonstrate a number of important elements which humans and rodents have in common with regard to regulation of energy homeostasis: (1) weight gain and the development of obesity are dependent upon the interaction of genetic background with a number of environmental factors such as perinatal environment, diet composition and length of exposure; (2) when fed energy-dense diets, there is a great deal of heterogeneity in weight gain patterns among outbred (and even inbred) individuals with common genetic backgrounds suggesting important genetic–environmental interactions; (3) in obesity-prone individuals obesity cannot be reversed simply by lowering the caloric density of the diet or by chronic caloric restriction, i.e. the defended body weight can be moved upwards but rarely downwards in such individuals.

The major exception to this rule occurs when rodents are fed highly palatable (especially liquid) diets which produce profound hyperphagia and obesity even in obesity-resistant individuals (Ramirez, 1987; Levin & Dunn-Meynell, 2002b). Such "non-homeostatic" intake is driven by reward pathways which can easily override metabolic cues involved in homeostatic regulation (Levin & Dunn-Meynell, 2002b). Slower accretion of adiposity on high caloric density diets which produce limited hyperphagia can produce permanent obesity in obesity-prone individuals. On the other hand, obesity which develops on highly palatable liquid diets or with forced overfeeding is not avidly defended and both obesity-prone and -resistant rats voluntarily reduce intake and rapidly lose weight when switched back to a solid diet of low palatability (Sims et al., 1973; Levin & Dunn-Meynell, 2002b). There is also clear evidence that non-homeostatic eating is regulated by different but overlapping sets of neural control mechanisms than those involved in homeostatic controls of energy balance (Will et al., 2003).

2.2   *Factors predisposing to DIO:why some individuals become obese*

Work in various outbred models of DIO has made it clear that there are major pre-existing differences between those who will become obese and those who will resist the development of obesity when the energy and fat density of their diets are increased. There is an extensive list of metabolic, hormonal, neural and physiologic characteristics which obesity-prone individuals possess before they are ever prodded to become obese by increasing the caloric density and fat content of their diets. The list of these characteristics enumerated in Table 6.1 is derived from studies in which obesity-prone and -resistant individuals were identified prior to exposure to a high fat diet or during the first week or so on such diets. Most studies demonstrate a common pattern when the caloric density of the diet is increased, usually by increasing the fat content. Both obesity-prone and -resistant rodents continue to eat the same weight of diet as they did on the lower density diet (Levin et al., 2003a). It appears that they monitor volume rather than calories during this time and the result is that they increase their caloric intake. However, obesity-resistant individuals are able to respond to the increased caloric density of the diet and reduce their caloric intake back to what it was on the lower density diet (Levin et al., 2003b). Even in obesity-resistant individuals, this adjustment often takes 3 days or more to occur. This suggests that it may take that long for them to increase signals such as leptin and insulin to levels which can be detected by their central metabolic sensing neurons. If so, such down-regulation of intake occurs before such increases in adiposity signals are readily detectable by standard assays (Levin et al., 2003c). On the other hand, obesity-prone rodents eat larger meals (Drewnowski et al., 1984) and many have an increased preference for and eat more of diets high in either fat (Smith et al., 1998) or sucrose (Grinker & Block, 1991; but see Levin, 1993). Such animals do not make the expected reduction in their caloric intake for up to 2–4 weeks on such diets despite early increases in inhibitory hormones like leptin and insulin (Chang et al., 1990; Levin & Dunn-Meynell, 2002a; Levin et al., 2003a). This suggests, and we have confirmed, that some obesity-prone rats do have a raised threshold for detecting and responding to these inhibitory signals. Both outbred and selectively bred DIO rats show an

Table 6.1 *Characteristics of DIO rats prior to and during early exposure to a high fat diet.*

	Difference	References
SAS		
NE turnover in pancreas and heart	D	(Levin, 1995; Yoshida *et al.*, 1987)
24h urine NE levels	I	(Levin & Planas, 1993; Levin, 1995; West *et al.*, 1991; Levin & Dunn-Meynell, 1997b)
Epi response to hypoglycemia	D	(Tkacs & Levin, 2004)
Central Monoamines		
NE turnover in ARC/ME	I	(Levin, 1995)
NE turnover VMN, DMN, LH	D	(Levin, 1995)
DA turnover in ARC/ME	D	(Levin & Dunn-Meynell, 1997a; Levin *et al.*, 1986)
Plasma NE and insulin response to PVN NE infusion	D	(Levin, 1996)
Forebrain a_2-adrenoceptor binding		(Levin, 1990b; Levin, 1996)
5HT turnover diurnal rhythms ARC, PVN	D	(Hassanain & Levin, 2002)
Central Neuropeptides		
ARC NPY mRNA in outbred	I	(Levin & Dunn-Meynell, 1997a; Levin, 1999)
ARC NPY mRNA in selectively bred	N	(Ricci & Levin, 2003)
GH release	D	(Lauterio & Perez, 1997)
Glucosensing		
Plasma NE response to i.v. glucose	I	(Levin & Sullivan, 1987)
Plasma NE response to intracarotid glucose	I	(Levin, 1992)
Hypothalamic c-Fos response to intracarotid glucose	D	(Levin *et al.*, 1998)
Epi response to insulin-induced hypoglycemia	D	(Tkacs & Levin, 2004)
Binding to hypothalamic low affinity sulfonylurea receptors	D	(Levin & Dunn-Meynell, 1997a)
VMN K_{ATP} channel sulfonylurea sensitivity	D	(Routh *et al.*, 1998)
VMN K_{ATP} channel ATP sensitivity	D	(Routh *et al.*, 1998)
Glucose regulation of a_2- adrenoceptors	D	(Levin & Planas, 1993)
Number and function of VMN glucosensing neurons	D	(Song *et al.*, 2001)
ARC and PVN GK mRNA expression	I	(Dunn-Meynell *et al.*, 2002)
Leptin signaling		
ARC, VMN, DMN Lepr-b mRNA expression	D	(Levin *et al.*, 2003a)
ARC, VMN, DMN leptin-induced pSTAT3 expression	D	(Levin *et al.*, 2003a)

Table 6.1 (*cont.*)

	Difference	References
Anorectic response to leptin (i.c.v. and i.p.)	D	(Levin & Dunn-Meynell, 2002a; Levin *et al.*, 2003c)
Early increase in plasma leptin levels on high fat diet	I/D	(Levin *et al.*, 2003a; Boozer & Lauterio, 1998; Harrold *et al.*, 2000; Surwit *et al.*, 1997)
Blood–brain barrier leptin transport	N	(Levin *et al.*, 2003a)
Insulin signaling		
Skeletal muscle glucose uptake and disposal	D	(Pagliassotti *et al.*, 1993)
Hepatic glucose production on low fat diet	I	(Pagliassotti *et al.*, 1997; Pagliassotti *et al.*, 1995; Levin *et al.*, 2005)
Generalized insulin sensitivity	D	(Levin *et al.*, 2003b; Levin *et al.*, 2005)
Anorectic response to i.c.v. insulin	D	(Clegg *et al.*, 2005)
Melanocortin signaling		
Central response to agonist	I	(Chandler *et al.*, 2005)
Metabolic		
Muscle UCP3 response to high fat diet	D	(Weigle & Levin, 2000)
Type I muscles (oxidative)	D	(Abou *et al.*,1992; Mrad *et al.*, 1992)
Skeletal muscle LPL activity at 1wk on high fat diet	D	(Pagliassotti *et al.*, 1994)
Adipose LPL at 1wk on high fat diet	I	(Pagliassotti *et al.*, 1994)
Plasma ghrelin levels	D	(Levin *et al.*, 2003)
Resting energy expenditure on low fat diet	N	(Gayles *et al.*, 1997)
Resting energy expenditure 1wk high fat diet	D	(Boozer & Lauterio, 1998)
Early increase in carbohydrate oxidation on high fat diet	I/N	(Chang *et al.*, 1990; Gayles *et al.*, 1997) but Commerford *et al.* (2000)
Early weight gain associated with hyperphagia	I	(Levin *et al.*, 2003; Gayles *et al.*, 1997)
Epi-induced lipolysis *in vitro*		(Landerholm & Stern, 1992)
Serum pyruvate and lactate	I	(Nagase *et al.*, 1996)
Ingestive		
Larger meals (gorgers)	I	(Drewnowski *et al.*, 1984; Farley *et al.*, 2003)
Sucrose preference	I/N	(Grinker & Block, 1991) vs (Levin & Planas, 1993)
High fat preference	I	(Shor-Posner *et al.*, 1991; Smith, *et al.*, 1998)

Table 6.1 (*cont.*)

	Difference	References
Miscellaneous		
Sensitivity and binding to anorectic drugs	I	(Levin *et al.*, 1994; Camacho *et al.*, 1999)
Size of VMN	D	(Levin, 1996; Mohan *et al.*, 1990)
Basal glucose utilization (neuronal activity) in VMN	D	(Levin & Sullivan, 1989b)
Neuronal activation to conditioned reward in NTS, DMNX, ACe	D	(Levin & Sullivan, 1989a)
Exercise-induced loss of body and adipose pad weight	I	(Mayer *et al.*, 1954; Levin & Dunn-Meynell, 2005)
Stress		
Stress-induced weight gain on high fat diet	I	(Michel *et al.*, 2003)
ACe CRH and hippocampal GR mRNA expression	D	(Michel *et al.*, 2004)
Anxiety in an open field	D	(Michel *et al.*, 2003)

Notes: D = decreased; I = increased; N = no difference; SAS, sympathoadrenal; NE, norepinephrine; Epi, epinephrine; ARC, arcuate nucleus; ME, median eminence; LH, lateral hypothalamus; VMN, ventromedial nucleus; DMN, dorsomedial nucleus; DA, dopamine; PVN, paraventricular nucleus; 5HT, serotonin; NPY, neuropeptide Y; GH, growth hormone; Lepr-b, long form of leptin receptor; K_{ATP}, ATP-sensitive K^+ channel; GK, glucokinase; icv, intracerebroventricular; i.p., intraperitoneal; UCP3, uncoupling protein 3; LPL, lipoprotein lipase; NTS, nucleus tractus solitarius; DMNX, dorsal motor nucleus of the vagus; ACe, central nucleus of the amygdala; CRH, corticotrophin-releasing hormone; GR, glucocorticoid receptor.

attenuated anorectic response to leptin before they are ever made obese on high energy diets. Their diminished sensitivity to leptin is not due to reduced transport across the blood–brain barrier but rather to a raised central detection threshold (Levin & Dunn-Meynell, 2002a; Levin *et al.*, 2003a). They have reduced hypothalamic expression of the leptin receptor and leptin-induced phosphorylation of the downstream signaling molecule, STAT3 is greatly attenuated (Levin *et al.*, 2003a). Similarly, DIO rats have a pre-existing reduction in their responsiveness to the anorectic effects of centrally administered insulin (Clegg *et al.*, 2005) and a raised threshold for responding to glucose (Levin & Sullivan, 1989a; Levin, 1992; Levin & Planas, 1993; Levin *et al.*, 1998; Song, *et al.*, 2001; Dunn-Meynell *et al.*, 2002) (Table 6.1).

Depending upon strain and species, there are also a number of other pre-existing characteristics of obesity-prone rodents before they become obese which may predispose them to become obese when fed high fat diets. Some overexpress NPY in ARC neurons (Levin & Dunn-Meynell, 1997b; Levin, 1999), a trait seen in other obese rodents such as the leptin-resistant obese Zucker rats (Kowalski et al., 1998) and db/db mice and the leptin-deficient ob/ob mice (Schwartz et al., 1996). Obesity-prone rodents also have pre-existing disorders of central neurotransmitter regulation such as norepinephrine and serotonin (Levin et al., 1983, 1986; Wilmot et al., 1988; Levin, 1990a, 1995; Hassanain & Levin, 2002).

Other characteristics which may or may not be unrelated to leptin sensitivity include an exaggerated cephalic phase insulin response in anticipation of highly palatable meals (Berthoud, 1985), reduced anxiety in an open field (Michel et al., 2003) and reduced amygdalar corticotrophin-releasing hormone and glucocorticoid receptor expression in their hippocampus (Michel et al., 2004). Some obesity-prone rodents also have a raised threshold for monitoring and responding to raised glucose levels which may predispose them to develop abnormal glucose homeostasis (Levin & Sullivan, 1989; Levin, 1992; Levin & Planas, 1993; Levin & Dunn-Meynell, 1997a; Levin et al., 1998; Song et al., 2001, Dunn-Meynell et al., 2002). In fact, obesity-prone rats have pre-existing hepatic (Pagliassotti et al., 1993; Levin et al., 2005) and total body insulin resistance (Levin et al., 2003b, 2005). Some have reduced pancreatic sympathetic activity (Levin et al., 1983; Levin, 1995) which would reduce their ability to inhibit insulin release (Porte, 1969). This defect is also seen in obese Zucker rats (Levin et al., 1982) and may be partly responsible for their early increase in plasma insulin levels when they are fed high-fat diets. Most obesity-prone rodents have relatively normal resting metabolic rates (Hill et al., 1983; Corbett et al., 1986; Chang et al., 1990) but some do not appear to increase their oxidation of fatty acids appropriately when the fat content of their diet is increased (Chang et al., 1990). This may be due to failure to upregulate muscle UCP-3 on high energy diets (Weigle & Levin, 2000) and to a reduced complement of oxidative muscle fibers (Mrad et al., 1992; Pagliassotti et al., 1993).

Once obesity starts to develop on high-energy diets, a large number of physiologic, metabolic and neural changes and progressive upward re-setting of the defended body weight occur (Levin et al., 1983, 2000; Levin, 1999). Whereas obesity-prone rats differ in many neural and metabolic characteristics from obesity-resistant rats before they become obese (Table 6.1), some of these differences gradually disappear as obesity develops. Hypothalamic norepinephrine (Levin, 1995) and serotonin turnover (Hassanain & Levin, 2002), a_2-adrenoceptor binding (Wilmot et al., 1988; Levin, 1990b; Levin & Hamm, 1994), ARC NPY expression (Levin & Dunn-Meynell, 1997b; Levin, 1999) and some aspects of central glucosensing (Levin et al., 1996) and cardiac and pancreatic sympathetic activity (Levin et al., 1985) all differ between obesity-prone and -resistant rats when both are fed low fat diets but disappear once DIO develops on high energy diets. The long list of pre-existing differences between obesity-prone and -resistant individuals and the "normalization" of some of these as obesity develops on high energy diets suggests that the neural mechanisms regulating energy homeostasis are preset to promote the development of obesity on high energy diets and only function normally (or at least at the same level as obesity-resistant rats) once obesity develops.

There are a number of changes in metabolic, physiologic, hormonal and neural functions which occur in obese individuals regardless of whether they carry the thrifty genotype or phenotype. Like humans (Reaven, 1988; Bjorntorp, 1991), DOI rats exhibit many of the characteristics of what has been called the metabolic syndrome. Aside from hyperinsulinemia and insulin resistance, hyperlipidemia and hypertension (Triscari et al., 1985; Davies et al., 1999; Levin et al., 2003b, 2005), obese rodents also develop hyperleptinemia associated with defects in leptin transport across the blood–brain barrier (Banks et al., 1999; El-Haschimi et al., 2000) and reduced central leptin signaling and responsiveness (Van Heek et al., 1997; El-Haschimi et al., 2000). Some DIO rodents have reduced ARC NPY expression (Levin, 1999) and dopamine metabolism (Levin et al., 1986), decreased growth hormone secretion (Lauterio & Perez, 1997) and altered basal neuronal activity in the amygdala (Levin, 1991b). Depending on diet, strain and genetic predisposition, responsivity of DIO rodents to stress may be either increased (Balkan et al., 1993) or decreased (Levin, 1991a; Levin et al., 2000).

One of the most common problems in the interpretation of functional changes associated with obesity is the ability to separate the effects of obesity per se from those resulting from the diets used to produce obesity. This is particularly true of high fat diets which may have many effects which are independent of the presence of obesity. A number of strategies have been used to separate the effects of these two interrelated variables in the DIO model. One is to control for dietary content by using inbred, selectively bred or outbred strains in which only obesity-prone animals become obese on a common high fat diet. Another is to assess various metabolic and physiologic changes which occur during the first few days after exposure to a high fat diet. Alternatively, all animals can be switched to a common low fat diet after one has developed obesity or intake of high fat diet in obese rodents can be restricted to that of resistant animals long enough to reduce their adiposity to the level of resistant animals. Studies utilizing variations on these strategies have clearly shown that high fat diets have independent effects on systems involved in the regulation of energy homeostasis. These effects are likely due to alterations in the fatty acid composition of cellular membranes where ion channels, receptors and transporters reside. Changes in fatty acids can alter membrane fluidity and thereby the function of these various effectors. Diets high in cholesterol alter the formation of lipid rafts and thereby insulin signaling in peripheral (Bickel, 2002) and central systems (Taghibiglou et al., 2004). Intake of high fat diets can alter the fatty acid composition of axon terminal membranes although this varies as a function of genetic predisposition towards obesity and the specific brain area in which the terminals are located (Levin & Hamm, 1994). Intake of high-fat diets also alters leptin transport across the blood–brain barrier (Banks et al., 1999; Levin et al., 2003a) as well as central insulin (Kaiyala et al., 2000) and melanocortin signaling (Clegg et al., 2005) independently of obesity. There are also independent effects of high-fat diets on hypothalamic norepinephrine and dopamine turnover (Levin et al., 1986), a_2-adrenoceptor (Wilmot et al., 1988) and sulfonylurea binding (Levin et al., 1996).

2.3   Conclusion

Studies of DIO in rodents have shown that obesity-prone individuals have pre-existing characteristics which may predispose them to become obese when the caloric density and/or fat content of their diets are increased. Some of these traits "normalize" upon development of obesity suggesting that the obese state is the desired one for these animals. At least one major predisposing factor in some rodents is a raised threshold for sensing and responding to inhibitory signals from the periphery which tend to limit upward movement of the defended body weight in lean individuals. While DIO in rodents has many of the same adverse metabolic consequences as does obesity in human beings, some of these may be more a consequence of dietary composition than of obesity per se.

3.   Diet-induced obesity in non-rodent species

Studies with non-rodent species attempt to bridge the differences in energy balance characteristics of rodents and humans. Notably, dogs and primates are well studied, have disease sequelae more closely associated with obesity of humans than rodents do and lack a dependence on brown adipose tissue as a component for energy expenditure. Genetic similarity between primates and humans make the primate a particularly attractive model despite the challenges involved in working with these higher order species. Primate species are perhaps the most relevant animal models for the study of human disease although clearly the most difficult to study. Dogs and the two non-human primates for which the greatest amount of work has been done, the rhesus macaque and the baboon, will be discussed below.

3.1   Dogs

Most studies addressing obesity in dog models use either beagles or mongrel dogs. As pets, a great deal is understood regarding the extent of different diet compositions and the onset of obesity as well as the extent to which caloric restriction can decrease body weight (Butterwick & Hawthorne, 1998). Molecular tools are now providing even greater advantages of the dog as a model for obesity since the dog genome has now been sequenced (Lindblad-Toh et al., 2005). More than 60 cardiac genes have been identified which are differentially expressed with DIO, hypertension and time on a high fat diet (Philip-Couderc et al., 2004). Most often in dogs, DIO is generated by the addition of lard or other saturated fats into the diet. As in humans, chronic obesity in dogs is associated with lowered plasma ghrelin and increased leptin levels, both of which are reversed by a maintained weight loss (Jeusette et al., 2005). However, little has been done to systematically study energy expenditure or to look at large enough populations to understand the extent to which genetic influences are a component of obesity in dogs.

Dogs are a particularly fruitful model with which to study the comorbidities associated with obesity which share many of the same characteristics as obese humans (Truett et al., 1998; Kaiyala et al., 1999), including endocrine, autonomic, and renal shifts that lead to insulin resistance, dyslipidemia and hypertension. The extent to which the comorbidities are observed depends on the model, with differences including gender, castration, type and length of time on diet. From a practical perspective, dogs are large enough to provide relatively easy surgical access and blood volume to permit detailed, intricate studies allowing study of indices of insulin sensitivity, hypertension and potential interactions with fatty acids and dyslipidemia.

Diet-induced obesity in the dog results in both increased circulating insulin and insulin resistance peripherally (Kaiyala et al., 1999). The brain depends on insulin as a negative feedback signal for food intake and autonomic signaling. Kaiyala et al. (2000) demonstrated that the extent of obesity produced in the obese dog is correlated with both circulating insulin levels and the extent to which insulin is able to cross into the brain. The dogs gaining the greatest amount of weight had the largest decrease in CNS insulin delivery after 7 weeks of high-fat feeding. Thus the extent of obesity generated appears to depend partly on an individual's ability to maintain insulin sensitivity and insulin transport across the brain.

Again, mirroring the human situation, insulin resistance associated with obesity in dogs correlates best with visceral obesity and link free fatty acid levels to hepatic glucose output. In chow fed dogs, insulin sensitivity inversely correlates with the insulin response to glucose. By contrast, high-fat feeding for 7 weeks in the dog leads to a decrease in insulin sensitivity without a concomitant increase in the insulin response to glucose. This effect correlates best with high-fat feeding and circulating free fatty acids rather than generalized adiposity per se (Kaiyala et al., 1999). In vitro studies show that omental adipocytes are relatively resistant to insulin suppression of lipolysis (Zierath et al., 1998). Euglycemic clamp studies in the obese dog confirm insulin resistance of their omental fat (Mittelman et al., 2002) where increased portal fatty acid flux from omental fat tissue perfusing the liver is associated with increased hepatic glucose output (Bergman & Ader, 2000). Thus, DIO in dogs is associated with a combination of visceral adipose insulin resistance, impaired insulin suppression of hepatic glucose output and a failure of compensatory insulin secretion.

Obesity resulting from a high-fat diet in dogs also leads to altered cardiovascular function. Dogs placed on a saturated high-fat diet for 5 weeks have increased heart rate associated with impairment in tonic and reflex parasympathetic control (Van Vliet et al., 1995). The degree of fatty acid saturation also is an important factor. When dogs were made comparably obese after 6 weeks on saturated vs. unsaturated fat diets, parasympathetic tone was more impaired in the group fed saturated fat and they had higher blood pressures than those on unsaturated fat diets (Truett et al., 1998). Activation of the sympathetic nervous system is a major contributor to hypertension in obese dogs (Hall et al., 2000). Beagles, on a saturated high-fat diet for 21 weeks had increased plasma norepinephrine levels that peaked at week 2 and returned to normal after 4 weeks in one study (Verwaerde et al., 1999) but were elevated for a full 9 weeks of high-fat diet in another (Pelat et al., 2002). The contribution of increased sympathetic activity resulting from high-fat feeding was demonstrated by the finding that combined α- and β adrenergic blockade decreased blood pressure to a greater extent in those fed high rather than normal fat diets (Pelat et al., 2002). Thus, although the mechanism by which the effect occurs is unclear, obesity in dogs is associated with hypertension with underlying impaired parasympathetic and increased sympathetic tone.

3.2   Baboons

Baboons (genus Papio) share a high genetic similarity (96% identity) to humans (VandeBerg & Williams-Blangero, 1997) and obese baboons share many of the same comorbidities of obesity with humans (Comuzzie et al., 2003).

The best-studied group is a pedigreed colony at the Southwest Foundation for Biomedical Research in San Antonio, Texas. Careful longitudinal tracking of multiple measures in hundreds of animals fed a standard chow diet demonstrate a high degree of variation in the colony in terms of body weight and adiposity. The variability in obesity appears to stem simply from individual differences in caloric consumption or metabolic behavior in that all animals are provided identical ad libitum low-fat diet. The tendency to develop obesity is inherited with individual trait heritability ranging from ~20% (plasma leptin) to 60% (total body weight) (Comuzzie et al., 2003). Much like humans, a sexual dimorphism is observed in leptin levels, with a greater correlation between adiposity and leptin in females relative to males (Cole et al., 2003). Also similar to humans (Zamboni et al., 1994), the baboons show a positive correlation between insulin resistance and omental fat depot triglyceride concentrations (Cai et al., 2004). Conversely, baboons and humans both show discordance between obesity and insulin sensitivity in that not all obese baboons become insulin resistant.

The effects of diet and physical activity have been carefully tracked in a population of wild baboons that feed regularly from abundant, easily obtainable, energy-dense foods at a local garbage dump and compared with that of others which gather all of their food in the wild (Altmann et al., 1993; Banks et al., 2003). Females feeding at the dump were particularly prone to develop obesity. Their estimated caloric intake was similar to baboons feeding in the wild but the composition of the food was skewed towards a higher fat intake. In addition, their estimated energy expenditure was also lower. In animals that fed in the wild, leptin levels and BMI were both low and showed little variance. In contrast, half the animals foraging in the garbage dump had leptin and BMI levels similar to those feeding in the wild while the other half had markedly higher levels of both (Banks et al., 2003). These data suggest that these animals, much like the well-studied rodent models, have a split of DIO-resistant versus DIO-prone phenotypes. Interestingly, the high leptin group of baboons had increased insulin and glucose levels, suggesting insulin resistance and some had frank diabetes mellitus. Social ranking and age were eliminated as reasons for this split in the population. As with the well-characterized bimodal predisposition to develop DIO in outbred rodents, it is likely that the bimodal pattern in these outbred baboons also reflects an underlying genetic predisposition. Both groups were derived from a single genetic population and significant male transfer occurred between the garbage-eating and wild groups of females. Thus, like rodents and humans, baboons share the characteristic of having DIO-prone and DIO-resistant phenotypes.

Other long-term studies in baboons of overfeeding in early life and caloric restriction demonstrate important epigenetic influences on the regulation of energy homeostasis similar to those seen in both humans and rodents (Lewis *et al.*, 1991). When overfed during infancy, female baboons in particular developed obesity after puberty but not during adolescence. Effects of over-feeding included increases in insulin, thyroxin and cortisol, suggesting that increased exposure to these early metabolic cues may be possible drivers of the subsequent obesity (Lewis *et al.*, 1992). Interestingly, in a small experiment examining the effects of infant overfeeding on adipocyte cell volume in several baboon families, the resulting variability was accounted for by paternal lineage and the weight of the mothers (Lewis *et al.*, 1991). At the time of weaning, the infants fed a higher caloric load were 14% heavier than their normally fed counterparts but genetic background of the animals also had an important influence on the total adiposity of the offspring (Lewis *et al.*, 1991). Thus, the adult weight of the baboon is driven by both genetic and early environmental influences.

3.3   *Rhesus macaques*

Both in the wild and in captivity, rhesus macaques (*Macaca mulatta*) become spontaneously obese. Obesity in captivity was initially noted in the 1970s (Hamilton *et al.*, 1972) and has been characterized extensively by two groups since then (Kemnitz *et al.*, 1989; Bodkin *et al.*, 1993; Wolden-Hanson *et al.*, 1993). Rhesus monkeys fed a standard rhesus chow diet supplemented by fruit, most often develop obesity at middle age. Broadly, the obesity is gener-ally of abdominal origin. Consequences of the obesity are very similar to those observed in humans and are characterized by hyperinsulinemia leading ultimately to type II diabetes, hyperlipidemia and hypertension. Much like humans, these comorbidities of obesity in the rhesus can be ameliorated by caloric restriction (Hansen *et al.*, 1999; Lane *et al.*, 1999).

Unlike captive animals, free-ranging obese rhesus monkeys do not develop significant diabetes or hyperlipidemia. The rhesus colony in the Cayo Santiago, Puerto Rico, while free-ranging, has free access to commercial primate chow which it supplements by foraging for wild vegetation. In this colony, 7–10% of the adults were obese by measures of weight, BMI, abdominal circumference and fat distribution. However, there were no differences in cholesterol and triglycerides (Schwartz, 1989), fasting glucose, insulin or responses to an intravenous glucose tolerance test (Schwartz *et al.*, 1993). Only the obese males had a trend towards increased insulin secretion. The increased physical activity of free-ranging animals is the most likely explanation for the lack of comor-bidities associated with the obesity in contrast to those seen in the captive populations. Interestingly, the obese animals were found in 5 of 11 matrilines

(Schwartz, 1989; Schwartz et al., 1993). These families had high social ranking within the colony. One explanation for this separation is that the higher ranking animals have preferential access to food and thereby require less physical activity to acquire food. Most likely, genetic factors provide an additional component to account for the differential obesity between families.

The chow provided to both the captive and the free-ranging obese rhesus does not have a particularly high caloric density of fat content (Marriott et al., 1989). However, both populations have the benefit of a caloric supply that does not have a physical cost associated with its acquisition, suggesting that in either case the "spontaneity" of the obesity is not a natural consequence but instead a result of the balance of intake and expenditure being skewed by the changed environment, specifically, the decreased expenditure associated with caging in the captive population and the easy access to food for the wild population of rhesus.

4.   Summary and conclusions

Both animals and humans can develop obesity given the proper confluence of genetic background and environmental inputs. In truly feral animals which have little contact with humans and their detritus, true obesity is a rare occurrence save for hibernators and estivators. In fact, obesity would likely have a negative impact on survival because of an inability to flee predators. In man, obesity was a rare occurrence until the development of agricultural societies which allowed some individuals to obtain food with little expenditure of energy because of their elevated social status. Although the subject remains controversial, the idea that there is a "thrifty genotype" or "thrifty phenotype" which favors survival in times of feast and famine may explain why there are certain individuals in human and non-human populations who will become obese when the energy density and fat content of the diet are increased. It is likely that reduced energy expenditure is a necessary addition to the list of factors which promote obesity in such individuals. Thus, the interaction of genetic predisposition and environmental factors likely underlies much of human obesity. Since most human obesity is polygenic in origin, polygenic animal models serve as important experimental surrogates for discovery of the multitude of factors which contribute to the development of obesity and its comorbidities.

Non-rodent models of obesity such as the dog are often polygenic in nature and allow investigators to carry out somewhat more sophisticated physiological studies than can be accomplished in rodents. But size, expense and ethical considerations prevent more thorough study in free-living animals. Non-human primates, because of their genetic similarity to humans, may provide important insights into the genetic bases for obesity but their size, difficulty of handling and expense make them difficult subjects from which to obtain reliable physiological and neural functional data. This makes rodent models of DIO a reasonable compromise as a surrogate for human obesity. The relative ease with which their genotypes and phenotypes can be determined has provided invaluable information about the identity of peptides, transmitters, hormones, signaling and metabolic pathways involved in the central and peripheral systems responsible for the regulation of energy homeostasis. Such information has been gained because of the ease with which we can assess many behavioral, physiological and metabolic functions in vivo and then obtain access to both peripheral and central nervous system tissues for in vitro studies. There is no question that ability to generate transgenic animals has and will continue to provide important information about various critical pathways involved in the propensity to develop and sustain obesity. However, because most human obesity is polygenic in nature, the various models of DIO in outbred or selectively bred strains of animals may provide an excellent surrogate for the study of human obesity. As shown in Table 6.1, these models share a large number of commonalities with most human obesity and its pathological consequences. Thus, these models provide powerful tools which may eventually allow us to determine the molecular, metabolic and physiological underpinnings of human obesity.

References

Abou, M. J., Yakubu, F., Lin, D., Peters, J. C., Atkinson, J. B. & Hill, J. O. (1992). Skeletal muscle composition in dietary obesity-susceptible and dietary obesity-resistant rats. *Am. J. Physiol.* **262**, 1-8.

Adachi, A., Shimizu, N., Oomura, Y. & Kobashi, M. (1984). Convergence of heptoportal glucose-sensitive afferent signals to glucose-sensitive units within the nucleus of the solitary tract. *Neurosci. Lett.* **46**, 215-18.

Altmann, J., Schoeller, D., Altmann, S. A., Muruthi, P. & Sapolsky, R. M. (1993). Body size and fatness of free-living baboons reflect food availability and activity levels. *Am. J. Primatol.* **30**, 149-61.

Anand, B. K., Chhina, G. S., Sharma, K. N., Dua, S. & Singh, B. (1964). Activity of single neurons in the hypothalamus feeding centers: effect of glucose. *Am. J. Physiol.* **207**, 1146-54.

Archer, Z. A., Rayner, D. V., Rozman, J., Klingenspor, M. & Mercer, J. G. (2003). Normal distribution of body weight gain in male Sprague–Dawley rats fed a high-energy diet. *Obes. Res.* **11**, 1376-83.

Bai, F., Sozen, M. A., Lukiw, W. J. & Argyropoulos, G. (2005). Expression of AgRP, NPY, POMC and CART in human fetal and adult hippocampus. *Neuropeptides* **39**, 439-43.

Balkan, B., Strubbe, J. H., Bruggink, J. E. & Steffens, A. B. (1993). Overfeeding-induced obesity in rats: insulin sensitivity and autonomic regulation of metabolism *Metabolism.* **42**, 1509–18.

Banks, W. A. & Farrell, C. L. (2003). Impaired transport of leptin across the blood-brain barrier in obesity is acquired and reversible. *Am. J. Physiol.* **285**, E10–15.

Banks, W. A., DiPalma, C. R. & Farrell, C. L. (1999). Impaired transport of leptin across the blood-brain barrier in obesity. *Peptides* **20**, 1341–5.

Banks, W. A., Altmann, J., Sapolsky, R. M., Phillips-Conroy, J. E. & Morley, J. E. (2003). Serum leptin levels as a marker for a syndrome X-like condition in wild baboons. *J. Clin. Endocrinol. Metab.* **88**, 1234–40.

Bellinger, L. L. & Bernardis, L. L. (2002). The dorsomedial hypothalamic nucleus and its role in ingestive behavior and body weight regulation: lessons learned from lesioning studies. *Physiol Behav.* **76**, 431–42.

Bergman, R. N. & Ader, M. (2000). Free fatty acids and pathogenesis of type 2 diabetes mellitus. *TEM* **11**, 351–6.

Berthoud, H.-R. (1985). Cephalic phase insulin response as a predictor of body weight gain and obesity induced by a palatable cafeteria diet. *J. Obes. Weight Reg.* **4**, 120–8.

Bickel, P. E. (2002). Lipid rafts and insulin signaling. *Am. J. Physiol. Endocrinol. Metab.* **282**, E1–10.

Bjorntorp, P. (1991). Metabolic implications of body fat distribution. *Diabetes Care* **14**, 1132–43.

Bodkin, N. L. Hannah, J. S., Ortmeyer, H. K. & Hansen, B. C. (1993). Central obesity in rhesus monkeys: association with hyperinsulinemia, insulin resistance and hypertriglyceridemia? *Int. J. Obes. Relat. Metab. Disord.* **17**, 53–61.

Boozer, C. N. & Lauterio, T. J. (1998). High initial levels of plasma leptin predict diet-induced obesity in rats. *Int. J. Ob.* **22**, S166.

Bouchard, C. & Perusse, L. (1993). Genetics of obesity. *Ann. Rev. Nutr.* **13**, 337–54.

Burcelin, R., Crivelli, V., Dacosta, A., Roy-Tirelli, A. & Thorens, B. (2002). Heterogeneous metabolic adaptation of C57BL/6J mice to high-fat diet. *Am. J. Physiol.* **282**, E834–42.

Butterwick, R. F. & Hawthorne, A. J. (1998). Advances in dietary management of obesity in dogs and cats. *J. Nutr.* **128**, 2771s–5s.

Cai, G., Cole, S. A., Tejero, M. E. *et al.* (2004). Pleiotropic effects of genes for insulin resistance on adiposity in baboons. *Obes. Res.* **12**, 1766–72.

Camacho, R. E., Forrest, M. J., MacIntyre, D. E. & Strack, A. M. (1999). Increased sensitivity to dexfenfluramine in rats on high fat diet. *FASEB J.* **13**, A751.

Caro, J. F., Kolaczynski, J. W., Nyce, M. R. *et al.* (1996). Decreased cerebrospinal-fluid/serum leptin ratio in obesity: a possible mechanism for leptin resistance. *Lancet* **348**, 159–61.

Chandler, P., Viana, J., Oswald, K., Wauford, P. & Boggiano, M. (2005). Feeding response to melanocortin agonist predicts preference for and obesity from a high-fat diet. *Physiol. Behav.* **85**, 221–30.

Chang, S., Graham, B., Yakubu, F., Lin, D., Peters, J. C. & Hill, J. O. (1990). Metabolic differences between obesity-prone and obesity-resistant rats. *Am. J. Physiol. Regul. Integr. Comp. Physiol.* **259**, R1103–10.

Clark, F. M., Yeomans, D. C. & Proudfit, H. K. (1991). The noradrenergic innervation of the spinal cord: differences between two substrains of Sprague-Dawley rats determined using retrograde tracers combined with immunocytochemistry. *Neurosci. Lett.* **125**, 155–8.

Clegg, D. J., Riedy, C. A., Smith, K. A., Benoit, S. C. & Woods, S. C. (2003). Differential sensitivity to central leptin and insulin in male and female rats. *Diabetes* **52**, 682–7.

Clegg, D. J., Benoit, S. C., Reed, J. A., Woods, S. C. & Levin, B. E. (2005). Reduced anorexic effects of insulin in obesity-prone rats and rats fed a moderate fat diet. *Am. J. Physiol.* **288**, R981–6.

Cohn, C., Joseph, D. & Shrago, E. (1957). Effect of diet on body composition. I. The production of increased body fat without overweight (nonobese obesity) by force feeding the normal rat. *Metabolism* **6**, 381–7.

Cole, S. A., Martin, L. J., Peebles, K. W. *et al.* (2003). Genetics of leptin expression in baboons. *Int. J. Obes.* **27**, 778–83.

Commerford, S. R., Pagliassotti, M. J., Melby, C. L., Wei, Y., Gayles, E. C. & Hill, J. O. (2000). Fat oxidation, lipolysis, and free fatty acid cycling in obesity-prone and obesity-resistant rats. *Am. J. Physiol.* **279**, E875–85.

Comuzzie, A. G., Cole, S. A., Martin, L. *et al.* (2003). The baboon as a nonhuman primate model for the study of the genetics of obesity. *Obes. Res.* **11**, 75–80.

Corbett, S. W., Stern, J. S. & Keesey, R. E. (1986). Energy expenditure in rats with diet-induced obesity. *Am. J. Clin. Nutr.* **44**, 173–80.

Dallaporta, M., Himmi, T., Perrin, J. & Orsini, J. C. (1999). Solitary tract nucleus sensitivity to moderate changes in glucose level. *NeuroReport* **10**, 2657–60.

Davies, A. D., Dobrian, R. L., Prewitt, R. L. & Lauterio, J. L. (1999). Metabolic syndrome in a diet-induced obesity model. *Obes. Res.* **7**, 127S.

Davis, J. D. & Wirtshafter, D. (1978). Set points or settling points for body weight?: A reply to Mrosovsky and Powley. *Behav. Biol.* **24**, 405–11.

Drewnowski, A., Cohen, A. E., Faust, I. M. & Grinker, J. A. (1984). Meal-taking behavior is related to predisposition to dietary obesity in the rat. *Physiol. Behav.* **32**, 61–7.

Dunn-Meynell, A. A., Routh, V. H., Kang, L., Gaspers, L. & Levin, B. E. (2002). Glucokinase is the likely mediator of glucosensing in both glucose excited and glucose inhibited central neurons. *Diabetes* **51**, 2056–65.

El-Haschimi, K., Pierroz, D. D., Hileman, S. M., Bjorbaek, C. & Flier, J. S. (2000). Two defects contribute to hypothalamic leptin resistance in mice with diet-induced obesity. *J. Clin. Invest.* **105**, 1827–32.

Farley, C., Cook, J. A., Spar, B. D., Austin, T. M. & Kowalski, T. J. (2003). Meal pattern analysis of diet-induced obesity in susceptible and resistant rats. *Obes. Res.* **11**, 845–51.

Foster, D. O. & Frydman, M. L. (1978). Nonshivering thermogenesis in the rat. II. Measurement of blood flow with microspheres points to brown adipose tissue as the dominant site of calorigenesis induced by noradrenaline. *Can. J. Physiol. Pharmacol.* **56**, 110–22.

Gayles, E. C., Pagliassotti, M. J., Prach, P. A., Koppenhafer, T. A. & Hill, J. O. (1997). Contribution of energy intake and tissue enzymatic profile to body weight in high-fat-fed rats. *Am. J. Physiol.* **272**, R188–94.

Grill, H. J., Schwartz, M. W., Kaplan, J. M., Foxhall, J. S., Breininger, J. & Baskin, D. G. (2002). Evidence that the caudal brainstem is a target for the inhibitory effect of leptin on food intake. *Endocrinology* **143**, 239–46.

Grinker, J. A. & Block, W. D. (1991). Sensory responses, dietary-induced obesity and biochemical values in Sprague–Dawley rats. *Brain Res. Bull.* **27**, 535–40.

Guo, F. & Jen, K.-L. (1995). High-fat feeding during pregnancy and lactation affects offspring metabolism in rats. *Physiol. Behav.* **57**, 681–6.

Hales, C. N. & Barker, D. J. (1992). Type 2 (non-insulin-dependent) diabetes mellitus: the thrifty phenotype hypothesis. *Diabetologia* **35**, 595–601.

Hall, J. E., Brands, M. W., Hildebrandt, D. A., Kuo, J. & Fitzgerald, S. (2000). Role of sympathetic nervous system and neuropeptides in obesity hypertension. *Braz. J. Med. Biol. Res.* **33**, 605–18.

Hamilton, C. L., Kuo, P. T. & Fenge, L. Y. (1972). Experimental production of syndrome of obesity, hyperinsulinemia and hyperlipidemia in monkeys. *Proc. Soc. Exp. Biol. Med.* **140**, 1005–8.

Hansen, B. C., Bodkin, N. L. & Ortmeyer, H. K. (1999). Calorie restriction in nonhuman primates: mechanisms of reduced morbidity and mortality. *Toxicol. Sci.* **52**, 56–60.

Harrold, J. A., Williams, G. & Widdowson, P. S. (2000). Early leptin response to a palatable diet predicts dietary obesity in rats: key role of melanocortin-4 receptors in the ventromedial hypothalamic nucleus. *J. Neurochem.* **74**, 1224–8.

Hassanain, M. & Levin, B. E. (2002). Dysregulation of hypothalamic serotonin turnover in diet-induced obese rats. *Brain Res.* **929**, 175–80.

Helies, J. M., Diane, A., Langlois, A. *et al.* (2005). Comparison of fat storage between Fischer 344 and obesity-resistant Lou/C rats fed different diets. *Obes. Res.* **13**, 3–10.

Hill, J. O., Fried, S. K. & Digirolamo, M. (1983). Effects of a high-fat diet on energy intake and expenditure in rats. *Life Sci.* **33**, 141–9.

Hill, J. O., Dorton, J., Sykes, M. N. & Digirolamo, M. (1989). Reversal of dietary obesity is influenced by its duration and severity. *Int. J. Obes.* **13**, 711–22.

Hollifield, G. & Parson, W. (1962). Metabolic adaptations to a "stuff and starve" feeding program. II. Obesity and the persistence of adaptive changes in adipose tissue and liver occurring in rats limited to a short daily feeding period. *J. Clin. Invest.* **41**, 250–3.

Ingle, D. J. (1949). A simple means of producing obesity in the rat. *Proc. Soc. Exp. Biol. Med.* **72**, 604.

Jeusette, I. C., Detilleux, J., Shibata, H. et al. (2005). Effects of chronic obesity and weight loss on plasma ghrelin and leptin concentrations in dogs. Res. Vet. Sci. **79**, 169–75.

Jones, A. P., Simson, E. L. & Friedman, M. I. (1984). Gestational undernutrition and the development of obesity in rats. J. Nutr. **114**, 1484–92.

Kaiyala, K. J., Prigeon, R. L., Kahn, S. E., Woods, S. C., Porte, D. & Schwartz, M. W. (1999). Reduced β-cell function contributes to impaired glucose tolerance in dogs made obese by high-fat feeding. Am. J. Physiol. **277**, E659–67.

Kaiyala, K. J., Prigeon, R. L., Kahn, S. E., Woods, S. C. & Schwartz, M. W. (2000). Obesity induced by a high-fat diet is associated with reduced brain insulin transport in dogs. Diabetes **49**, 1525–33.

Kang, L., Routh, V. H., Kuzhikandathil, E. V., Gaspers, L. & Levin, B. E. (2004). Physiological and molecular characteristics of rat hypothalamic ventromedial nucleus glucosensing neurons. Diabetes **53**, 549–59.

Keesey, R. E., Mitchel, J. S. & Kemnitz, J. W. (1979). Body weight and body composition of male rats following hypothalamic lesions. Am. J. Physiol. **237**, R68–73.

Kemnitz, J. W., Goy, R. W., Flitsch, T. J., Lohmiller, J. J. & Robinson, J. A. (1989). Obesity in male and female rhesus monkeys: fat distribution, glucoregulation, and serum androgen levels. J. Clin. Endocrinol. Metab. **69**, 287–93.

Kennedy, G. C. (1953). The role of depot fat in the hypothalamic control of food intake in the rat. Proc. R. Soc. Lond. B. Biol. Sci. **611**, 221–35.

Kennedy, G. C. (1957). The development with age of hypothalamic restraint upon the appetite of the rat. J. Endocrinol. **16**, 9–17.

King, B. M. Kass, J. M., Neville, K. L., Sam, H., Tatford, A. C. I. & Zansler, A. C. (1993). Abnormal weight gain in rats with amygdaloid lesions. Physiol. Behav. **54**, 467–70.

Kowalski, T. J., Houpt, T. A., Jahng, J., Okada, N., Chua Jr., S. C. & Smith, G. P. (1998). Ontogeny of neuropeptide Y expression in response to deprivation in lean Zucker rat pups. Am. J. Physiol. **275**, R466–70.

Kramer, F. M., Jeffery, R. W., Forster, J. L. & Snell, M. K. (1989). Long-term follow-up of behavioral treatment for obesity: patterns of weight regain among men and women. Int. J. Obes. **13**, 123–36.

Landerholm, T. E. & Stern, J. S. (1992). Adipose tissue lipolysis in vitro: a predictor of diet-induced obesity in female rats. Am. J. Physiol. Regul. Integr. Comp. Physiol. **263**, R1248–53.

Lane, M. A., Ingram, D. K. & Roth, G. S. (1999). Calorie restriction in nonhuman primates: effects on diabetes and cardiovascular disease risk. Toxicol. Sci. **52**, 41–8.

Lauterio, T. J. & Perez, F. M. (1997). Growth hormone secretion and synthesis are depressed in obesity-susceptible compared with obesity-resistant rats. Metabolism **46**, 210–16.

Leibel, R. L. & Hirsch, J. (1984). Diminished energy requirements in reduced-obese patients. Metabolism **33**, 164–70.

Levin, B. E. (1990a). Obesity-prone and -resistant rats differ in their brain ^{3}H paraminoclonidine binding. *Brain Res.* **512**, 54–9.

Levin, B. E. (1990b). Increased brain ^{3}H paraminoclonidine (a_2-adrenoceptor) binding associated with perpetuation of diet-induced obesity in rats. *Int. J. Obes.* **14**, 689–700.

Levin, B. E. (1991a). Defective cerebral glucose utilization in diet-induced obese rats. *Am. J. Physiol.* **261**, R787–92.

Levin, B. E. (1991b). Spontaneous motor activity during the development and maintenance of diet-induced obesity in the rat. *Physiol. Behav.* **50**, 573–81.

Levin, B. E. (1992). Intracarotid glucose-induced norepinephrine response and the development of diet-induced obesity. *Int. J. Obesity.* **16**, 451–7.

Levin, B. E. (1994). Diet cycling and age alter weight gain and insulin levels in rats. *Am. J. Physiol.* **267**, R527–35.

Levin, B. E. (1995). Reduced norepinephrine turnover in organs and brains of obesity-prone rats. *Am. J. Physiol.* **268**, R389–94.

Levin, B. E. (1996). Reduced paraventricular nucleus norepinephrine responsiveness in obesity-prone rats. *Am. J. Physiol.* **270**, R456–61.

Levin, B. E. (1999). Arcuate NPY neurons and energy homeostasis in diet-induced obese and resistant rats. *Am. J. Physiol.* **276**, R382–7.

Levin, B. E. (2000). Metabolic imprinting on genetically predisposed neural circuits perpetuates obesity. *Nutrition.***16**, 909–15.

Levin, B. E. (2001). Glucosensing neurons do more than just sense glucose. *Int. J. Obes. Relat. Metab. Disord.* **25**, S68–72.

Levin, B. E. (2002a). Glucosensing neurons: the metabolic sensors of the brain? *Diab. Nutr. Metab.* **15**, 274–80.

Levin, B. E. (2002b). Metabolic sensors: viewing glucosensing neurons from a broader perspective. *Physiol. Behav.* **76**, 397–401.

Levin, B. E. (2004). The drive to regain is mainly in the brain. *Am. J. Physiol.* **287**, R1297–300.

Levin, B. E. & Dunn-Meynell, A. A. (1997a). In vivo and in vitro regulation of [^{3}H]glyburide binding to brain sulfonylurea receptors in obesity-prone and resistant rats by glucose. *Brain Res.* **776**, 146–53.

Levin, B. E. & Dunn-Meynell, A. A. (1997b). Dysregulation of arcuate nucleus preproneuropeptide Y mRNA in diet-induced obese rats. *Am. J. Physiol.* **272**, R1365–70.

Levin, B. E. & Dunn-Meynell, A. A. (2000). Defense of body weight against chronic caloric restriction in obesity-prone and -resistant rats. *Am. J. Physiol.* **278**, R231–7.

Levin, B. E. & Dunn-Meynell, A. A. (2002a). Reduced central leptin sensitivity in rats with diet-induced obesity. *Am. J. Physiol.* **283**, R941–8.

Levin, B. E. & Dunn-Meynell, A. A. (2002b). Defense of body weight depends on dietary composition and palatability in rats with diet-induced obesity. *Am. J. Physiol.* **282**, R46–54.

Levin, B. E. & Dunn-Meynell, A. A. (2002c) Maternal obesity alters adiposity and monoamine function in genetically predisposed offspring. *Am. J. Physiol.* **283**, R1087–93.

Levin, B. E. & Dunn-Meynell, A. A. (2005). Differential effects of exercise on body weight gain in obesity-prone and -resistant rats. *Int. J. Obes.* **30**, 722–7.

Levin, B. E. & Govek, E. (1998). Gestational obesity accentuates obesity in obesity-prone progeny. *Am. J. Physiol.* **275**, R1374–9.

Levin, B. E. & Hamm, M. W. (1994). Plasticity of brain a-adrenoceptors during the development of diet-induced obesity in the rat. *Obes Res.* **2**, 230–8.

Levin, B. E. & Keesey, R. E. (1998). Defense of differing body weight set-points in diet-induced obese and resistant rats. *Am. J. Physiol.* **274**, R412–19.

Levin, B. E. & Planas, B. (1993). Defective glucoregulation of brain a_2-adrenoceptors in obesity-prone rats. *Am. J. Physiol.* **264**, R305–11.

Levin, B. E. & Sullivan, A. C. (1987). Glucose-induced norepinephrine levels and obesity resistance. *Am. J. Physiol.* **253**, R475–81.

Levin, B. E. & Sullivan, A. C. (1989a). Glucose-induced sympathetic activation in obesity-prone and resistant rats. *Int. J. Obesity.* **13**, 235–46.

Levin, B. E. & Sullivan, A. C. (1989b). Differences in saccharin-induced cerebral glucose utilization between obesity-prone and resistant rats. *Brain Res.* **488**, 221–32.

Levin, B. E., Triscari, J. & Sullivan, A. C. (1982). Sympathetic activity in thyroid-treated Zucker rats. *Am. J. Physiol.* **243**, R170–8.

Levin, B. E., Triscari, J. & Sullivan, A. C. (1983). Relationship between sympathetic activity and diet-induced obesity in two rat strains. *Am. J. Physiol.* **245**, R367–71.

Levin, B. E., Finnegan, M., Triscari, J. & Sullivan, A. C. (1985). Brown adipose and metabolic features of chronic diet-induced obesity. *Am. J. Physiol.* **248**, R717–23.

Levin, B. E., Triscari, J. & Sullivan, A. C. (1986). The effect of diet and chronic obesity on brain catecholamine turnover in the rat. *Pharmacol. Biochem. Behav.* **24**, 299–304.

Levin, B. E., Brown, K. L. & Vincent, D. G. (1994). Increased potency and binding of mazindol to putative brain anorectic receptors in obesity-prone rats. *Brain Res.* **668**, 171–9.

Levin, B. E., Brown, K. L. & Dunn-Meynell, A. A. (1996). Differential effects of diet and obesity on high and low affinity sulfonylurea binding sites in the rat brain. *Brain Res.* **739**, 293–300.

Levin, B. E., Dunn-Meynell, A. A., Balkan, B. & Keesey, R. E. (1997). Selective breeding for diet-induced obesity and resistance in Sprague–Dawley rats. *Am. J. Physiol.* **273**, R725–30.

Levin, B. E., Govek, E. K. & Dunn-Meynell, A. A. (1998). Reduced glucose-induced neuronal activation in the hypothalamus of diet-induced obese rats. *Brain Res.* **808**, 317–19.

Levin, B. E., Richard, D., Michel, C. & Servatius, R. (2000). Differential stress responsivity in diet-induced obese and resistant rats. *Am. J. Physiol.* **279**, R1357–64.

Levin, B. E., Dunn-Meynell, A. A. & Banks, W. A. (2003a). Obesity-prone rats have normal blood-brain barrier transport but defective central leptin signaling prior to obesity onset. *Am. J. Physiol.* **286**, R143–50.

Levin, B. E., Dunn-Meynell, A. A., McMinn, J. E., Cunningham-Bussel, A. & Chua, S. C. Jr. (2003b). A new obesity-prone, glucose intolerant rat strain (F.DIO). *Am. J. Physiol.* **285**, R1184–91.

Levin, B. E., Dunn-Meynell, A. A., Ricci, M. R. & Cummings, D. E. (2003c). Abnormalities of leptin and ghrelin regulation in obesity-prone juvenile rats. *Am. J. Physiol.* **285**, E949–57.

Levin, B. E., Routh, V. H., Kang, L., Sanders, K. L. & Dunn-Meynell, A. A. (2004). Neuronal glucosensing: what do we know after 50 years? *Diabetes* **53**, 2521–8.

Levin, B. E., Magnan, C., Migrenne, S., Chua, S. C. Jr. & Dunn-Meynell, A. A. (2005). The F-DIO obesity-prone rat is insulin resistant prior to obesity onset. *Am. J. Physiol.* **289**, R704–11.

Lewis, D. S., Coelho, A. M. J. & Jackson, E. M. (1991). Maternal weight and sire group, not caloric intake, influence adipocyte volume in infant female baboons. *Pediatr. Res.* **30**, 534–40.

Lewis, D. S., Jackson, E. M. & Mott, G. E. (1992). Effect of energy intake on postprandial plasma hormones and triglyceride concentrations in infant female baboons (Papio species). *J. Clin. Endocrinol. Metab.* **74**, 920–6.

Li, A. J. & Ritter, S. (2004). Glucoprivation increases expression of neuropeptide Y mRNA in hindbrain neurons that innervate the hypothalamus. *Eur. J. Neurosci.* **19**, 2147–54.

Lin, X., Chavez, M. R., Bruch, R. C. et al. (1998). The effects of a high fat diet on leptin mRNA, serum leptin and the response to leptin are not altered in a rat strain susceptible to high fat diet–induced obesity. *J. Nutr.* **128**, 1606–13.

Lindblad-Toh, T. K., Wade, C. M., Mikkelsen, T. S. et al. (2005). Genome sequence, comparative analysis and haplotype structure of the domestic dog. *Nature* **438**, 803–19.

MacLean, P. S., Higgins, J. A., Johnson, G. C. et al. (2004). Enhanced metabolic efficiency contributes to weight regain after weight loss in obesity-prone rats. *Am. J. Physiol.* **287**, R1306–15.

Mahankali, S., Liu, Y., Pu, Y. et al. (2000). In vivo fMRI demonstration of hypothalamic function following intraperitoneal glucose administration in a rat model. *Magn. Reson. Med.* **43**, 155–9.

Marriott, B. M., Roemer, J. & Sultana, C. (1989). An overview of the food intake patterns of the Cayo Santiago rhesus monkeys (*Macaca mulatta*): report of a pilot study. *P R Health Sci. J.* **8**, 87–94.

Matsuda, M., Liu, Y., Mahankali, S. et al. (1999). Altered hypothalamic function in response to glucose ingestion in obese humans. *Diabetes* **48**, 1801–6.

Mayer, J., Marshall, N. B., Vitale, J. J., Christensen, J. H., Mashayekhi, M. B. & Stare, F. J. (1954). Exercise, food intake and body weight in normal rats and genetically obese adult mice. *Am. J. Physiol.* **177**, 544–8.

Michel, C., Levin, B. E. & Dunn-Meynell, A. A. (2003). Stress facilitates body weight gain in genetically predisposed rats on medium fat diet. *Am. J. Physiol.* **285**, R791-9.

Michel, C., Dunn-Meynell, A. A. & Levin, B. E. (2004). Reduced brain CRH and GR mRNA expression precedes obesity in juvenile rats bred for diet-induced obesity. *Behav. Brain Res.* **154**, 511-17.

Minami, T., Shimizu, N., Duan, S. & Oomura, Y. (1990). Hypothalamic neuronal activity responses to 3-hydroxybutyric acid, an endogenous organic acid. *Brain Res.* **509**, 351-4.

Mittelman, S. D., Van Citters, V. W., Kirkman, E. L. & Bergman, R. N. (2002). Extreme insulin resistance of the central adipose depot *in vivo. Diabetes* **51**, 755-61.

Mohan, P. F., Ihnen, J. S., Levin, B. E. & Cleary, M. P. (1990). Effects of dehydroepiandrosterone treatment in rats with diet-induced obesity. *J. Nutr.* **120**, 1103-14.

Mrad, J. A., Yakubu, F., Lin, D., Peters, J. C., Atkinson, J. B. & Hill, J. O. (1992). Skeletal muscle composition in dietary obesity-susceptible and dietary obesity-resistant rats. *Am. J. Physiol.* **262**, R684-8.

Nagase, H., Bray, G. A. & York, D. A. (1996). Pyruvate and hepatic pyruvate dehydrogenase levels in rat strains sensitive and resistant to dietary obesity. *Am. J. Physiol.* **270**, R485-95.

Neel, V. (1962). In diabetes mellitus: a "thrifty" genotype rendered detrimental by progress. *Am. J. Hum. Genet.* **14**, 353-62.

Niijima, A. (1969). Afferent impulse discharges from glucoreceptors in the liver of the guinea pig. *Ann. N.Y. Acad. Sci.* **157**, 690-700.

Oomura, Y., Kimura, K., Ooyama, H., Maeo, T., Iki, M. & Kuniyoshi, N. (1964). Reciprocal activities of the ventromedial and lateral hypothalamic area of cats. *Science* **143**, 484-5.

Oomura, Y., Nakamura, T., Sugimori, M. & Yamada, Y. (1975). Effect of free fatty acid on the rat lateral hypothalamic neurons. *Physiol. Behav.* **14**, 483-6.

Pagliassotti, M. J., Shahrokhi, K. A. & Hill, J. O. (1993). Skeletal muscle glucose metabolism in obesity-prone and obesity-resistant rats. *Am. J. Physiol.* **264**, R1224-8.

Pagliassotti, M. J., Knobel, S. M., Shahrokhi, K. A., Manzo, A. M. & Hill, J. O. (1994). Time course adaptation to a high-fat diet in obesity-resistant and obesity-prone rats. *Am. J. Physiol.* **267**, R659-64.

Pagliassotti, M. J., Pan, D. A., Prach, P. A., Koppenhafer, T. A., Storlien, L. H. & Hill, J. O. (1995). Tissue oxidative capacity, fuel stores and skeletal muscle fatty acid composition in obesity-prone and obesity-resistant rats. *Obes. Res.* **3**, 459-64.

Pagliassotti, M. J., Horton, T. J., Gayles, E. C., Koppenhafer, T. A., Rosenzweig, T. D. & Hill, J. O. (1997). Reduced insulin suppression of glucose appearance is related to susceptibility to dietary obesity in rats. *Am. J. Physiol.* **272**, R1264-70.

Pelat, M., Verwaerde, P., Tran, M.-A., Montastruc, J.-L. & Senard, J. M. (2002). Alpha$_2$-adrenoceptor function in arterial hypertension associated with obesity in dogs fed a high-fat diet. *J Hypertens.* **20**, 957-64.

Philip-Couderc, P., Smih, F., Hall, J. E. *et al.* (2004). Kinetic analysis of cardiac transcriptome regulation during chronic high-fat diet in dogs. *Physiol. Genomics.* **19**, 32-40.

Plagemann, A., Heidrich, I., Gotz, F., Rohde, W. & Dorner, G. (1992). Lifelong enhanced diabetes susceptibility and obesity after temporary intrahypothalamic hyperinsulinism during brain organization. *Exp. Clin. Endocrinol.* **99**, 91-5.

Popkin, B. M. & Doak, C. M. (1999). The obesity epidemic is a worldwide phenomenon. *Nutr. Rev.* **56**, 106-14.

Porte, D. Jr. (1969). Sympathetic regulation of insulin secretion. Its relation to diabetes mellitus. *Arch. Intern. Med.* **123**, 252-60.

Ramirez, I. (1987). Feeding a liquid diet increases energy intake, weight gain and body fat in rats. *J. Nutr.* **117**, 2127-34.

Reaven, G. M. (1988). Banting Lecture 1988: role of insulin resistance in human disease. *Diabetes* **37**, 1595-607.

Reifsnyder, P. C., Churchill, G. & Leiter, E. H. (2000). Maternal environment and genotype interact to establish diabesity in mice. *Genome Res.* **10**, 1568-78.

Ricardo, J. A. & Koh, E. T. (1978). Anatomical evidence of direct projections from the nucleus of the solitary tract to the hypothalamus, amygdala, and other forebrain structures in the rat. *Brain Res.* **153**, 1-26.

Ricci, M. M. & Levin, B. E. (2003). Ontogeny of diet-induced obesity in selectively-bred Sprague-Dawley rats. *Am. J. Physiol.* **285**, R610-18.

Ritter, S., Dinh, T. T. & Zhang, Y. (2000). Localization of hindbrain glucoreceptive sites controlling food intake and blood glucose. *Brain Res.* **856**, 37-47.

Ritter, S., Bugarith, K. & Dinh, T. T. (2001). Immunotoxic destruction of distinct catecholamine subgroups produces selective impairment of glucoregulatory responses and neuronal activation. *J. Comp. Neurol.* **432**, 197-216.

Rolls, B. A. & Rowe, E. A. (1979). Exercise and the development and persistence of dietary obesity in male and female rats. *Physiol. Behav.* **23**, 241-7.

Rolls, B. A., Rowe, E. A. & Turner, R. C. (1980). Persistent obesity in rats following a period of consumption of a mixed, high energy diet. *J. Physiol.* **298**, 415-27.

Routh, V. H., Levin, B. E. & McArdle, J. J. (1998). Defective ATP-sensitive K$^+$ (K$_{ATP}$) channel in ventromedial hypothalamic nucleus (VMN) of obesity-prone (DIO) rats. *FASEB J.* **12**, A864.

Rowland, N. E. & Carlton, J. (1986). Tolerance to fenfluramine anorexia: fact or fiction?. *Appetite.* **7**, Suppl. 71-83.

Sanders, N. M., Dunn-Meynell, A. A. & Levin, B. E. (2004). Third ventricular alloxan reversibly impairs glucose counterregulatory responses. *Diabetes* **53**, 1230-6.

Schemmel, R., Mickelsen, O. & Tolgay, Z. (1969). Dietary obesity in rats: influence of diet, weight, age, and sex on body composition. *Am. J. Physiol.* **216**, 373-9.

Schemmel, R., Mickelsen, O. & Gill, J. L. (1970). Dietary obesity in rats: body weight and body fat accretion in seven strains of rats. *J. Nutr.* **100**, 1041–8.

Schwartz, M. W., Baskin, D. G., Bukowski, T. R. *et al.* (1996). Specificity of leptin action on elevated blood glucose levels and hypothalamic neuropeptide Y gene expression in ob/ob mice. *Diabetes* **45**, 531–5.

Schwartz, S. M. (1989). Characteristics of spontaneous obesity in the Cayo Santiago rhesus macaque: preliminary report. *P. R. Health Sci. J.* **8**, 103–6.

Schwartz, S. M., Kemnitz, J. W. & Howard, C. F. J. (1993). Obesity in free-ranging rhesus macaques. *Int. J. Obes.* **17**, 1–9.

Sclafani, A. & Springer, D. (1976). Dietary obesity in adult rats: similarities to hypothalamic and human obesity syndromes. *Physiol. Behav.* **17**, 461–71.

Shor-Posner, G., Ian, C., Brennan, G. *et al.* (1991). Self-selecting albino rats exhibit differential preferences for pure macronutrient diets: characterization of three subpopulations. *Physiol. Behav.* **50**, 1187–95.

Sims, E. A. H., Danforth, E., Jr., Bray, G. A., Glennon, J. A. & Salans, L. B. (1973). Endocrine and metabolic effects of experimental obesity in man. *Recent Progr. Horm. Res.* **29**, 457–87.

Smith, B. K., Kelly, L. A., Pina, R., York, D. A. & Bray, G. A. (1998). Preferential fat intake increases adiposity but not body weight in Sprague-Dawley rats. *Appetite* **31**, 127–39.

Song, Z. & Routh, V. H. (2005). Differential effects of glucose and lactate on glucosensing neurons in the ventromedial hypothalamic nucleus. *Diabetes* **54**, 15–22.

Song, Z., Levin, B. E., McArdle, J. J., Bakhos, N. & Routh, V. H. (2001). Convergence of pre- and postsynaptic influences on glucosensing neurons in the ventromedial hypothalamic nucleus (VMN). *Diabetes* **50**, 2673–81.

Spanswick, D., Smith, M. A., Groppi, V. E., Logan, S. D. & Ashford, M. L. (1997). Leptin inhibits hypothalamic neurons by activation of ATP- sensitive potassium channels. *Nature* **390**, 521–5.

Stunkard, A. J. (1982). Anorectic agents lower a body weight set point. *Life Sci.* **30**, 2043–55.

Stunkard, A. J., Harris, J. R., Pedersen, N. L. & McClearn, G. E. (1990). The body-mass index of twins who have been reared apart. *N. Engl. J. Med.* **322**, 1483–7.

Surwit, R. S., Petro, A. E., Parekh, P. & Collins, S. (1997). Low plasma leptin in response to dietary fat in diabetes- and obesity-prone mice. *Diabetes* **46**, 1516–20.

Taghibiglou, C., Bradley, C. A., Wang, Y. & Wang, Y. (2004). High cholesterol levels in neuronal cells impair the insulin signaling pathway and interfere with insulin's neuromodulatory action. *Soc. Neurosci. Abst.* **24**, 633.13.

Tang-Christensen, M., Larsen, P. J., Thulesen, J., Romer, J. & Vrang, N. (2000). The proglucagon-derived peptide, glucagon-like peptide-2, is a neurotransmitter involved in the regulation of food intake. *Nat. Med.* **6**, 802–7.

Tkacs, N. C. & Levin, B. E. (2004). Obesity-prone rats have pre-existing defects in their counterregulatory response to insulin-induced hypoglycemia. *Am. J. Physiol.* **287**, R1110–15.

Triscari, J., Nauss-Karol, C., Levin, B. E. & Sullivan, A. C. (1985). Changes in lipid metabolism in diet-induced obesity. *Metabolism* **34**, 580–7.

Truett, A. A., Borne, A. T., Monteiro, M. P. & West, D. B. (1998). Composition of dietary fat affects blood pressure and insulin responses to dietary obesity in the dog. *Obes. Res.* **6**, 137–46.

Tschop, M., Weyer, C., Tataranni, P. A., Devanarayan, V., Ravussin, E. & Heiman, M. L. (2001). Circulating ghrelin levels are decreased in human obesity. *Diabetes* **50**, 707–9.

Vainio, S., Heino, S., Mansson, J. E. *et al.* (2002). Dynamic association of human insulin receptor with lipid rafts in cells lacking caveolae. *EMBO Rep.* **3**, 95–100.

VandeBerg, J. L. & Williams-Blangero, S. (1997). Advantages and limitations of nonhuman primates as animal models in genetic resesarch on complex diseases. *J. Med. Primatol.* **26**, 113–19.

Van Heek, M., Compton, D. S., France, C. F. *et al.* (1997). Diet-induced obese mice develop peripheral, but not central, resistance to leptin. *J. Clin. Invest.* **99**, 385–90.

Van Vliet, B. N., Hall, J. E., Mizelle, H. L., Montani, J. P. & Smith, M. J., Jr. (1995). Reduced parasympathetic control of heart rate in obese dogs. *Am. J. Physiol.* **269**, H629–37.

Verwaerde, P., Senard, J. M., Galinier, M. *et al.* (1999). Changes in short-term variability of blood pressure and heart rate during the development of obesity-associated hypertension in high-fat fed dogs. *J. Hypertens.* **17**, 1135–43.

Vilberg, T. R. & Keesey, R. E. (1990). Ventromedial hypothalamic lesions abolish compensatory reduction in energy expenditure to weight loss. *Am. J. Physiol.* **258**, R476–80.

Wang, R., Liu, X., Hentges, S. T. *et al.* (2004). The regulation of glucose-excited neurons in the hypothalamic arcuate nucleus by glucose and feeding-relevant peptides. *Diabetes* **53**, 1959–65.

Wang, R., Cruciani-Guglielmacci, C., Migrenne, S., Magnan, C., Cotero, V. & Routh, V. H. (2005). The effects of oleic-acid (OA) on distinct populations of neurons in the hypothalamic arcuate nucleus (ARC) are dependent on extracellular glucose levels. *J. Neurophysiol.* **95**, 1491–8.

Weigle, D. S. & Levin, B. E. (2000). Defective dietary induction of uncoupling protein 3 in skeletal muscle of obesity-prone rats. *Obes. Res.* **8**, 385–91.

Weinsier, R. L., Nelson, K. M., Hensrud, K. M., Darnell, B. E., Hunter, G. R. & Schutz, Y. (1995). Metabolic predictors of obesity: contribution of resting energy expenditure, thermic effect of food, and fuel utilization to four-year weight gain of post-obese and never-obese women. *J. Clin. Invest.* **95**, 980–5.

West, D. B., Moody, D. L., Boozer, C. N., Atkinson, R. L. & Levin, B. E. (1991). Differential catecholamine response to intraperitoneal glucose injection in inbred mice susceptible or resistant to dietary obesity. *Int. J. Obes.* **15**, 16.

West, D. B., Boozer, C. N., Moody, D. L. & Atkinson, R. L. (1992). Dietary obesity in nine inbred mouse strains. *Am. J. Physiol.* **262**, R1025–32.

West, D. B., Goudey-Lefevre, J., York, B. & Truett, G. E. (1994). Dietary obesity linked to genetic loci on chromosomes 9 and 15 in a polygenic mouse model. *J. Clin. Invest.* **94**, 1410–16.

Will, M. J., Franzblau, E. B. & Kelley, A. E. (2003). Nucleus accumbens mu-opioids regulate intake of a high-fat diet via activation of a distributed brain network. *J. Neurosci.* **23**, 2882–8.

Williams, T., Berelowitz, M., Joffe, S. N. *et al.* (1984). Impaired growth hormone responses to growth hormone-releasing factor in obesity. *N. Engl. J. Med.* **311**, 1403–7.

Wilmot, C. A., Sullivan, A. C. & Levin, B. E. (1988). Effects of diet and obesity on brain a_1- and a_2-noradrenergic receptors in the rat. *Brain Res.* **453**, 157–66.

Wolden-Hanson, T., Davis, G. A., Baum, S. T. & Kemnitz, J. W. (1993). Insulin levels, physical activity, and urinary catecholamine excretion of obese and non-obese rhesus monkeys. *Obes. Res.* **1**, 5–17.

Woods, S. C., Seeley, R. J., Rushing, P. A., D'Alessio, D. & Tso, P. (2003). A controlled high-fat diet induces an obese syndrome in rats. *J. Nutr.* **133**, 1081–7.

Yang, X., Kow, L. M., Funabashi, T. & Mobbs, C. V. (1999). Hypothalamic glucose sensor. Similarities to and differences from pancreatic β-cell mechanisms. *Diabetes* **48**, 1763–72.

Yang, X. J., Kow, L. M., Pfaff, D. W. & Mobbs, C. V. (2004). Metabolic pathways that mediate inhibition of hypothalamic neurons by glucose. *Diabetes* **53**, 67–73.

Yoshida, T., Fisler, J. S., Fukushima, M., Bray, G. A. & Schemmel, R. A. (1987). Diet, lighting, and food intake affect norepinephrine turnover in dietary obesity. *Am. J. Physiol.* **252**, R402–8.

Zamboni, M., Armellini, F., Turcato, E. *et al.* (1994). Relationship between visceral fat, steroid hormones and insulin sensitivity in premenopausal obese women. *J. Intern. Med.* **236**, 521–7.

Zierath, J. R., Livingston, J., Thorne, A., Bolinder, J. & Reynisdottir, S. (1998). Regional difference in insulin inhibition of non-esterified fatty acid release from human adipocytes: relation to insulin receptor phosphorylation and intracellular signalling through the insulin receptor substrate-1 pathway. *Diabetologia* **41**, 1343–54.

7

Melanocortins and the control of body weight

VIRGINIE TOLLE AND MALCOLM J. LOW

1.   Introduction

The initial report that melanocortin peptides potently inhibit food intake after central administration was published in 1986 (Poggioli *et al.*, 1986). Because the melanocortin receptors had not yet been cloned or shown to be expressed in the brain, there was no physiological context to fully appreciate the significance of these data. In the two decades since that first publication, a remarkable web of experimental findings has firmly established the melano-cortin system as a critical component in the brain's control of energy homeo-stasis. A key breakthrough was the cloning and characterization of the agouti gene from the "obese yellow" mouse (Lu *et al.*, 1994). This spontaneous mutant strain expresses a dominant agouti A^Y allele and has an obesity phenotype in addition to a yellow coat color. The demonstration that agouti is an antagonist of melanocortin receptors (MCR), together with the findings of ectopic brain expression of the peptide and expression of MC3R and MC4R in the brain was the genesis of the "agouti-melanocortin" hypothesis for the mechanism of obesity in A^Y mice. Critical elements of this hypothesis were substantiated in 1997 by a trilogy of publications. First, targeted inactivation of the gene encoding the brain-specific MC4R caused an obesity phenotype similar to that of A^Y mice (Huszar *et al.*, 1997). Second, novel agonists and antagonists of the MC3/4R inhibited or stimulated feeding, respectively, when injected into the 3rd ventricle in rodents (Fan *et al.*, 1997). Finally, a homologue of agouti named

Neurobiology and Obesity, ed. Jenni Harvey and Dominic J. Withers. Published by Cambridge University Press. © Cambridge University Press 2008

agouti-related peptide (AGRP) was cloned, shown to be an MC4R antagonist normally expressed in hypothalamic neurons, and demonstrated to induce an obesity syndrome after transgenic overexpression in brain (Graham *et al.*, 1997; Ollmann *et al.*, 1997).

This chapter summarizes our knowledge of the melanocortin system accumulated since the seminal discoveries noted above, and attempts to identify the major lacunae for which additional experimental work is required to answer. By necessity, it focuses on the connection between melanocortins and regulation of energy balance while ignoring many other fascinating aspects of this pleiotropic peptide-receptor system in the mediation of pigmentation, adrenal steroidogenesis, immune function, neuromuscular regeneration and non-feeding related behaviors.

2.   Anatomy and neurochemistry of the melanocortin system

2.1   POMC and AGRP neurons

The central melanocortin system includes distinct neuronal subpopulations expressing the genes encoding either proopiomelanocortin (POMC) or AGRP and the second-order target neurons that express melanocortin receptors. There are approximately 3000–4000 neurons that strongly express POMC in the mouse hypothalamus, distributed along the rostral-caudal extent of the arcuate nucleus (ArcN) (Cowley *et al.*, 2001). Less than a tenth of that number, with much lower mRNA and peptide expression, are located in the caudal nucleus of the solitary tract (NTS) of the medulla (Palkovits *et al.*, 1987). Cell-specific transcription of *Pomc* in the brain is mediated by distal neuronal enhancer sequences that work independently from the proximal, pituitary-specific promoter elements in the gene (de Souza *et al.*, 2005b). Although POMC mRNA levels vary about two-fold in response to the extremes of anabolic and catabolic states, probably the more functionally relevant control step in POMC biosynthesis is at the level of posttranslational processing of the prohormone to biologically active peptides (Pritchard *et al.*, 2002). In the rodent brain, POMC is processed to a complex mixture of signaling molecules including γ3-MSH, des-acetyl-α-MSH, α-MSH, ACTH, and β-endorphin by the combined actions of prohormone convertases 1 and 2 (PC1, PC2), carboxypeptidase E (CPE), peptidyl α-amidating mono-oxygenase (PAM) and N-acetyltransferase (N-AT). The stoichiometry of these biologically active peptides and their intermediate processing precursor peptides may be dynamically regulated to influence the net functional synaptic read-out from POMC nerve terminals.

An intriguing feature of POMC neurons is their simultaneous production of the anorectic melanocortin peptides and the potent opioid peptide, β-endorphin.

As discussed in detail in Chapter 8, opioids generally are orexigenic and mediate increased consumption of palatable foods. Furthermore, almost all arcuate POMC neurons co-express another anorectic neuropeptide, cocaine- and amphetamine-responsive transcript (CART). A smaller number of POMC neurons also express galanin-like peptide (GALP) and our laboratory recently demonstrated that at least a third of POMC neurons produce and release the fast inhibitory neurotransmitter gamma-aminobutyric acid (GABA) from pre-synaptic terminals (Hentges *et al.*, 2004). The functional significance of each component in this complex mix of synaptically released signaling molecules is still under active investigation, but it seems likely that different levels of POMC neuron activity can result in finely nuanced communication with downstream targets in other brain areas.

POMC/CART neurons in the ArcN innervate multiple brain areas of potential or proven relevance to their role in control of body weight. A dense plexus of POMC fibers is present in most subdivisions of the hypothalamus including the medial preoptic nucleus (MePO), supraoptic nucleus (SON), periventricular nucleus (PeVN), paraventricular nucleus (PVN), ArcN, lateral hypothalamic (LH) and perifornical areas, and dorsal medial nucleus (DMN). The phenotypic identity of many hypothalamic target neurons has been established by double-label immunohistochemistry and immuno-electron microscopy and includes gonadotropin-releasing hormone (GnRH) neurons in the MePO, magnocellular oxytocin neurons in the SON, dopamine neurons in the PeVH, parvicellular thyrotropin-releasing hormone (TRH) and corticotropin-releasing hormone (CRH) neurons in the PVH, and melanin-concentrating hormone (MCH) and orexin neurons in the LH. Conversely, POMC fibers are almost totally excluded from the suprachiasmatic and most subdivisions of the ventral medial nucleus (VMH). Within the forebrain there are also dense projections to all subdivisions of the bed nucleus of the stria terminalis (BNST), nucleus accumbens (NAc), central nucleus of the amygdala (CeA) and paraventricular nucleus of the thalamus. Descending efferent fibers reach the ventral tegmental area (VTA), periaqueductal gray, and medullary nuclei including the parabrachial, ventral and dorsal raphe, NTS, and dorsal vagal complex. NTS POMC neurons apparently only make local efferent connections to an overlapping set of medullary nuclei (Palkovits *et al.*, 1987).

Important afferents onto arcuate POMC/CART neurons include inhibitory GABAergic terminals from limbic forebrain areas, excitatory glutamatergic terminals, intrahypothalamic projections from the LH, ArcN (including POMC neurons), and DMN, and 5-HT terminals from the raphe. Individual POMC neurons possess only a fraction of all these possible efferent and afferent connections, although the exact distribution, degree of axonal bifurcation, and extent of overlap remain the subject of investigation. For this reason, together with the demonstrated individual differences in transmitter co-expression and gradients of intracellular signaling molecules, POMC neurons should be viewed as a heterogeneous group subserving distinct functions rather than a blandly homogenous unit.

AGRP expression in the brain is predominantly localized to the ArcN of the hypothalamus in a subpopulation of neuropeptide Y (NPY) positive neurons distinct from, but in close spatial association to, POMC/CART neurons. At least a third of AGRP/NPY neurons utilize GABA as a fast, inhibitory neurotransmitter and there is a prominent synaptic innervation from this subpopulation onto POMC neurons in the ArcN (Cowley et al., 2001). Conversely, AGRP/NPY neurons express MC3R and are probably reciprocally innervated by local POMC neurons (Mounien et al., 2005; Menyhert et al., 2006). Both AGRP/NPY and POMC/CART neurons are prominent sites of leptin receptor expression in the hypothalamus. As described in other chapters, these first-order neurons respond to numerous circulating hormonal and nutrient signals that access the ArcN due to its lack of a blood–brain barrier. Intimate cross-talk between the two subpopulations of arcuate neurons would further fine tune their integration of humoral and synaptic signals.

Steady-state levels of AGRP mRNA vary over a much wider range than those of POMC in response to feeding state and pharmacological manipulation, suggesting a prominent role for transcriptional regulation in setting AGRP tone. However, a recent study demonstrated that most of the AGRP released in the brain is the biologically active carboxy-terminal peptide AGRP(83-132), which is cleaved from full-length AGRP predominantly by PC1, and therefore regulation of posttranslational processing may also be important in the cell biology of AGRP (Creemers et al., 2006). A prominent feature of AGRP/NPY neurons is that they project heavily to many, but not all, of the forebrain sites innervated by POMC fibers (Haskell-Luevano et al., 1999). This parallel distribution of POMC and AGRP terminals to the same neural targets is the neuroanatomical foundation supporting the unique agonist/antagonist relationship of melanocortin peptides and AGRP peptides at central MCRs.

2.2   Melanocortin receptors

Of the five known subtypes, MC4R is the most widely expressed in brain structures (Mountjoy et al., 1994; Kishi et al., 2003) and accounts for the majority of autoradiographic binding by radioligands. However, MC3R is relatively heavily expressed in medial brain structures including the ArcN, shell of the NAc, lateral septum, and ventral tegmental area (VTA) (Roselli-Rehfuss et al.,

1993; Lindblom et al., 1998) as well as several peripheral tissues including the heart and gastrointestinal tract. Together, these two MCR subtypes likely account for all the central effects of melanocortin ligands. Each binds the natural agonists α-MSH, β-MSH, and ACTH with approximately the same high affinity (Schioth et al., 2005). In contrast, only the MC3R exhibits high affinity binding and activation by γ-MSH. MC1R is the classical MSH receptor expressed in dermal structures and responsible for regulating melanin biosynthesis (Robbins et al., 1993). MC2R is the only subtype with an absolute selectivity for activation by ACTH and is expressed in the adrenal cortex and fat cells (Schioth et al., 2005). MC5R is highly expressed in exocrine glands and regulates their production and secretion of lipids (Chen et al., 1997).

All MCR are G-protein coupled seven transmembrane receptors that signal through G_{sa} to stimulate adenylyl cylase and increase intracellular cAMP concentrations. MSH increases cAMP in striatal brain slices (Florijn et al., 1993), consistent with physiological activation in primary neurons via this biochemical pathway. A recent investigation utilizing microinjections of the potent melanocortin agonist MTII into the 4th ventricle of rats demonstrated dose-responsive elevations in both phosphorylated extracellular-signal regulated kinase (ERK) and cAMP-response element binding protein (CREB), which were partially attenuated by antagonism of either protein kinase A (PKA) or mitogen-activated protein kinase (MAPK) upstream effector pathways (Sutton et al., 2005). Therefore, MC4R stimulated increases in cAMP are postulated to activate the MAPK-ERK signaling pathway through the Ras homologue Rap-1 in select neurons. Melanocortin peptides can mobilize intracellular Ca^{++} stores in transfected HEK293 cells by an alternative signaling pathway that does not involve PKA or an increase in inositol triphosphate (Mountjoy et al., 2003), but the relevance of this pathway to primary neurons is unknown. Further investigation is necessary to characterize the full range of intracellular signaling pathways utilized by both MC3R and MC4R in different populations of neurons that are the natural synaptic targets of POMC neurons.

An important aspect of melanocortin signaling is the constitutive activity exhibited by MC4R to elevate intracellular cAMP levels (Adan, 2006). Although this phenomenon was initially demonstrated in transfected heterologous cell lines, N-terminal mutations of MC4R isolated from obese individuals lacked constitutive activity while retaining normal responsiveness to MSH, suggesting that constitutive activity of the wild-type MC4R is critical for normal weight regulation in humans (Srinivasan et al., 2004). A postulated basis for the constitutive activity is that the extracellular N-terminal domain of MC4R acts as a tethered partial agonist of the receptor. Furthermore, in vitro studies have clearly demonstrated that AGRP acts as both a competitive antagonist and an inverse agonist at MC4R to modulate cAMP levels (Haskell-Luevano & Monck, 2001; Nijenhuis *et al.*, 2001). The extracellular N-terminus of the receptor is also important for mediating AGRPs action as an inverse agonist, while intracellular C-terminal truncations blocked inverse agonism but not competitive antagonism by AGRP (Chen *et al.*, 2006). More recently, AGRP was shown to exhibit agonistic properties on both MC3R and MC4R expressed in HEK293 cells by inducing arrestin-mediated endocytosis (Breit *et al.*, 2006). Therefore, AGRP could also counteract agonist actions of MSH by reducing the availability of melanocortin receptor binding sites. Rigorous assessment of the relative contributions of each of these proposed AGRP mechanisms in vivo is still required.

Two epistatic modifiers of MC1R and MC4R signaling were identified based on their suppression of yellow coat color and obesity in A^y mice (Phan *et al.*, 2006). These are the attractin (ATRN) and mahogunin (MGRN1) proteins inactivated by the mouse *mahogany* (*mg*) and *mahoganoid* (*md*) mutations, respectively. Although there is still debate about the mechanism of action of these proteins, ATRN being a transmembrane protein and MGRN1 an intracellular E3 ubiquitin ligase, they clearly illustrate the molecular complexity of signaling by the melanocortin system and suggest the existence of other unidentified modifier genes.

3.   Comparative vertebrate physiology of the melanocortin system

Melanocyte-stimulating hormone (MSH) is a phylogenetically ancient peptide whose primary amino acid sequence has been virtually unchanged over 400 million years of evolution. Similarly, POMC gene structure and the dual pattern of expression in the pituitary gland and medial basal hypothalamus have been essentially conserved (de Souza *et al.*, 2005a). Of the MCR, MC2R is likely closest to the primordial receptor from which the others evolved by gene duplication events and divergent mutations (Schioth *et al.*, 2005). Interestingly, all teleost fish lack the coding sequence for γ-MSH in their amino-terminal POMC peptide and some also have no discernable MC3R homologue, consistent with the proposal that γ-MSH is the physiological ligand for MC3R.

Functional homology in the melanocortin system occurs across the range of vertebrate classes in the control of body weight and adiposity as well as regulation of adrenal steroidogenesis and pigmentation. As discussed in Chapter 2, there is a significant amount of convergent genetic evidence implicating similar roles for the melanocortin system in weight regulation between humans and rodents. However, it is not known to what extent these similarities apply across all orders of mammals. For example, in the pig, melanocortin agonists suppressed food intake but centrally administered antagonists did not stimulate intake (Barb *et al.*, 2004). More limited evidence is available from distant vertebrate classes, nevertheless it appears that essential features of the melanocortin system relevant to body weight are remarkably conserved in both birds and fish (Song *et al.*, 2003; Strader *et al.*, 2003). In particular, the conservation of functional homologies mediated via POMC, AGRP, and MC4R signaling is the basis for ongoing, forward genetic screening by saturation mutagenesis in zebrafish to identify additional molecular components of the neural circuitry regulating body weight.

4.   Rodent genetic models of altered melanocortin function

Molecular characterization of metabolic defects in mouse strains with spontaneous genetic mutations led to many of the critical early insights concerning the relationship of the melanocortin system to regulation of energy homeostasis. Subsequently, increasingly sophisticated strategies to generate genetically modified animal models have been employed to assess the role of the melanocortin system in the regulation of energy homeostasis and metabolism. These models are summarized in Table 7.1 and focus on the function of the *Pomc* and *AGRP* genes, POMC/CART and NPY/AGRP neurons, the five receptor subtypes mediating the effects of melanocortins, and the enzymes responsible for the cleavage of prohormones, including POMC (PC1, PC2 and its associated protein 7B2).

The importance of POMC pathways in the regulation of energy balance was highlighted by the observations that null mutations in the genes encoding mouse or human POMC result in early-onset obesity (Krude *et al.*, 1998; Yaswen *et al.*, 1999; Challis *et al.*, 2004). *Pomc*-null mutants also exhibit adrenal insufficiency due to the lack of ACTH production from the pituitary gland and, conceivably, their obese phenotype may be partly a consequence of deficient pituitary MSH. To differentiate the contribution of central versus pituitary POMC, Smart and colleagues introduced a POMC transgene that selectively restores peripheral melanocortins, including ACTH and α-MSH, in *Pomc*-null mice, creating a neural-selective POMC-deficient mouse model (Smart *et al.*, 2006). The genetic replacement aggravated the obesity and metabolic syndrome by increasing caloric intake, reducing energy expenditure, increasing subcutaneous, visceral and hepatic fat and inducing severe insulin resistance, suggesting a key role of CNS-derived POMC that cannot be substituted by endogenous peripheral POMC (Figure 7.1).

Consistent with the phenotype of *Pomc*-null mice, ablation of POMC neurons by transgenic expression of diphtheria toxin receptor (DTR), induced hyperphagia

Table 7.1 *Phenotype of mice or rats with genetic alterations of the melanocortin system.*

Animal model	Phenotype	Reference
Global POMC KO	Moderate obesity and hyperphagia; normal plasma insulin, fasting glucose, and glucose clearance in glucose tolerance tests, but increased insulin sensitivity	(Yaswen et al., 1999) (Hochgeschwender et al., 2003) (Brennan et al., 2003)
Neural-selective POMC KO	Extreme obesity and hyperphagia; increased caloric intake and fat depots, insulin resistance, hyperleptinemia, and reduced energy expenditure	(Smart et al., 2006)
Diphtheria toxin-induced ablation of POMC neurons	Delayed hyperphagia, mild obesity and hypocortisolism; unaltered blood glucose	(Gropp et al., 2005)
Recombinant adeno-associated virus (rAAV) encoding POMC in rats	12-fold increase in POMC expression; transient reduction in food intake, body weight and visceral adiposity; improved glucose metabolism and insulin sensitivity; induction of UCP-1 in brown adipose tissue	(Li et al., 2005)
Transgenic overexpression of POMC from a neuron-specific enolase promoter	Attenuated fasting-induced hyperphagia; partially reversed obesity and hyperphagia; normalized hyperglycemia, glucose intolerance, and insulin resistance in *ob/ob* leptin-deficient mice	(Mizuno et al., 2003)
Transgenic α and γ3-MSH ubiquitous overexpression	Reduced weight gain and adiposity; improved glucose tolerance and decreased insulin; attenuation of obesity in *db/db* mice and improved glucose tolerance in A^y mice	(Savontaus et al., 2004)
AGRP KO	Normal body weight, body composition, growth rate and food intake; normal response to fasting and diet-induced obesity in young adults; age-related lean phenotype associated with increased metabolic rate, locomotor activity, thyroid hormones and BAT UCP1 expression	(Qian et al., 2002) (Wortley et al., 2005)
AGRP/NPY double KO	Normal body weight and food intake, normal response to fasting	(Qian et al., 2002)
Transgenic AGRP overexpression	Increased body weight, food intake, and body length	(Graham et al., 1997) (Ollmann et al., 1997)
Ablation of AGRP expressing neurons	47% loss of AGRP neurons; reduced body weight, food intake, total body fat, plasma insulin, and increased brown adipose tissue UCP1 expression	(Bewick et al., 2005)

Table 7.1 (cont.)

Animal model	Phenotype	Reference
Diphtheria toxin-induced ablation of AGRP neurons	Immediate reduction of body weight, food intake, blood glucose, plasma insulin and leptin (adults); temporal ablation in neonates has little effect	(Gropp et al., 2005; Luquet et al., 2005)
AGRP RNA interference	Decreased BW; increased metabolic rate; food intake unchanged	(Makimura et al., 2002)
MC4R KO	Obesity and hyperphagia; reduced oxygen consumption; impaired metabolic response to dietary fat; hyperinsulinemia and hyperleptinemia; impaired insulin tolerance	(Huszar et al., 1997) (Ste Marie et al., 2000) (Chen et al., 2000b) (Fan et al., 2000; Butler et al., 2001; Butler, 2006)
Conditional re-expression of MC4R from a floxed allele	Cross to a Sim1-Cre transgenic strain reveals a spatial dissociation between MC4R mediated actions on food intake and energy expenditure	(Balthasar et al., 2005)
MC3R KO	No excess weight and absence of hyperphagia; increased adiposity and increased feed efficiency; increased body weight in females on HF diet	(Chen et al., 2000a; Butler et al., 2001)
MC3/4R double KO	Heavier than MC4 or MC3R single KO mice	(Chen et al., 2000a)
MC1R mutations	Altered coat color and unaltered body weight	(Robbins et al., 1993)
MC5R KO	Altered lipid production; defects in thermoregulation when wet; unaltered body weight	(Chen et al., 1997)
PC1/3 KO	Growth retardation; normal corticosterone; no ACTH	(Zhu et al., 2002)
Point mutation in the coding sequence of PC1	Decreased α-MSH content (Hypothalamus); maturity onset obesity, increased energy intake, decreased metabolic rate, increased fat mass and plasma leptin, decreased lean mass, increased plasma insulin, hyperproinsulinemic, normal plasma glucose, normal insulin sensitivity, glucose intolerant, normal corticosterone	(Lloyd et al., 2006)
PC2 KO	High pituitary ACTH; lack of brain and pituitary α-MSH, energy balance phenotype not reported	(Laurent et al., 2004)

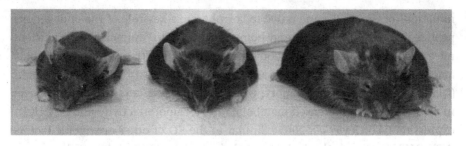

Figure 7.1 Relative body size of 6-month-old female mice on a predominant C57BL/6 genetic background. Left, wild-type; center, global *Pomc* null; right, neuronal-specific *Pomc* null (Smart *et al.*, 2006). (Photograph courtesy of JL Smart.)

and mild obesity. This phenotype may not be exclusively due to destruction of POMC cells in the CNS because the mice also developed adrenal insufficiency secondary to POMC cell death in the pituitary gland and probable ACTH deficiency (Gropp *et al.*, 2005). Conversely, overexpression of POMC in the hypothalamus of rats by a recombinant adeno-associated virus encoding POMC was associated with decreased body weight, food intake, and visceral adiposity as well as improved glucose metabolism and insulin sensitivity (Li *et al.*, 2005). Furthermore, selective overexpression of a POMC transgene under the control of a neuron-specific enolase promoter attenuated fasting-induced hyperphagia in wild-type mice and partially reversed obesity, hyperphagia, and hypothermia and effectively normalized hyperglycemia, glucose intolerance, and insulin resistance in leptin-deficient mice (Mizuno *et al.*, 2003). Together, these data indicate that central POMC is a key modulator of feeding, energy expenditure and glucose homeostasis. However, these studies did not differentiate among the roles of the different POMC-derived peptides or identify whether the ArcN or NTS is the relevant source of the peptides.

According to pharmacological studies discussed later in this chapter, the catabolic effects of POMC are largely mediated by α-MSH. Transgenic overexpression of α- and γ3-MSH in the medial basal hypothalamus and brainstem, but also in different peripheral tissues, led to reduced weight gain and adiposity and improved glucose tolerance in lean male mice and a significant decrease in insulin levels in females. The MSH transgene also attenuated obesity in *db/db* male and female mice and improved glucose tolerance in male A^y mice, animal models with reduced α-MSH tone (Savontaus *et al.*, 2004).

Although pharmacological studies have demonstrated a powerful orexigenic effect of exogenous AGRP and transgenic overexpression of AGRP increased body weight, food intake and body length (Graham *et al.*, 1997; Ollmann *et al.*, 1997) similar to the phenotype observed in obese A^y mice, null mutations of the *AGRP* gene failed to corroborate a key role of the endogenous peptide in the regulation of energy homeostasis in young animals. AGRP-deficient mice had normal body weight, body composition, growth rate and food intake, and normal responses to fasting and diet-induced obesity up to age 20 weeks (Qian *et al.*, 2002). A lean phenotype was only observed after 6 months of age, in association with increased metabolic rate, locomotor activity and BAT UCP1 expression (Wortley *et al.*, 2005). Similar to the KO of other orexigenic factors (NPY, MCH, ghrelin), the lack of an obvious phenotype in *Agrp*-null mice or *AGRP/Npy* double KO mice suggests that compensatory mechanisms occur during development to mitigate the fetal absence of AGRP. Consistent with those observations, two recent studies revealed that AGRP expressing neurons are essential to regulate energy homeostasis in adult but not neonatal mice. Indeed, reduced body weight, food intake, total body fat, plasma glucose, insulin, leptin and increased brown adipose tissue UCP1 expression were observed after ablation of AGRP/NPY neurons by transgenic cell type-specific expression of a diphtheria toxin receptor and intraperitoneal administration of the toxin to adult mice (Bewick *et al.*, 2005; Gropp *et al.*, 2005). However, no phenotype was observed if the cell ablation was induced during the neonatal period (Luquet *et al.*, 2005).

To determine which MCR mediates the effects of melanocortins on food intake and metabolism, genes encoding each receptor subtype have been invalidated. Consistent with their respective roles in pigmentation and exocrine function, spontaneous *Mc1r*-null mice have altered coat color (Robbins *et al.*, 1993) and gene-targeted *Mc5r*-null mice have altered lipid production and defects in thermoregulation when wet (Chen *et al.*, 1997), but body weights are unchanged in the two mutants.

In contrast, *Mc4r*-null mice are obese and hyperphagic, have reduced energy expenditure, impaired metabolic response to dietary fat, hyperinsulinemia, hyperleptinemia and impaired insulin tolerance (Huszar *et al.*, 1997; Chen *et al.*, 2000b; Fan *et al.*, 2000; Ste Marie *et al.*, 2000; Butler *et al.*, 2001). *Mc3r*-null mice have no excess weight and are not hyperphagic, but have increased adiposity and feed efficiency on a mixed genetic background (Butler *et al.*, 2000; Chen *et al.*, 2000a). Males on a C57BL/6 background were slightly hyperphagic when placed on a high-fat diet (Butler, 2006). These data suggest primary roles of MC4R in energy intake, energy expenditure and glucose homeostasis and a distinct role of MC3R in fat metabolism, which are complementary to each other. Interestingly, *Mc3/4r* double KO mice are heavier than *Mc4r*-null mice, further suggesting that function of the two receptors is not redundant (Chen *et al.*, 2000a). Although *a*-MSH can bind and activate both MC3 and MC4R, it is thought that *a*-MSH inhibits food intake mostly through

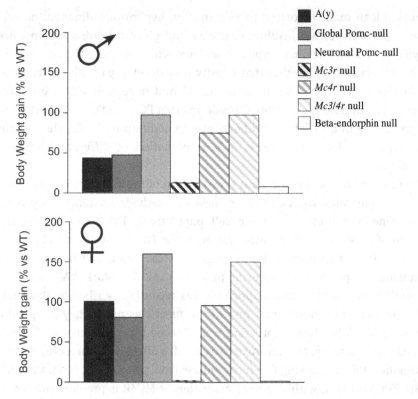

Figure 7.2 Percentage body weight increase relative to wild-type controls at age 26 weeks of mouse models deficient in melanocortin or beta-endorphin signaling [Data adapted from: A^Y mice (Savontaus *et al.*, 2004); Global *Pomc* null and neuronal-specific *Pomc* null mice (Smart *et al.*, 2006); *Mc4r* null, *Mc3r* null and *Mc3/4r* null mice (Chen *et al.*, 2000a); Beta-endorphin-deficient mice (Appleyard *et al.*, 2003)].

modulation of MC4R as *Mc3r*- but not *Mc4r*-null mice respond to the anorectic effects of MTII (Marsh *et al.*, 1999; Chen *et al.*, 2000a). Figure 7.2 compares the percentage increase of body weight relative to wild-type, age- and sex-matched animals of several mutant mouse models, illustrating the additive effect of combined MC3R and MC4R deletion and greater similarity to the neuronal-specific *Pomc*-null mice than either global *Pomc*-nulls or A^y mice.

Other evidence for a role of melanocortins and more specifically α-MSH in the obesity syndromes comes from mice deficient in PC1/3 and PC2. Although *Pc1/3*-null mice do not display any phenotype related to positive energy balance, they are growth retarded probably due to a defect in processing of growth hormone-releasing hormone (GHRH) (Zhu *et al.*, 2002). A point mutation in the coding sequence of PC1 induces maturity onset obesity, increased energy intake, decreased metabolic rate, increased fat mass and plasma leptin, decreased lean mass, increased plasma insulin, hyperproinsulinemia, normal plasma glucose, normal insulin sensitivity and glucose intolerance in mice (Lloyd et al., 2006). The phenotype is associated with reduced a-MSH content in the hypothalamus, suggesting that obesity may develop partially via reduced a-MSH signaling in the CNS. In addition, Pc2-null mice lack a-MSH but have intact ACTH (Laurent et al., 2004). Considering that PC1 and PC2 are involved in the processing of a variety of prohormones in addition to POMC, the mutant phenotypes are likely the result of a combination of different hormonal alterations.

Despite the advances made from investigation of these animal models, they have also illustrated the necessity to develop methods for temporally regulating gene mutations in specific cell populations. Examples include the ablation of POMC neurons or inactivation of the Pomc gene selectively in the ArcN or NTS, inactivation of the Agrp gene in the adult, and transgenic re-expression of specific melanocortin peptides (a-MSH, γ-MSH, β-MSH) in the Pomc-null background. A novel approach was recently described by Balthasar and colleagues that shows great promise to meet this need. They designed a mutant Mc4r allele whose expression was silenced by the inclusion of a loxP-flanked stop sequence. Mutant mice carrying this allele were then crossed to a transgenic strain expressing Cre recombinase from a Sim1 gene promoter only in the PVH and CeA, with resultant activation of MC4R expression limited to the same hypothalamic nuclei. The compound mutant mice had significantly less obesity and completely normalized food intake compared with global Mc4r-null mice, but they still exhibited a reduction in energy expenditure, suggesting that distinct MC4R-expressing populations of neurons regulate food intake and thermogenesis (Balthasar et al., 2005).

5.   Central actions of melanocortins in the regulation of energy balance

5.1   Regulation of appetite and food intake

The anorectic effects of POMC neurons are potentially mediated by a-MSH, β-MSH and/or γ-MSH. However, pharmacological studies have shown that a-MSH in the CNS is the most powerful anorectic melanocortin peptide. Intracerebroventricular (icv) administration of a-MSH or MTII, a synthetic MC3/4R agonist, reduces food intake and body weight in lean and obese rodents (Shimizu et al., 1989; Fan et al., 1997; Thiele et al., 1998; McMinn et al., 2000). The action of a-MSH is antagonized by AGRP, the endogenous MC3/4R antagonist (Ollmann et al., 1997; Pritchard et al., 2004) and SHU9119, a synthetic competitive antagonist. AGRP has been shown to stimulate food intake for a prolonged period of time (Rossi *et al.*, 1998) but this long-lasting hyperphagia cannot be reproduced by the antagonist activity of SHU9119 (Grill *et al.*, 1998; Hwa *et al.*, 2001). Based on the absence of antagonist action of AGRP when given 24h prior to MTII, and c-Fos activation of differential brain nuclei 2h and 24h post-injection of AGRP, several studies suggest that the short-term and long-term effects of AGRP involve two different pathways. The short-term effects may be due to interactions with MC4R whereas the prolonged action may involve agonist-independent pathways (Hagan *et al.*, 2000, 2001). A possible explanation could be the property of AGRP to act as an inverse agonist at MC3/4R to induce sustained increases in food consumption (Haskell-Luevano & Monck, 2001; Nijenhuis *et al.*, 2001; Adan & Kas, 2003; Srinivasan *et al.*, 2004; Breit *et al.*, 2006; Smith *et al.*, 2006), but this still needs to be demonstrated in animal models.

Considering that β-MSH binds with equivalent or even higher affinity than α-MSH to MC4R, β-MSH/γ-LPH-immunoreactive fibers are found in several nuclei involved in the regulation of feeding, and β-MSH-like peptides but not α-MSH levels in several hypothalamic nuclei are increased in food-restricted rats (Harrold & Williams, 2006), it was postulated that β-MSH and its precursor, γ-LPH, are important components of energy homeostasis in situations of underfeeding (Harrold *et al.*, 2003).

However, pharmacological data on the feeding effects of β-MSH are inconsistent. Although rodents, unlike humans, do not process β-MSH from γ-LPH because of an altered proteolytic processing site, icv administration of human β-MSH has been reported to reduce food intake to the same extent as α-MSH in fed and fasted rats (Abbott *et al.*, 2000; Kask *et al.*, 2000). This contrasts, however, with another study showing that central administration of α-MSH and γ2-MSH but not β-MSH significantly reduced food intake in 48h fasted rats (Millington *et al.*, 2001). A recent study comparing the effects of individual POMC-derived peptides in POMC-deficient animals demonstrated that α-MSH, β-MSH and γ-MSH all had short-term anorectic effects after a single icv injection at the onset of the dark cycle in ad libitum fed animals (Tung *et al.*, 2006). However, α-MSH had the most potent effect and was the only one of the peptides to induce loss of body weight and fat mass after long-term treatment. Interestingly, the effects of α-MSH were primarily due to reduced food intake rather than increased energy expenditure. Together these data do not conclusively support a key role of β-MSH or γ-MSH in the long-term regulation of body weight in rodents.

Recently, two independent genetic studies provided convincing evidence for a physiological role of β-MSH in human body-weight regulation. The researchers identified polymorphisms in the region of POMC encoding β-MSH that impair the ability of the peptide to bind to and activate MC4R (Biebermann et al., 2006; Lee et al., 2006). The mutations were associated with hyperphagia and obesity despite the apparently unaltered production of α-MSH.

The role of γ-MSH, which binds preferentially to MC3R, is still unclear but might be expected to have a role in fat deposition rather than food consumption (Millington et al., 2001; Tung et al., 2006). γ-MSH peptides have been mostly involved in other functions, including cardiovascular responses (Humphreys, 2007). (See Section 5.3 on regulation of the autonomic nervous system.)

5.2   Dissection of the component processes underlying melanocortin effects on intake

Feeding behavior can be divided heuristically into a number of sequential or overlapping component processes that differ in their neurochemical and neuroanatomical substrates (reviewed in Adan et al., 2006). For example, it is well established that supracollicular decerebrate rats are capable of responding acutely to satiety signals with appropriate termination of feeding and that these phenomena are integrated within the medulla independently of any descending neural influences from forebrain structures (Grill & Norgren, 1978). However, the same surgical preparation abolishes the long-term control over energy homeostasis in response to chronic caloric imbalance. Higher limbic forebrain structures including the extended amygdala are necessary for evaluation and prioritization of competing appetitive drives while the hypothalamic nuclei are essential for monitoring and responding to adipostatic and other signals that reflect stored energy depots. Brainstem nuclei respond rapidly to neuronal afferents that are stimulated by the contact of direct satiety factors with the gut mucosa. Furthermore, the medulla contains the central pattern generator controlling oral–lingual–pharyngeal motor activity.

Meal pattern analysis is the experimental procedure used to quantify meal size, meal number, meal frequency, latencies to initiate intake, and the length of intervals separating individual meals. This procedure in combination with pharmacological or genetic manipulations can test the role of specific neurochemical systems to regulate either hunger and feeding initiation or satiation and feeding termination. The central administration of MTII in rats decreased meal size without disruption of motor performance in meal pattern experiments (Azzara et al., 2002; Williams et al., 2002; Zheng et al., 2005). Conversely, selective injection of AGRP in the 4th ventricle increased meal size, but not meal number or frequency (Zheng et al., 2005). These results are consistent with a role of the melanocortin system to modulate the sensitivity of medullary nuclei to either detect or respond to endogenous satiety signals. However, a different type of behavioral analysis that measured extinction responding of rats to a conditioned stimulus previously paired with food deprivation suggested that MTII influenced intake by a mechanism distinct from that of natural satiation by pre-feeding (Benoit et al., 2001). In addition, melanocortin agonists preferentially decrease intake of high energy density foods while antagonists increase the preference of rodents for high-fat foods (reviewed in Adan et al., 2006). Alterations of food choice are suggestive of melanocortin actions in the CeA, parabrachial nucleus, and LH because of the established roles of these brain areas in taste perception and reward.

In addition to modulation of satiety and homeostasis-driven food intake, melanocortins might also influence intake via the brain's reward circuitry and mesolimbic dopamine system. Melanocortin receptors are abundantly expressed in the VTA, NAc shell, and ventral striatum and site-specific injections of melanocortin agonists into the VTA increased the extracellular levels of dopamine in the NAc measured by microdialysis (Lindblom et al., 2001). In other studies, VTA injection of a-MSH and γ1-MSH produced a marked increase in grooming behavior and rearing of rats, while γ2-MSH had the opposite effect and blocked γ1-MSH (Klusa et al., 1999). Finally, dopamine D1R agonists increased MC4R expression in the striatum (Alvaro et al., 2003). A possible functional role of reward circuits in melanocortin regulation of intake was suggested from operant studies using MC4-deficient mice (Vaughan et al., 2006). These animals are hyperphagic and emitted twice as many lever presses to receive food pellets on a progressive ratio schedule, indicative of increased motivation to support larger meal sizes.

There are parallels between the potential role of melanocortins to regulate food intake and the influence of the melanocortin system on the ingestion of drugs of abuse. For example, administration of MTII significantly augmented the rewarding effect of amphetamine (Cabeza de Vaca et al., 2002) and reduced voluntary ethanol consumption in wild-type but not MC4R-deficient mice (Navarro et al., 2005), suggesting that the effect is mediated via MC4R and not MC3R. Finally, a melanocortin antagonist infused directly into the NAc blocked the rewarding effects of cocaine (Hsu et al., 2005).

5.3   *Regulation of the autonomic nervous system*

Melanocortins modulate the activities of the sympathetic and parasympathetic nervous systems that innervate many organs involved in energy homeostasis and metabolism. Among the target organs, the brown adipose tissue (BAT) regulates energy expenditure and diet-induced thermogenesis, the white adipose tissue (WAT) participates in glucose uptake, lipid metabolism and adipokine secretion, the liver in glucose production, and the pancreas in glucose homeostasis. Melanocortins also mediate cardiovascular responses at the brainstem level. Both a-MSH and γ-MSH have been shown to increase blood pressure and heart rate through central stimulation of sympathetic nervous outflow (reviewed in Humphreys, 2007).

MC4R is expressed in the dorsal motor nucleus of the vagus (DMX), where parasympathetic motor neurons are located, and in the sympathetic preganglionic neurons in the intermediolateral cell column (IML) of the spinal cord (Fliers *et al.*, 2003; Kishi *et al.*, 2003; Romijn & Fliers, 2005). A subset of POMC neurons in the ArcN projects to the IML, suggesting a direct control of sympathetic activity by melanocortins. In addition, POMC neurons in the NTS project to the DMX (Palkovits *et al.*, 1987) suggesting a potential direct control of parasympathetic activity by melanocortin peptides. MC4R mRNA is also localized in the PVH and DMH, which receive afferent inputs from ArcN POMC and AGRP neurons and project to the DMX and the IML in the spinal cord. Thus, the effects of melanocortins on the autonomic nervous system are mediated by a combination of direct projections from melanocortin-producing neurons and projections from second-order neurons in the hypothalamus. The sympathetic nervous system in general mediates catabolic effects (e.g. activation of lipolysis) while the parasympathetic nervous system mediates anabolic responses (e.g. increased insulin sensitivity of the adipose tissue) (reviewed in Romijn & Fliers, 2005).

Control of brown adipose tissue and thermogenesis

Animal models with a disrupted melanocortin signal not only have dysregulated energy intake but also perturbations in regulation of thermogenesis and markers of BAT activity, including uncoupling protein 1 (UCP-1) (see Table 7.1). The effects of melanocortin agonists on thermogenesis are manifested by increased BAT sympathetic nerve activity and BAT temperature after a-MSH injection in the 3rd ventricle (Yasuda *et al.*, 2004) and increased BAT UCP-1 levels in rats, fed either chow or high-fat diets, after central MTII administration (Li *et al.*, 2004). The synthetic agonist MTII has also been shown to increase oxygen consumption and elevate BAT UCP-1 in lean and obese rodents (Hwa *et al.*, 2001; Hamilton & Doods, 2002; Li *et al.*, 2004; Zhang *et al.*, 2004; Kim *et al.*, 2005). These effects were abolished in surgically denervated BAT, suggesting a role for the sympathetic nervous system (Williams *et al.*, 2003). Similar effects of MTII on UCP-1 expression were observed after injection into the 3rd or the 4th ventricle of the brain (Williams *et al.*, 2003; Yasuda *et al.*, 2004) and were still present in decerebrate rats, demonstrating that the brainstem can control BAT metabolism independently of forebrain input.

Complementary studies have demonstrated that antagonizing the effects of a-MSH with AGRP reduces oxygen consumption (Goto et al., 2003; Small et al., 2003). Central infusion of AGRP into the 3rd cerebral ventricle gradually suppressed sympathetic nerve activity, decreased BAT temperature and reduced UCP-1 content (Small et al., 2001; Yasuda et al., 2004). Chronic icv infusion of HS014, a MC4R antagonist, similarly suppressed the expression of BAT UCP-1 (Baran et al., 2002). Despite their absence of orexigenic actions, amino-terminal AGRP peptides that lack antagonist activity at MC-R decreased oxygen consumption, and increased body weight and epididymal/mesenteric fat pad weight (Goto et al., 2003), further suggesting that AGRP can modulate thermogenesis in an agonist-independent manner. Endogenous AGRP is involved in the regulation of metabolic rate as well, because reducing AGRP by RNA interference increases metabolic rate and decreases body weight without affecting food intake (Makimura et al., 2002).

Control of white adipose tissue metabolism

ACTH, a-MSH and β-LPH all have lipolytic properties and their effects on WAT are mediated at least partly through the central nervous system. Chronic icv treatment with MTII reduced WAT mass in ad libitum fed or pair-fed animals, showing that these effects are independent of the anorectic action of the peptide (Raposinho et al., 2003). In addition, reduction of the respiratory quotient after icv injections of MTII has been observed and suggests that MSH preferentially increases the oxidation of lipids over carbohydrates (Hwa et al., 2001). Chronic icv infusion of a-MSH decreased intra-abdominal fat while antagonizing MSH tone with AGRP or SHU9119 induced opposite effects (Obici et al., 2001). Chronic AGRP infusion increased body weight and plasma leptin in the absence of hyperphagia, suggesting that the effects of the peptide on metabolism and food intake can be dissociated (Korner et al., 2003).

White adipose tissue is innervated by the sympathetic and parasympathetic nervous systems, which modulate metabolic and endocrine functions of adipose tissue including lipolysis and lipogenesis, glucose and fatty acid uptake, adipokine biosynthesis, and insulin sensitivity (reviewed in Romijn & Fliers, 2005). Recent anatomical evidence demonstrating the expression of MC4R in the sympathetic nervous system outflow neurons to inguinal WAT in Siberian Hamster (Song et al., 2005) supports a role of central melanocortins to regulate lipolysis via the sympathetic nervous system. These effects are likely mediated by a-MSH or β-MSH as they bind MC4R with high affinity. However, there may also be a role of γ3-MSH activation of MC3R in the control of fat metabolism as γ3-MSH reduces total fat mass, Mc3r-null mice have increased adiposity, and γ-MSH has the ability to modulate the activity of the sympathetic nervous system, as evidenced by its action on cardiovascular functions.

Control of insulin secretion and glucose homeostasis

A role of melanocortin peptides and receptors in the regulation of glucose homeostasis is manifested by dysregulation of glucose homeostasis in animal models with disruption of the melanocortin pathway (see Table 7.1). In addition, centrally administered melanocortin agonists inhibit basal insulin release and alter glucose tolerance, effects which are completely abolished by *a*-adrenergic receptor blockade (Fan *et al.*, 2000). Chronic AGRP infusion increases plasma insulin and glucose and these effects are abolished in pair-fed animals, suggesting that insulin resistance may be secondary to hyperphagia (Tallam *et al.*, 2004). In contrast, another study showed that the increased insulin concentration was maintained in pair-fed rats (Korner *et al.*, 2003). The central melanocortin system may thus directly modulate pancreatic function.

The pancreas receives innervation from both the sympathetic and parasympathetic nervous systems (Buijs *et al.*, 2001) and the above data suggest that melanocortin agonists inhibit insulin secretion by increasing sympathetic activity (Fan *et al.*, 2000). Central MC4R may also play an important role in the sensitivity of peripheral organs to insulin actions. Stimulation of central MC3/4R modulates insulin sensitivity, independently of any effect on food intake and body weight (Heijboer *et al.*, 2005). Chronic icv infusion of *a*-MSH markedly enhanced the actions of insulin on both glucose uptake and glucose production from the liver, while SHU9119 exerted opposite effects (Obici *et al.*, 2001). These effects are likely mediated by the sympathetic nervous system that innervates the liver and modulates both hepatic glucose production and glucose uptake in peripheral tissues (reviewed in Nonogaki, 2000). The adipose tissue also participates in glucose uptake, and parasympathetic nerve activity increases the insulin sensitivity of white adipose tissue (WAT) (Romijn & Fliers, 2005). Recent evidence of an interaction between liver and adipose tissue via neuronal pathways has also been demonstrated (Uno *et al.*, 2006).

The implication of *γ*-MSH in sodium metabolism and insulin resistance through the sympathetic nervous system has been reviewed (Humphreys, 2007). In addition, *γ*-MSH seems to be involved in glucose homeostasis as demonstrated by the observations that insulin resistance and hypertension develop in PC2 and *Mc3r* null mice lacking *γ*-MSH signaling.

6.   Electrophysiologic actions of melanocortins

A key issue at the current juncture in our understanding of the melanocortin system and control of energy balance is to characterize the downstream cellular events invoked by melanocortin release in specific populations of neurons and relate those events to the recruitment of neural networks and eventually to the relevant behavioral and autonomic motor outputs. Electro-physiological studies dissect the short-term effects of melanocortins on the spontaneous and synaptic membrane properties of target neurons and complement the biochemical identification of intracellular signaling pathways coupled to MCR. Because MCR are not ion channels, and therefore incapable of directly conducting charge across plasma membranes, they must indirectly modulate neuronal excitability and action potentials by other mechanisms.

A limited number of studies investigating the electrophysiological actions of melanocortins from brain slice recordings have been published, and they include contradictory results due in part to heterogenous neuronal responses. The MC3R agonist DTrp^8-γ-MSH hyperpolarized the majority of POMC neurons in the first of these studies and led to the suggestion that the MC3R functions as an autoinhibitory receptor (Cowley et al., 2001). Later, MTII was reported to depolarize MC4R positive neurons in the DMH and PVH (Liu et al., 2003). Mixed effects of MTII to either stimulate or inhibit unidentified neurons of the rat VMH have been demonstrated, but AGRP suppressed the firing of the majority of VMH neurons even in the presence or absence of exogenous agonist (Li & Davidowa, 2004). The most recent and thorough investigation demonstrated that both MC3R and MC4R agonists depolarized the majority of arcuate POMC neurons and a distinct population of non-POMC neurons largely via decreases of both I_A and K_{IR} K^+ conductances (Smith et al., 2006). Moreover, AGRP generally hyperpolarized the same cells, even in the absence of exogenously applied agonists, consistent with inverse agonism by AGRP. It should be noted that arcuate neurons have high input resistances due to very low resting conductances, thus only small changes in resting K^+ currents are required to produce mV changes in resting membrane potential and alter the excitability of the neurons and probability of firing action potentials. The exact mechanism by which MCR activation actually alters K^+ conductances through elevation of intracellular cAMP remains to be determined.

7.   Peripheral actions of melanocortins relevant for energy balance

The non-neuronal effects of melanocortins in the control of energy homeostasis and metabolism have not been fully evaluated. A few studies have indicated a potential role of melanocortins to regulate WAT metabolism and glucose homeostasis by a direct action on fat cells. Initial anatomical evidence for a role of melanocortins in peripheral tissues was the demonstration of melanocortin binding sites by NDP-MSH radioligand autoradiography on differentiated adipocytes (reviewed in Boston, 1999). Later, expression of MC2R and MC5R were demonstrated in mouse adipose tissue and MC4R in rat adipocytes by RT-PCR (Boston, 1999; Hoggard *et al.*, 2004a). Furthermore, melanocortin agonists pharmacologically increase cAMP levels in adipocytes.

ACTH has been shown to be the most potent lipolytic melanocortin peptide in rats. The hormone circulates in the plasma and primarily stimulates corticosterone production and secretion via activation of MC2R located on the adrenal gland. Because MC2R is also expressed in adipocytes and exclusively binds ACTH, it is likely that the POMC-derived hormone produced by the pituitary gland can mediate lipolysis via a direct action on MC2R in the adipose tissue, as demonstrated by in vitro studies with primary rat adipocytes. The physiologic role of ACTH on adipose tissue might be to increase the release of energy stores into the circulation in periods of energy demand. a-MSH and β-LPH also have lipolytic actions in vitro but with marked species-dependent differences in potency (Boston, 1999; Hoggard *et al.*, 2004a). In addition, both a-MSH and MTII stimulate free fatty acid release from differentiated adipocytes (Bradley *et al.*, 2005). Potential direct effects of ACTH and a-MSH to increase thermogenesis have also been described (Rothwell & Stock, 1985).

More recent studies suggest that a-MSH and AGRP can modulate metabolism via a direct peripheral action. a-MSH and AGRP are produced in the periphery (a-MSH in the pituitary gland, pancreas and skin; AGRP in the adrenal cortex, testes, lung and kidneys, among other sites), where they may exert paracrine functions on these organs. Although the relevant sources are unclear, a-MSH and AGRP also circulate in the blood and are regulated by nutritional state. Plasma AGRP is increased during fasting while plasma a-MSH is decreased. Leptin secretion and gene expression by differentiated adipocytes in culture are inhibited by a-MSH and this effect is antagonized by AGRP (Hoggard *et al.*, 2004a). These effects are likely independent of MC2R but could potentially be mediated through MC4R, which binds both a-MSH and AGRP. The physiological significance of this action still needs to be determined, but a hypothesis is that melanocortin control of WAT metabolism may regulate energy storage in fat during prolonged caloric restriction.

Direct peripheral effects of a-MSH in the regulation of glucose homeostasis are also suggested by the fact that a-MSH inhibits insulin secretion of insulin-secreting tumor cell lines, HIT-T 15 (Shimizu *et al.*, 1995). Expression of MC5R and a-MSH immunoreactivity in rat pancreas (Hirsch & O'Donohue, 1985) suggests a possible paracrine role of melanocortins to regulate insulin secretion. In addition, a-MSH and β-MSH but not γ-MSH increase plasma insulin and FFA in rabbits after intravenous injection (Knudtzon, 1984).

In vivo experiments have not conclusively demonstrated physiologically relevant CNS-independent actions of MSH on lipid metabolism, thermogenesis and glucose homeostasis. Intraperitoneal administration of the a-MSH synthetic analogues, NDP-MSH or MTII, decreased body weight gain in POMC-deficient mice (Yaswen et al., 1999), attenuated the POMC mutant's hypoglycemia during insulin tolerance test (Brennan et al., 2003) and attenuated the temperature drop during a cold challenge in ob/ob mice (Forbes et al., 2001). In addition, peripheral administration of MTII modulated the expression of UCP-1 and UCP-3, markers for energy expenditure in BAT and muscle (Cettour-Rose & Rohner-Jeanrenaud, 2002). Although NDP-MSH and MTII may poorly cross the blood–brain barrier, the possibility that the analogues interact with melanocortin receptors at sites in the CNS involved in the control of energy homeostasis with a relatively permeable blood–brain barrier is likely. Thus, it cannot be concluded whether MSH influences body weight partly by a direct effect of melanocortins on adipocytes to stimulate lipolysis or exclusively through central modulation of food intake and the autonomic nervous system. Similarly problematic are conclusions for the effects of peripherally administered NDP-MSH on glucose homeostasis (Cettour-Rose & Rohner-Jeanrenaud, 2002), metabolic rate (Hoggard et al., 2004b) and thermoregulation (Forbes et al., 2001). A recent study demonstrating that re-expression of peripheral POMC in the Pomc-null background did not attenuate the obesity phenotype of the mice suggests that peripheral a-MSH cannot substitute for lack of central a-MSH (Smart et al., 2006). Instead, it exacerbated the obese phenotype by restoration of peripheral ACTH secretion and stimulation of glucocorticoid production by the adrenal glands (Smart et al., 2007).

Conversely, a recent study demonstrated that a MC3R agonist, d-Trp(8)-γ-MSH, increased food intake after peripheral injection (Marks et al., 2006). Although the authors concluded that the effects were likely mediated through MC3R localized on POMC neurons in the ArcN, which lacks a blood–brain barrier, the study did not exclude interactions with MC3R on AGRP/NPY neurons or a peripheral effect on MC3R in the gastrointestinal tract.

Therefore, to definitively establish critical direct effects of melanocortins on energy homeostasis in vivo that are mediated by MCR outside of the CNS, it will be essential to analyze mutant mice with site-selective inactivation of MC3/4R in both the CNS and/or relevant peripheral tissues.

8.   Pharmacotherapy

Because of the key role played by melanocortin peptides in the regulation of feeding, energy expenditure, insulin secretion and insulin sensitivity, drugs that target central MC3/4R may be beneficial not only for the treatment of obesity and obesity-related syndromes like type II diabetes but also for the treatment of cachexia (Marks et al., 2001).

Agonists have reliably decreased food intake and body weight and improved glucose tolerance in several genetic and diet-induced obese rodent models. In most cases, icv administration of either aMSH or the synthetic MC3/4R agonist MTII is at least as efficacious to reduce food intake and body weight in obese rodents (Shimizu et al., 1989; Fan et al., 1997), if not more so, than in lean rodents (Thiele et al., 1998; McMinn et al., 2000). These data suggest increased functional activity of MC3/4R in the CNS of obese rodents and rationalize the development of melanocortin agonists to treat obesity. In diet-induced obese (DIO) Sprague–Dawley rats, a 6-day central infusion of MTII decreased food intake and reduced body weight and visceral adiposity (Chandler et al., 2005). MTII increased fat catabolism in the muscle of DIO rats and also improved glucose and cholesterol metabolism in both groups (Li et al., 2004). In diabetic-prone Otsuka Long-Evans Tokushima Fatty (OLETF) rats, subcutaneous administration of MTII increased insulin sensitivity and improved glucose tolerance independently of food intake (Banno et al., 2004). In Zucker fa/fa rats, a 3-day peripheral administration of MTII decreased food intake and body weight, with a more pronounced effect in obese rats (Cettour-Rose & Rohner-Jeanrenaud, 2002). Central administration of MTII for 4 days (10 nmol/day) in DIO mice significantly suppressed food intake, induced weight loss, and increased energy expenditure. However, after repeated intraperitoneal injections of MTII, feeding was no longer suppressed after 4 days and body weight nadir reached a plateau (Pierroz et al., 2002). In POMC-deficient mice, peripheral administration of the long-acting MSH analogue NDP-MSH attenuated the severe hypoglycemia observed after insulin administration in mutant mice (Brennan et al., 2003).

A major goal for the development of therapeutically useful melanocortins is the selective modulation of MCR subtypes to target specific biological functions. According to pharmacological and genetic studies outlined previously, MC4R is probably a better target than MC3R for modulation of energy homeostasis (reviewed in MacNeil et al., 2002; Nargund et al., 2006). First, the role of MC3R is not as well characterized and may be limited to the modulation of fat metabolism. Second, whereas MC4R is almost exclusively expressed in the CNS, MC3R is expressed in the CNS and also in many peripheral tissues (placenta, gut, heart, stomach, pancreas, testis, ovary, muscle and kidney) where its activation may produce unwanted side effects.

A variety of melanocortin analogues have been developed (MacNeil et al., 2002; Nargund et al., 2006) in attempts to fulfill the criteria of oral availability, once-daily dosing, adequate receptor occupancy in the CNS, functional receptor activation, maintenance of biological response after chronic stimulation, and lack of adverse effects (including modulation of cardiovascular, immunological and neurological function). Linear peptides like a-MSH are rapidly degraded in vivo. Common strategies to improve the potency and in vivo stability of peptidyl analogues are cyclization and the inclusion of modified amino acids. A family of melanocortin compounds that includes the core message sequence of MSH (His-Phe-Arg-Trp) has been developed based on these design principles (Table 7.2). Among the first of these analogues, which are still frequently used in research studies, are melanotan II (MTII) and SHU9119. MTII is a potent but non-selective MC1, MC3, MC4 and MC5R agonist and SHU9119 is an MC1/5R agonist but MC3/4R antagonist. Additional modifications of MTII have led to the development of potent agonists and antagonists with better selectivity for MC4R (reviewed in Irani & Haskell-Luevano, 2005). For example, HS014 and HS024, with disulfide bridges, are MC4R antagonists with moderate selectivity over MC3R and have been shown to increase food intake and body weight in rats (MacNeil et al., 2002; Nargund et al., 2006). Linear tetrapeptide and small molecule analogues have also been developed (reviewed in Irani & Haskell-Luevano, 2005). Additionally, analogues of β-MSH with selectivity for MC4R have been developed and one demonstrated strong efficacy (short-term anorectic effect but sustained body weight loss) when administered subcutaneously at doses less than 1 mg/kg to diet-induced obese rats for 14 days (Hsiung et al., 2005; Mayer et al., 2005).

Although there have been early-stage clinical trials to test the safety and short-term efficacy of MC4R agonists in humans, there are no approved drugs in this class for the treatment of obesity or overweight. However, the development of melanocortin agonists may meet other therapeutic needs. For example, activation of MCR has been associated with improved erectile function and agonists are being evaluated in pre-clinical stages for the treatment of male and female sexual dysfunctions (Martin & MacIntyre, 2004).

Two lines of evidence concerning the mechanism of action of AGRP in the regulation of body weight suggest novel strategies for the treatment of obesity. First is the inhibition of endogenous AGRP tone by RNA interference to improve agonist efficacy at MC3/4R. Indeed inhibition of AGRP tone by RNA interference in rodents decreased body weight and increased oxygen consumption (Makimura et al., 2002). A second possible strategy is to increase the constitutive activity of MC4R in combination with MCR agonists. Recent evidence showing that specific domains in the MC4R play an important role in the mediation of AGRP inverse agonism, but not NDP-MSH mediated receptor activation (Chen et al., 2006), suggest the possibility of developing effectors

Table 7.2 *Structure of selected melanocortin agonists and antagonists.*

Linear analogue	α-MSH	Ac-Ser-Tyr-Ser-Met-Glu-**His-l-Phe-Arg-Trp**-Gly-Lys-Pro-Val-NH$_2$
	NDP-α-MSH	[Nle^4,DPhe^7]-α-MSH Ac-Ser-Tyr-Ser-Nle-Glu-**His-DPhe-Arg-Trp**-Gly-Lys-Pro-Val-NH$_2$
Cyclic analogues	MTII	Ac-Nle^4-cyclo[Asp^5-**His^6-DPhe^7-Arg^8-Trp^9**-Lys^{10}]-NH$_2$
	SHU9119	Ac-Nle^4-cyclo[Asp^5-**His^6-DNal(2')^7-Arg^8-Trp^9**-Lys^{10}]-NH$_2$
	HS014	Ac-cyclo(S-S)[Cys^4-Glu^5-**His^6-DNal(2')^7-Arg^8-Trp^9**-Gly^{10}-Cys^{11}]-Pro^{12}- Pro^{13}-Lys^{14}-Asp^{15}-NH$_2$
Linear tetrapeptide analogue	JRH420-12	Ac-**Anc^6-DPhe^7-Arg^8-Trp^9**-NH$_2$
Small molecule	THIQ	1,2,3R,4-tetrahydro-3-isoquinolinecarboxylic acid[1R-(4-chloro-benzyl)]-2-(4-cyclohexyl-4-[1,2,4]triazol-1-ylmethyl-piperidin-1-yl)-2-oxo-ethyl]-amide
β-MSH and analogue	β-MSH (5-22)	Asp-Glu-Gly-Pro-Tyr-LArg-Met-Glu-**His-l-Phe-Arg-Trp**-Gly-Ser-Pro-Pro-Lys-Asp
	Compound 18	Ac-DArg-cyclo(S-S)[Cys-Glu-**His-DPhe-Arg-Trp**-Cys]-NH$_2$

Notes: The putative tetrapeptide message sequence common to all melanocortin agonists is shown in bold font (**His-Phe-Arg-Trp**). Abbreviations for substituted amino acids: Anc, amino-2-naphthylcarboxylic acid; Nal, β-naphthylalanine; Nle, norleucine.

that enhance the MCR constitutive activity at a site different than the a-MSH binding sites.

Utilization of MC4R antagonists may be a promising tool for the treatment of cachexia, which is often associated with cancer, renal failure or heart failure. In rodent models of cancer and renal failure, administration of MC4R antagonists resulted in an attenuation of cachexia by maintenance of appetite, and lean body mass with a reduction in basal energy expenditure (reviewed in DeBoer & Marks, 2006).

9.   Conclusion

The commonly held viewpoint that melanocortin agonists are anorexigenic peptides, and conversely melanocortin antagonists are orexigenic peptides, short-changes the complexity of the brain's melanocortin system and its interaction with other neuronal circuits to regulate energy balance. As discussed in this chapter, melanocortins prominently influence the activity of the autonomic nervous system independently of appetite. The diverse sites of MCR expression in the CNS are consistent with these two functions, but also suggest discrete roles for melanocortins in mediating aspects of satiety, taste perception, rewarding properties of food, and habit formation. Therefore, melanocortins act at multiple points within an interconnected neuronal network to bias its motor outputs in favor of either positive or negative energy balance. The question remains as to precisely how MCR signaling from the plasma membrane of neurons in multiple neural substrates alters the activity of this neuronal network.

Acknowledgements

VT was the recipient of an ASPET/Merck postdoctoral fellowship in integrative pharmacology. Research support for MJL was from NIH grants DK066604 and DK068400.

References

Abbott, C. R., Rossi, M., Kim, M. *et al.* (2000). Investigation of the melanocyte stimulating hormones on food intake. Lack of evidence to support a role for the melanocortin-3-receptor. *Brain Res.* **869**, 203–10.

Adan, R. A. (2006). Constitutive receptor activity series: endogenous inverse agonists and constitutive receptor activity in the melanocortin system. *Trends Pharmacol. Sci.* **27**, 183–6.

Adan, R. A. & Kas, M. J. (2003). Inverse agonism gains weight. *Trends Pharmacol. Sci.* **24**, 315–21.

Adan, R. A., Tiesjema, B., Hillebrand, J. J., la Fleur, S. E., Kas, M. J. & de Krom, M. (2006). The MC4 receptor and control of appetite. *Br. J. Pharmacol.* **149**, 815–27.

Alvaro, J. D., Taylor, J. R. & Duman, R. S. (2003). Molecular and behavioral interactions between central melanocortins and cocaine. *J. Pharmacol. Exp. Ther.* **304**, 391–9.

Appleyard, S. M., Hayward, M., Young, J. I. *et al.* (2003). A role for the endogenous opioid beta-endorphin in energy homeostasis. *Endocrinology* **144**, 1753–60.

Azzara, A. V., Sokolnicki, J. P. & Schwartz, G. J. (2002). Central melanocortin receptor agonist reduces spontaneous and scheduled meal size but does not augment duodenal preload-induced feeding inhibition. *Physiol. Behav.* **77**, 411–16.

Balthasar, N., Dalgaard, L. T., Lee, C. E. *et al.* (2005). Divergence of melanocortin pathways in the control of food intake and energy expenditure. *Cell* **123**, 493–505.

Banno, R., Arima, H., Sato, I. *et al.* (2004). The melanocortin agonist melanotan II increases insulin sensitivity in OLETF rats. *Peptides* **25**, 1279–86.

Baran, K., Preston, E., Wilks, D., Cooney, G. J., Kraegen, E. W. & Sainsbury, A. (2002). Chronic central melanocortin-4 receptor antagonism and central neuropeptide-Y infusion in rats produce increased adiposity by divergent pathways. *Diabetes* **51**, 152–8.

Barb, C. R., Robertson, A. S., Barrett, J. B., Kraeling, R. R. & Houseknecht, K. L. (2004). The role of melanocortin-3 and -4 receptor in regulating appetite, energy homeostasis and neuroendocrine function in the pig. *J. Endocrinol.* **181**, 39–52.

Benoit, S. C., Tracy, A. L., Air, E. L., Kinzig, K., Seeley, R. J. & Davidson, T. L. (2001). The role of the hypothalamic melanocortin system in behavioral appetitive processes. *Pharmacol. Biochem. Behav.* **69**, 603–9.

Bewick, G. A., Gardiner, J. V., Dhillo, W. S. *et al.* (2005). Post-embryonic ablation of AgRP neurons in mice leads to a lean, hypophagic phenotype. *Faseb J.* **19**, 1680–2.

Biebermann, H., Castaneda, T. R., van Landeghem, F. *et al.* (2006). A role for beta-melanocyte-stimulating hormone in human body-weight regulation. *Cell Metab.* **3**, 141–6.

Boston, B. A. (1999). The role of melanocortins in adipocyte function. *Ann. N. Y. Acad. Sci.* **885**, 75–84.

Bradley, R. L., Mansfield, J. P. & Maratos-Flier, E. (2005). Neuropeptides, including neuropeptide Y and melanocortins, mediate lipolysis in murine adipocytes. *Obes. Res.* **13**, 653–61.

Breit, A., Wolff, K., Kalwa, H., Jarry, H., Buch, T. & Gudermann, T. (2006). The natural inverse agonist agouti-related protein induces arrestin-mediated endocytosis of melanocortin-3 and -4 receptors. *J. Biol. Chem.* **281**, 37447–56.

Brennan, M. B., Costa, J. L., Forbes, S., Reed, P., Bui, S. & Hochgeschwender, U. (2003). Alpha-melanocyte-stimulating hormone is a peripheral, integrative regulator of glucose and fat metabolism. *Ann. N. Y. Acad. Sci.* **994**, 282–7.

Buijs, R. M., Chun, S. J., Niijima, A., Romijn, H. J. & Nagai, K. (2001). Parasympathetic and sympathetic control of the pancreas: a role for the suprachiasmatic nucleus and other hypothalamic centers that are involved in the regulation of food intake. *J. Comp. Neurol.* **431**, 405–23.

Butler, A. A. (2006). The melanocortin system and energy balance. *Peptides* **27**, 281–90.

Butler, A. A., Kesterson, R. A., Khong, K. et al. (2000). A unique metabolic syndrome causes obesity in the melanocortin-3 receptor-deficient mouse. *Endocrinology* **141**, 3518–21.

Butler, A. A., Marks, D. L., Fan, W., Kuhn, C. M. Bartolome, M. & Cone, R. D. (2001). Melanocortin-4 receptor is required for acute homeostatic responses to increased dietary fat. *Nat. Neurosci.* **4**, 605–11.

Cabeza de Vaca, S., Kim, G. Y. & Carr, K. D. (2002). The melanocortin receptor agonist MTII augments the rewarding effect of amphetamine in ad-libitum-fed and food restricted rats. *Psychopharmacology (Berl.)* **161**, 77–85.

Cettour-Rose, P. & Rohner-Jeanrenaud, F. (2002). The leptin-like effects of 3-d peripheral administration of a melanocortin agonist are more marked in genetically obese Zucker (fa/fa) than in lean rats. *Endocrinology* **143**, 2277–83.

Challis, B. G., Coll, A. P., Yeo, G. S. et al. (2004). Mice lacking pro-opiomelanocortin are sensitive to high-fat feeding but respond normally to the acute anorectic effects of peptide-YY(3-36). *Proc. Natl. Acad. Sci. USA* **101**, 4695–700.

Chandler, P. C., Viana, J. B., Oswald, K. D., Wauford, P. K. & Boggiano, M. M. (2005). Feeding response to melanocortin agonist predicts preference for and obesity from a high-fat diet. *Physiol. Behav.* **85**, 221–30.

Chen, A. S., Marsh, D. J., Trumbauer, M. E. et al. (2000a). Inactivation of the mouse melanocortin-3 receptor results in increased fat mass and reduced lean body mass. *Nat. Genet.* **26**, 97–102.

Chen, A. S., Metzger, J. M., Trumbauer, M. E. et al. (2000b). Role of the melanocortin-4 receptor in metabolic rate and food intake in mice. *Transgenic Res.* **9**, 145–54.

Chen, M., Celik, A., Georgeson, K. E., Harmon, C. M. & Yang, Y. (2006). Molecular basis of melanocortin-4 receptor for AGRP inverse agonism. *Regul. Pept.* **136**, 40–9.

Chen, W., Kelly, M. A., Opitz-Araya, X., Thomas, R. E., Low, M. J. & Cone, R. D. (1997). Exocrine gland dysfunction in MC5-R-deficient mice: evidence for coordinated regulation of exocrine gland function by melanocortin peptides. *Cell* **91**, 789–98.

Cowley, M. A., Smart, J. L., Rubinstein, M. et al. (2001). Leptin activates anorexigenic POMC neurons through a neural network in the arcuate nucleus. *Nature* **411**, 480–4.

Creemers, J. W., Pritchard, L. E., Gyte, A. et al. (2006). Agouti-related protein is posttranslationally cleaved by proprotein convertase 1 to generate agouti-related protein (AgRP)83-132: interaction between AGRP83-132 and melanocortin receptors cannot be influenced by syndecan-3. *Endocrinology* **147**, 1621–31.

de Souza, F. S., Bumaschny, V. F., Low, M. J. & Rubinstein, M. (2005a). Subfunctionalization of expression and peptide domains following the ancient duplication of the proopiomelanocortin gene in teleost fishes. *Mol. Biol. Evol.* **22**, 2417–27.

de Souza, F. S., Santangelo, A. M., Bumaschny, V. *et al.* (2005b). Identification of neuronal enhancers of the proopiomelanocortin gene by transgenic mouse analysis and phylogenetic footprinting. *Mol. Cell Biol.* **25**, 3076–86.

DeBoer, M. D. & Marks, D. L. (2006). Therapy insight: use of melanocortin antagonists in the treatment of cachexia in chronic disease. *Nat. Clin. Pract. Endocrinol. Metab.* **2**, 459–66.

Fan, W., Boston, B. A., Kesterson, R. A., Hruby, V. J. & Cone, R. D. (1997). Role of melanocortinergic neurons in feeding and the agouti obesity syndrome. *Nature* **385**, 165–8.

Fan, W., Dinulescu, D. M., Butler, A. A., Zhou, J., Marks, D. L. & Cone, R. D. (2000). The central melanocortin system can directly regulate serum insulin levels. *Endocrinology* **141**, 3072–9.

Fliers, E., Kreier, F., Voshol, P. J. *et al.* (2003). White adipose tissue: getting nervous. *J. Neuroendocrinol.* **15**, 1005–10.

Florijn, W. J., Mulder, A. H., Versteeg, D. H. & Gispen, W. H. (1993). Adrenocorticotropin/alpha-melanocyte-stimulating hormone (ACTH/MSH)-like peptides modulate adenylate cyclase activity in rat brain slices: evidence for an ACTH/MSH receptor-coupled mechanism. *J. Neurochem.* **60**, 2204–11.

Forbes, S., Bui, S., Robinson, B. R., Hochgeschwender, U. & Brennan, M. B. (2001). Integrated control of appetite and fat metabolism by the leptin-proopiomelanocortin pathway. *Proc. Natl. Acad. Sci. USA* **98**, 4233–7.

Goto, K., Inui, A., Takimoto, Y. *et al.* (2003). Acute intracerebroventricular administration of either carboxyl-terminal or amino-terminal fragments of agouti-related peptide produces a long-term decrease in energy expenditure in rats. *Int. J. Mol. Med.* **12**, 379–83.

Graham, M., Shutter, J. R., Sarmiento, U., Sarosi, I. & Stark, K. L. (1997). Overexpression of Agrt leads to obesity in transgenic mice. *Nat. Genet.* **17**, 273–4.

Grill, H. J. & Norgren, R. (1978). Chronically decerebrate rats demonstrate satiation but not bait shyness. *Science* **201**, 267–9.

Grill, H. J., Ginsberg, A. B., Seeley, R. J. & Kaplan, J. M. (1998). Brainstem application of melanocortin receptor ligands produces long-lasting effects on feeding and body weight. *J. Neurosci.* **18**, 10 128–35.

Gropp, E., Shanabrough, M., Borok, E. *et al.* (2005). Agouti-related peptide-expressing neurons are mandatory for feeding. *Nat. Neurosci.* **8**, 1289–91.

Hagan, M. M., Rushing, P. A., Pritchard, L. M. *et al.* (2000). Long-term orexigenic effects of AgRP-(83-132) involve mechanisms other than melanocortin receptor blockade. *Am. J. Physiol. Regul. Integr. Comp. Physiol.* **279**, R47–52.

Hagan, M. M., Benoit, S. C., Rushing, P. A., Pritchard, L. M., Woods, S. C. & Seeley, R. J. (2001). Immediate and prolonged patterns of Agouti-related peptide-(83-132)-induced c-Fos activation in hypothalamic and extrahypothalamic sites. *Endocrinology* **142**, 1050–6.

Hamilton, B. S. & Doods, H. N. (2002). Chronic application of MTII in a rat model of obesity results in sustained weight loss. *Obes. Res.* **10**, 182–7.

Harrold, J. A. & Williams, G. (2006). Melanocortin-4 receptors, beta-MSH and leptin: key elements in the satiety pathway. *Peptides* **27**, 365–71.

Harrold, J. A., Widdowson, P. S. & Williams, G. (2003). Beta-MSH: a functional ligand that regulated energy homeostasis via hypothalamic MC4-R? *Peptides* **24**, 397–405.

Haskell-Luevano, C. & Monck, E. K. (2001). Agouti-related protein functions as an inverse agonist at a constitutively active brain melanocortin-4 receptor. *Regul. Pept.* **99**, 1–7.

Haskell-Luevano, C., Chen, P., Li, C. *et al.* (1999). Characterization of the neuroanatomical distribution of agouti-related protein immunoreactivity in the rhesus monkey and the rat. *Endocrinology* **140**, 1408–15.

Heijboer, A. C., van den Hoek, A. M., Pijl, H. *et al.* (2005). Intracerebroventricular administration of melanotan II increases insulin sensitivity of glucose disposal in mice. *Diabetologia* **48**, 1621–6.

Hentges, S. T., Nishiyama, M., Overstreet, L. S., Stenzel-Poore, M., Williams, J. T. & Low, M. J. (2004). GABA release from proopiomelanocortin neurons. *J. Neurosci.* **24**, 1578–83.

Hirsch, M. D. & O'Donohue, T. L. (1985). Characterization of alpha-melanocyte-stimulating hormone in rat pancreas. *Peptides* **6**, 293–6.

Hochgeschwender, U., Costa, J. L., Reed, P., Bui, S. & Brennan, M. B. (2003). Altered glucose homeostasis in proopiomelanocortin-null mouse mutants lacking central and peripheral melanocortin. *Endocrinology* **144**, 5194–202.

Hoggard, N., Hunter, L., Duncan, J. S. & Rayner, D. V. (2004a). Regulation of adipose tissue leptin secretion by alpha-melanocyte-stimulating hormone and agouti-related protein: further evidence of an interaction between leptin and the melanocortin signalling system. *J. Mol. Endocrinol.* **32**, 145–53.

Hoggard, N., Rayner, D. V., Johnston, S. L. & Speakman, J. R. (2004b). Peripherally administered [Nle4,D-Phe7]-alpha-melanocyte stimulating hormone increases resting metabolic rate, while peripheral agouti-related protein has no effect, in wild type C57BL/6 and ob/ob mice. *J. Mol. Endocrinol.* **33**, 693–703.

Hsiung, H. M., Smiley, D. L., Zhang, X. Y. *et al.* (2005). Potent peptide agonists for human melanocortin 3 and 4 receptors derived from enzymatic cleavages of human beta-MSH(5-22) by dipeptidyl peptidase I and dipeptidyl peptidase IV. *Peptides* **26**, 1988–96.

Hsu, R., Taylor, J. R., Newton, S. S. *et al.* (2005). Blockade of melanocortin transmission inhibits cocaine reward. *Eur. J. Neurosci.* **21**, 2233–42.

Humphreys, M. H. (2007). Cardiovascular and renal actions of melanocyte-stimulating hormone peptides. *Curr. Opin. Nephrol. Hypertens.* **16**, 32–8.

Huszar, D., Lynch, C. A., Fairchild-Huntress, V. *et al.* (1997). Targeted disruption of the melanocortin-4 receptor results in obesity in mice. *Cell* **88**, 131–41.

Hwa, J. J., Ghibaudi, L., Gao, J. & Parker, E. M. (2001). Central melanocortin system modulates energy intake and expenditure of obese and lean Zucker rats. *Am. J. Physiol. Regul. Integr. Comp. Physiol.* **281**, R444–51.

Irani, B. G. & Haskell-Luevano, C. (2005). Feeding effects of melanocortin ligands – a historical perspective. *Peptides* **26**, 1788–99.

Kask, A., Rago, L., Wikberg, J. E. & Schioth, H. B. (2000). Differential effects of melanocortin peptides on ingestive behaviour in rats: evidence against the involvement of MC(3) receptor in the regulation of food intake. *Neurosci. Lett.* **283**, 1–4.

Kim, Y. W., Choi, D. W., Park, Y. H. *et al.* (2005). Leptin-like effects of MTII are augmented in MSG-obese rats. *Regul. Pept.* **127**, 63–70.

Kishi, T., Aschkenasi, C. J., Lee, C. E., Mountjoy, K. G., Saper, C. B. & Elmquist, J. K. (2003). Expression of melanocortin 4 receptor mRNA in the central nervous system of the rat. *J. Comp. Neurol.* **457**, 213–35.

Klusa, V., Svirskis, S., Opmane, B., Muceniece, R. & Wikberg, J. E. (1999). Behavioural responses of gamma-MSH peptides administered into the rat ventral tegmental area. *Acta Physiol. Scand.* **167**, 99–104.

Knudtzon, J. (1984). Alpha-melanocyte stimulating hormone increases plasma levels of glucagon and insulin in rabbits. *Life Sci.* **34**, 547–54.

Korner, J., Wissig, S., Kim, A., Conwell, I. M. & Wardlaw, S. L. (2003). Effects of agouti-related protein on metabolism and hypothalamic neuropeptide gene expression. *J. Neuroendocrinol.* **15**, 1116–21.

Krude, H., Biebermann, H., Luck, W., Horn, R., Brabant, G. & Gruters, A. (1998). Severe early-onset obesity, adrenal insufficiency and red hair pigmentation caused by POMC mutations in humans. *Nat. Genet.* **19**, 155–7.

Laurent, V., Jaubert-Miazza, L., Desjardins, R., Day, R. & Lindberg, I. (2004). Biosynthesis of proopiomelanocortin-derived peptides in prohormone convertase 2 and 7B2 null mice. *Endocrinology* **145**, 519–28.

Lee, Y. S., Challis, B. G., Thompson, D. A. *et al.* (2006). A POMC variant implicates beta-melanocyte-stimulating hormone in the control of human energy balance. *Cell Metab.* **3**, 135–40.

Li, G., Zhang, Y., Wilsey, J. T. & Scarpace, P. J. (2004). Unabated anorexic and enhanced thermogenic responses to melanotan II in diet-induced obese rats despite reduced melanocortin 3 and 4 receptor expression. *J. Endocrinol.* **182**, 123–32.

Li, G., Zhang, Y., Wilsey, J. T. & Scarpace, P. J. (2005). Hypothalamic pro-opiomelanocortin gene delivery ameliorates obesity and glucose intolerance in aged rats. *Diabetologia* **48**, 2376–85.

Li, Y. Z. & Davidowa, H. (2004). Food deprivation decreases responsiveness of ventromedial hypothalamic neurons to melanocortins. *J. Neurosci. Res.* **77**, 596–602.

Lindblom, J., Schioth, H. B., Larsson, A., Wikberg, J. E. & Bergstrom, L. (1998). Autoradiographic discrimination of melanocortin receptors indicates that the MC3 subtype dominates in the medial rat brain. *Brain Res.* **810**, 161–71.

Lindblom, J., Opmane, B., Mutulis, F. *et al.* (2001). The MC4 receptor mediates alpha-MSH induced release of nucleus accumbens dopamine. *Neuroreport* **12**, 2155–8.

Liu, H., Kishi, T., Roseberry, A. G. *et al.* (2003). Transgenic mice expressing green fluorescent protein under the control of the melanocortin-4 receptor promoter. *J. Neurosci.* **23**, 7143–54.

Lloyd, D. J., Bohan, S. & Gekakis, N. (2006). Obesity, hyperphagia and increased metabolic efficiency in Pc1 mutant mice. *Hum. Mol. Genet.* **15**, 1884–93.

Lu, D., Willard, D., Patel, I. R. *et al.* (1994). Agouti protein is an antagonist of the melanocyte-stimulating-hormone receptor. *Nature* **371**, 799–802.

Luquet, S., Perez, F. A., Hnasko, T. S. & Palmiter, R. D. (2005). NPY/AgRP neurons are essential for feeding in adult mice but can be ablated in neonates. *Science* **310**, 683–5.

MacNeil, D. J., Howard, A. D., Guan, X. *et al.* (2002). The role of melanocortins in body weight regulation: opportunities for the treatment of obesity. *Eur. J. Pharmacol.* **440**, 141–57.

Makimura, H., Mizuno, T. M., Mastaitis, J. W., Agami, R. & Mobbs, C. V. (2002). Reducing hypothalamic AGRP by RNA interference increases metabolic rate and decreases body weight without influencing food intake. *BMC Neurosci.* **3**, 18.

Marks, D. L., Ling, N. & Cone, R. D. (2001). Role of the central melanocortin system in cachexia. *Cancer Res.* **61**, 1432–8.

Marks, D. L., Hruby, V., Brookhart, G. & Cone, R. D. (2006). The regulation of food intake by selective stimulation of the type 3 melanocortin receptor (MC3R). *Peptides* **27**, 259–64.

Marsh, D. J., Hollopeter, G., Huszar, D. *et al.* (1999). Response of melanocortin-4 receptor-deficient mice to anorectic and orexigenic peptides. *Nat. Genet.* **21**, 119–22.

Martin, W. J. & MacIntyre, D. E. (2004). Melanocortin receptors and erectile function. *Eur. Urol.* **45**, 706–13.

Mayer, J. P., Hsiung, H. M., Flora, D. B. *et al.* (2005). Discovery of a beta-MSH-derived MC-4R selective agonist. *J. Med. Chem.* **48**, 3095–8.

McMinn, J. E., Wilkinson, C. W., Havel, P. J., Woods, S. C. & Schwartz, M. W. (2000). Effect of intracerebroventricular alpha-MSH on food intake, adiposity, c-Fos induction, and neuropeptide expression. *Am. J. Physiol. Regul. Integr. Comp. Physiol.* **279**, R695–703.

Menyhert, J., Wittmann, G., Hrabovszky, E., Keller, E., Liposits, Z. & Fekete, C. (2006). Interconnection between orexigenic neuropeptide Y- and anorexigenic alpha-melanocyte stimulating hormone-synthesizing neuronal systems of the human hypothalamus. *Brain Res.* **1076**, 101–5.

Millington, G. W., Tung, Y. C., Hewson, A. K., O'Rahilly, S. & Dickson, S. L. (2001). Differential effects of alpha-, beta- and gamma(2)-melanocyte-stimulating hormones on hypothalamic neuronal activation and feeding in the fasted rat. *Neuroscience* **108**, 437–45.

Mizuno, T. M., Kelley, K. A., Pasinetti, G. M., Roberts, J. L. & Mobbs, C. V. (2003). Transgenic neuronal expression of proopiomelanocortin attenuates hyperphagic response to fasting and reverses metabolic impairments in leptin-deficient obese mice. *Diabetes* **52**, 2675–83.

Mounien, L., Bizet, P., Boutelet, I., Vaudry, H. & Jegou, S. (2005). Expression of melanocortin MC3 and MC4 receptor mRNAs by neuropeptide Y neurons in the rat arcuate nucleus. *Neuroendocrinology* **82**, 164–70.

Mountjoy, K. G., Mortrud, M. T., Low, M. J., Simerly, R. B. & Cone, R. D. (1994). Localization of the melanocortin-4 receptor (MC4-R) in neuroendocrine and autonomic control circuits in the brain. *Mol. Endocrinol.* **8**, 1298–308.

Mountjoy, K. G., Wu, C. S., Cornish, J. & Callon, K. E. (2003). alpha-MSH and desacetyl-Alpha-MSH signaling through melanocortin receptors. *Ann. N. Y. Acad. Sci.* **994**, 58–65.

Nargund, R. P., Strack, A. M. & Fong, T. M. (2006). Melanocortin-4 receptor (MC4R) agonists for the treatment of obesity. *J. Med. Chem.* **49**, 4035–43.

Navarro, M., Cubero, I., Chen, A. S. *et al.* (2005). Effects of melanocortin receptor activation and blockade on ethanol intake: a possible role for the melanocortin-4 receptor. *Alcohol Clin. Exp. Res.* **29**, 949–57.

Nijenhuis, W. A., Oosterom, J. & Adan, R. A. (2001). AgRP(83-132) acts as an inverse agonist on the human-melanocortin-4 receptor. *Mol. Endocrinol.* **15**, 164–71.

Nonogaki, K. (2000). New insights into sympathetic regulation of glucose and fat metabolism. *Diabetologia* **43**, 533–49.

Obici, S., Feng, Z., Tan, J., Liu, L., Karkanias, G. & Rossetti, L. (2001). Central melanocortin receptors regulate insulin action. *J. Clin. Invest.* **108**, 1079–85.

Ollmann, M. M., Wilson, B. D., Yang, Y. K. *et al.* (1997). Antagonism of central melanocortin receptors in vitro and in vivo by agouti-related protein. *Science* **278**, 135–8.

Palkovits, M., Mezey, E. & Eskay, R. L. (1987). Pro-opiomelanocortin-derived peptides (ACTH/beta-endorphin/alpha-MSH) in brainstem baroreceptor areas of the rat. *Brain Res.* **436**, 323–38.

Phan, L. K., Chung, W. K. & Leibel, R. L. (2006). The mahoganoid mutation (Mgrn1md) improves insulin sensitivity in mice with mutations in the melanocortin signaling pathway independently of effects on adiposity. *Am. J. Physiol. Endocrinol. Metab.* **291**, E611–20.

Pierroz, D. D., Ziotopoulou, M., Ungsunan, L., Moschos, S., Flier, J. S. & Mantzoros, C. S. (2002). Effects of acute and chronic administration of the melanocortin agonist MTII in mice with diet-induced obesity. *Diabetes* **51**, 1337–45.

Poggioli, R., Vergoni, A. V. & Bertolini, A. (1986). ACTH-(1-24) and alpha-MSH antagonize feeding behavior stimulated by kappa opiate agonists. *Peptides* **7**, 843–8.

Pritchard, L. E., Turnbull, A. V. & White, A. (2002). Pro-opiomelanocortin processing in the hypothalamus: impact on melanocortin signalling and obesity. *J. Endocrinol.* **172**, 411–21.

Pritchard, L. E., Armstrong, D., Davies, N. *et al.* (2004). Agouti-related protein (83-132) is a competitive antagonist at the human melanocortin-4 receptor: no evidence for differential interactions with pro-opiomelanocortin-derived ligands. *J. Endocrinol.* **180**, 183–91.

Qian, S., Chen, H., Weingarth, D. *et al.* (2002). Neither agouti-related protein nor neuropeptide Y is critically required for the regulation of energy homeostasis in mice. *Mol. Cell Biol.* **22**, 5027–35.

Raposinho, P. D., White, R. B. & Aubert, M. L. (2003). The melanocortin agonist Melanotan-II reduces the orexigenic and adipogenic effects of neuropeptide Y (NPY) but does not affect the NPY-driven suppressive effects on the gonadotropic and somatotropic axes in the male rat. *J. Neuroendocrinol.* **15**, 173–81.

Robbins, L. S., Nadeau, J. H., Johnson, K. R. *et al.* (1993). Pigmentation phenotypes of variant extension locus alleles result from point mutations that alter MSH receptor function. *Cell* **72**, 827–34.

Romijn, J. A. & Fliers, E. (2005). Sympathetic and parasympathetic innervation of adipose tissue: metabolic implications. *Curr. Opin. Clin. Nutr. Metab. Care* **8**, 440–4.

Roselli-Rehfuss, L., Mountjoy, K. G., Robbins, L. S. *et al.* (1993). Identification of a receptor for gamma melanotropin and other proopiomelanocortin peptides in the hypothalamus and limbic system. *Proc. Natl. Acad. Sci. USA* **90**, 8856–60.

Rossi, M., Kim, M. S., Morgan, D. G. *et al.* (1998). A C-terminal fragment of Agouti-related protein increases feeding and antagonizes the effect of alpha-melanocyte stimulating hormone in vivo. *Endocrinology* **139**, 4428–31.

Rothwell, N. J. & Stock, M. J. (1985). Acute and chronic effects of ACTH on thermogenesis and brown adipose tissue in the rat. *Comp. Biochem. Physiol. A.* **81**, 99–102.

Savontaus, E., Breen, T. L., Kim, A., Yang, L. M., Chua, S. C. Jr. & Wardlaw, S. L. (2004). Metabolic effects of transgenic melanocyte-stimulating hormone overexpression in lean and obese mice. *Endocrinology* **145**, 3881–91.

Schioth, H. B., Haitina, T., Ling, M. K. *et al.* (2005). Evolutionary conservation of the structural, pharmacological, and genomic characteristics of the melanocortin receptor subtypes. *Peptides* **26**, 1886–900.

Shimizu, H., Shargill, N. S., Bray, G. A., Yen, T. T. & Gesellchen, P. D. (1989). Effects of MSH on food intake, body weight and coat color of the yellow obese mouse. *Life Sci.* **45**, 543–52.

Shimizu, H., Tanaka, Y., Sato, N. & Mori, M. (1995). Alpha-melanocyte-stimulating hormone (MSH) inhibits insulin secretion in HIT-T 15 cells. *Peptides* **16**, 605–8.

Small, C. J., Kim, M. S., Stanley, S. A. *et al.* (2001). Effects of chronic central nervous system administration of agouti-related protein in pair-fed animals. *Diabetes* **50**, 248–54.

Small, C. J., Liu, Y. L., Stanley, S. A. *et al.* (2003). Chronic CNS administration of Agouti-related protein (Agrp) reduces energy expenditure. *Int. J. Obes. Relat. Metab. Disord.* **27**, 530–3.

Smart, J. L., Tolle, V. & Low, M. J. (2006). Glucocorticoids exacerbate obesity and insulin resistance in neuron-specific proopiomelanocortin-deficient mice. *J. Clin. Invest.* **116**, 495–505.

Smart, J. L., Tolle, V., Otero-Corchon, V. & Low, M. J. (2007). Central dysregulation of the hypothalamic-pituitary-adrenal axis in neuron-specific proopiomelanocortin-deficient mice. *Endocrinology.* **148**, 647–59.

Smith, M. A., Hisadome, K., Al-Qassab, H., Heffron, H., Withers, D. J. & Ashford, M. L. (2006). Melanocortins and AGRP modulate mouse arcuate nucleus POMC and

RIPCre neuron excitability by alteration of resting potassium conductances. *J. Physiol.* (in press)

Song, C. K., Jackson, R. M., Harris, R. B., Richard, D. & Bartness, T. J. (2005). Melanocortin-4 receptor mRNA is expressed in sympathetic nervous system outflow neurons to white adipose tissue. *Am. J. Physiol. Regul. Integr. Comp. Physiol.* **289**, R1467–76.

Song, Y., Golling, G., Thacker, T. L. & Cone, R. D. (2003). Agouti-related protein (AGRP) is conserved and regulated by metabolic state in the zebrafish, *Danio rerio*. *Endocrine* **22**, 257–65.

Srinivasan, S., Lubrano-Berthelier, C., Govaerts, C. *et al.* (2004). Constitutive activity of the melanocortin-4 receptor is maintained by its N-terminal domain and plays a role in energy homeostasis in humans. *J. Clin. Invest.* **114**, 1158–64.

Ste Marie, L., Miura, G. I., Marsh, D. J., Yagaloff, K. & Palmiter, R. D. (2000). A metabolic defect promotes obesity in mice lacking melanocortin-4 receptors. *Proc. Natl. Acad. Sci. USA* **97**, 12 339–44.

Strader, A. D., Schioth, H. B. & Buntin, J. D. (2003). The role of the melanocortin system and the melanocortin-4 receptor in ring dove (*Streptopelia risoria*) feeding behavior. *Brain Res.* **960**, 112–21.

Sutton, G. M., Duos, B., Patterson, L. M. & Berthoud, H. R. (2005). Melanocortinergic modulation of cholecystokinin-induced suppression of feeding through extracellular signal-regulated kinase signaling in rat solitary nucleus. *Endocrinology* **146**, 3739–47.

Tallam, L. S., Kuo, J. J., da Silva, A. A. & Hall, J. E. (2004). Cardiovascular, renal, and metabolic responses to chronic central administration of agouti-related peptide. *Hypertension* **44**, 853–8.

Thiele, T. E., van Dijk, G., Yagaloff, K. A. *et al.* (1998). Central infusion of melanocortin agonist MTII in rats: assessment of c-Fos expression and taste aversion. *Am. J. Physiol.* **274**, R248–54.

Tung, Y. C., Piper, S. J., Yeung, D., O'Rahilly, S. & Coll, A. P. (2006). A comparative study of the central effects of specific proopiomelancortin (POMC)-derived melanocortin peptides on food intake and body weight in pomc null mice. *Endocrinology* **147**, 5940–7.

Uno, K., Katagiri, H., Yamada, T. *et al.* (2006). Neuronal pathway from the liver modulates energy expenditure and systemic insulin sensitivity. *Science* **312**, 1656–9.

Vaughan, C., Moore, M., Haskell-Luevano, C. & Rowland, N. E. (2006). Food motivated behavior of melanocortin-4 receptor knockout mice under a progressive ratio schedule. *Peptides* **27**, 2829–35.

Williams, D. L., Grill, H. J., Weiss, S. M., Baird, J. P. & Kaplan, J. M. (2002). Behavioral processes underlying the intake suppressive effects of melanocortin 3/4 receptor activation in the rat. *Psychopharmacology (Berl.)* **161**, 47–53.

Williams, D. L., Bowers, R. R., Bartness, T. J., Kaplan, J. M. & Grill, H. J. (2003). Brainstem melanocortin 3/4 receptor stimulation increases uncoupling protein gene expression in brown fat. *Endocrinology* **144**, 4692–7.

Wortley, K. E., Anderson, K. D., Yasenchak, J. et al. (2005). Agouti-related protein-deficient mice display an age-related lean phenotype. *Cell Metab.* **2**, 421-7.

Yasuda, T., Masaki, T., Kakuma, T. & Yoshimatsu, H. (2004). Hypothalamic melanocortin system regulates sympathetic nerve activity in brown adipose tissue. *Exp. Biol. Med. (Maywood)* **229**, 235-9.

Yaswen, L., Diehl, N., Brennan, M. B. & Hochgeschwender, U. (1999). Obesity in the mouse model of pro-opiomelanocortin deficiency responds to peripheral melanocortin. *Nat. Med.* **5**, 1066-70.

Zhang, Y., Matheny, M., Tumer, N. & Scarpace, P. J. (2004). Aged-obese rats exhibit robust responses to a melanocortin agonist and antagonist despite leptin resistance. *Neurobiol. Aging* **25**, 1349-60.

Zheng, H., Patterson, L. M., Phifer, C. B. & Berthoud, H. R. (2005). Brain stem melanocortinergic modulation of meal size and identification of hypothalamic POMC projections. *Am. J. Physiol. Regul. Integr. Comp. Physiol.* **289**, R247-58.

Zhu, X., Zhou, A., Dey, A. et al. (2002). Disruption of PC1/3 expression in mice causes dwarfism and multiple neuroendocrine peptide processing defects. *Proc. Natl. Acad. Sci. USA* **99**, 10293-8.

8

Role of opiate peptides in regulating energy balance

RICHARD J. BODNAR AND ALLEN S. LEVINE

The endogenous opioid system, initially characterized over 30 years ago, is a primary example of a multifunctional neural system involved in a wide range of basic homeostatic behaviors, including pain control, sexual behavior, learning and memory, reward, addiction and motivation, immune function, thermoregulatory, cardiovascular and respiratory processes, and as this review indicates, the regulation of energy balance through the modulation of food intake. Given the complexity and breadth of both the endogenous opioid system itself and the complex nature of energy regulation, this review is designed to inform the reader of the systematic steps taken by the field as a whole to understand their interaction. Thus, this review will focus on: (a) discovery and characterization of the endogenous opioids and their receptors, (b) early evidence involving the opioid system in ingestive behavior, (c) the role of opioids in rewarding aspects of food intake, (d) the role of macronutrient choice in opioid-induced feeding, (e) the specific roles of opiate receptor subtypes and specific brain sites in regulating opioid-induced feeding, (f) molecular mechanisms governing opioid-induced feeding, and (g) interactions of opioid-induced feeding with dopamine and other orexigenic neuropeptides.

1.   **Discovery and characterization of the endogenous opioids and their receptors**

The existence of an endogenous receptor in animals that bound opiates was reported in 1973 (Pert & Snyder, 1973; Simon *et al.*, 1973; Terenius, 1973).

Neurobiology and Obesity, ed. Jenni Harvey and Dominic J. Withers. Published by Cambridge University Press. © Cambridge University Press 2008

Shortly thereafter, it became apparent that multiple subtypes (mu, delta and kappa) of the receptor existed (Martin *et al.*, 1976; Lord *et al.*, 1977). Three corresponding classes of opioid peptides and their prohormone precursor genes were then characterized: endorphins (proopiomelanocortin; POMC: Mains *et al.*, 1977; Roberts *et al.*, 1979), enkephalins (pre-pro-enkephalin: Hughes *et al.*, 1975; Kimura *et al.*, 1980), and dynorphins (pre-pro-dynorphin: Goldstein *et al.*, 1981; Kangawa *et al.*, 1981). Although there were early attempts to describe three parallel opioid receptor and peptide systems (mu opioid receptor with beta-endorphin (BEND) and related peptides; delta opioid receptor with enkephalins and related peptides; kappa opioid receptor with dynorphin (DYN) and related peptides) (Akil *et al.*, 1984), it quickly became apparent that there was considerable cross-talk among these opioid peptide and receptor systems. Subsequently, in the early 1990s, the opioid receptors were cloned and sequenced: mu (MOP), delta (DOP) and kappa (KOP) (Uhl *et al.*, 1994; Kieffer, 1995), and indeed functional genomics identified a novel "orphan" opioid receptor (NOP) and its corresponding endogenous opioid peptide and prohormone, OFQ/N (pre-pro-orphanin: Meunier *et al.*, 1995; Reinscheid *et al.*, 1995). Finally, a new mu-selective opioid peptide group, the endomorphins were identified (Zadina *et al.*, 1997).

Classic opioid receptors were further subdivided based upon biochemical and pharmacological evidence: mu (mu-1 and mu-2; Wolozin & Pasternak, 1981; Pasternak & Wood, 1986), delta (delta-1 and delta-2; Jiang *et al.*, 1991; Mattia *et al.*, 1991) and kappa (kappa-1, kappa-2 and kappa-3; Nock *et al.*, 1988; Zukin *et al.*, 1988; Clark *et al.*, 1989) subtypes. Thus, in addition to more general non-peptide opioid antagonists (e.g., naloxone, naltrexone) and mu (morphine) and kappa (ketocyclazocine) agonists, receptor subtype characterization was aided in large part by the development of selective mu agonists (e.g., D-Ala2, M-Phe3, Gly-ol4-enkephalin (DAMGO)) and antagonists (e.g., beta-funaltrexamine (BFNA)), mu-1 antagonists (e.g., naloxonazine), delta-1 (e.g., D-Pen2, D-Pen5-enkephalin (DPDPE)) and delta-2 (e.g., Deltorphin (DELT)) agonists, delta antagonists (e.g., naltrindole), kappa-1 (e.g., U50488H) and kappa-3 (e.g., naloxone benzoylhydrazone (NalBzOH) agonists and kappa antagonists (e.g., nor-binaltorphamine (NBNI)).

2.   Opioids and feeding behaviour: early studies

The initial observation by Holtzman (1974) that systemic administration of the opioid antagonist, naloxone, significantly reduced food intake elicited by food deprivation supported earlier observations that chronic administration of morphine increased food intake after repeated injections

(Martin *et al.*, 1963; Kumar *et al.*, 1971). A direct role for endogenous opioid peptides was initially established by Grandison & Guidotti (1977) demonstrating that BEND administration directly into the ventromedial hypothalamus (VMH) stimulated food intake, and supported by the observation that BEND levels were associated with overeating in genetically obese *ob/ob* mice and *fa/fa* rats (Margules *et al.*, 1978). Early opiate agonist studies demonstrated that systemic administration of morphine increased feeding under both non-deprived and non-dependent conditions (Sanger & McCarthy, 1980; Sanger, 1981; Lowy & Yim, 1983) and also increased water intake (Cooper, 1981; Czech *et al.*, 1984). Ketocyclazocine and other kappa compounds increased food intake following systemic administration (Walker *et al.*, 1980; Morley & Levine, 1981, 1983; Sanger & McCarthy, 1981; Locke *et al.*, 1982; Morley *et al.*, 1982, 1985; Levine & Morley, 1983; Lowy & Yim, 1983; Cooper *et al.*, 1985b, 1985d; Jackson & Cooper, 1985, 1986; Gosnell *et al.*, 1986a). Further, intraventricular administration of enkephalin analogues increased feeding (Jackson & Sewell, 1985a; Gosnell *et al.*, 1986a; Gosnell & Majchrzak, 1989) and drinking (DeCaro *et al.*, 1979) in rats. Administration of mixed opioid agonists (e.g., methadone, buprenorphine and butorphanol) also increased free feeding (Rudski *et al.*, 1992, 1995).

Early opiate antagonist studies with naloxone and naltrexone demonstrated significant decreases in both food and water intake in deprived and non-deprived rats and mice (Holtzman, 1975; Maickel *et al.*, 1977; Brown & Holtzman, 1979; Frenk & Rogers, 1979; Cooper, 1980; Levine *et al.*, 1990a). In contrast, chronic systemic naltrexone treatment paradoxically increased body weight and food intake in Syrian hamsters, whereas acute naltrexone reduced intake in this species only in animals subjected to long durations of deprivation (Jones & Corp, 2003). Chronic administration of naloxone decreased food and water intake as well as weight in normal (Brands *et al.*, 1979; Jalowiec *et al.*, 1981; Ostrowski *et al.*, 1981; Shimomura *et al.*, 1982; Marks-Kaufman *et al.*, 1984; Olson *et al.*, 1985), hypothalamically lesioned obese (King *et al.*, 1979) and genetically obese (Recant *et al.*, 1980; Thornhill *et al.*, 1982; McLaughlin & Baile, 1983, 1984) mice and rats. The long-acting general opioid antagonists, beta-chlornaltrexamine and LY255582, also decreased intake, weight and opioid-induced feeding in normal (Gosnell *et al.*, 1987; Levine *et al.*, 1991b) and obese (Shaw *et al.*, 1990) rats. These inhibitory effects of general opioid antagonists were most apparent in potently reducing intake of palatable solutions and diets, including sucrose, saccharin and fats (e.g., Apfelbaum & Mandenoff, 1981; Mandenoff *et al.*, 1982; Lynch & Libby, 1983; Cooper *et al.*, 1985a, 1985c). General opioid antagonists also reduced all forms of fluid consumption in choice tests between sodium chloride solutions and water in both water-deprived and hypophysectomized rats (Brown & Holtzman, 1980; Brown et al., 1980; Czech & Stein, 1980; Siviy et al., 1981; Czech et al., 1983; Cooper & Gilbert, 1984; Ukai et al., 1988) as well as water intake following angiotensin II and hypertonic saline administration (Holtzman, 1975; Rowland, 1982).

Naloxone also reduced intake following glucodeprivation induced by 2-deoxy-D-glucose (2DG: Lowy et al., 1980) to a greater degree than insulin (Levine & Morley, 1981; Ostrowski et al., 1981; Rowland & Bartness, 1982). Indeed, diabetic rats displayed an enhanced inhibitory effect upon deprivation-induced feeding by naloxone (Levine et al., 1982a, 1985). Naloxone also decreased stress-induced feeding induced by tail-pinch (Lowy et al., 1980; Morley & Levine, 1980; Bertiere et al., 1984) and following electrical stimulation of the lateral hypo-thalamus (Carr & Simon, 1983; Jenck et al., 1986).

3.   Opioids and reward-related feeding

A large body of data has accumulated suggesting that opioids are involved in reward-related feeding behavior. For example, there seems to be a special connection between opioid ligands, their receptors and sweet tastants. Naloxone, an opioid antagonist, was shown to decrease the intake of sucrose solutions much more effectively than water intake (Levine et al., 1982b). Also, repeated injection of naltrexone decreases ingestion of laboratory chow plus a 32% sucrose solution more effectively than intake of chow alone (Marks-Kaufman et al., 1984). Mice that are deficient in opioid receptors prefer sac-charin less than do control mice (Yirmiya et al., 1988). Opioid blockade also inhibits the preference for an orange odor paired with intraoral sucrose infu-sion in 6-day-old rats (Shide & Blass, 1991). Levine and colleagues have reported that peripheral naloxone decreases intake of sweet diets more effectively than non-sweet diets (Levine et al., 1995). Zhang and Kelly found that the mu opioid DAMGO increased saccharin intake when injected into the nucleus accumbens (Zhang & Kelly, 2002). A variety of studies have attempted to find which opioid receptors are involved in intake of sweet diets. While central injection of mu and kappa opioid antagonists decrease intake of sweet diets, delta-1 opioid antagonists do not (Beczkowska et al., 1992). Similarly, sham-fed sucrose also is blocked by mu and kappa antagonists, but not by mu-1 or delta antagonists, suggesting a strong orosensory component (Leventhal et al., 1995). Yet, delta antagonists decrease saccharin intake, whereas mu and kappa antagonists do not (Beczkowska et al., 1993). Thus, opioid receptor subtypes may differentially affect intake of sweet tastants.

The rewarding properties of sucrose solutions, as reflected by facial expres-sions of rats in the taste reactivity test, are decreased by injection of naltrexone

(Parker *et al.*, 1992). Humans also report decreased pleasure from sweet solutions following opioid receptor blockade (Fantino *et al.*, 1986; Bertino *et al.*, 1991; Arbisi *et al.*, 1999). One reason for a decrease in the hedonic property of sucrose following opioid receptor blockade might be due to a change in the ability to discriminate or detect sweet taste. O'Hare *et al.* found that the opioid antagonist naloxone did not alter sucrose discrimination in rats trained to discriminate a 5% or 10% sucrose solution from water using an operant procedure (O'Hare *et al.*, 1997). Arbisi and co-workers found that oral naltrexone failed to affect sucrose taste discrimination in humans when compared with oral placebo (Arbisi *et al.*, 1999). Therefore, it is unlikely that opioids change pleasure derived from sweets by altering taste.

Several investigators have examined whether opioid receptor blockade alters the expression or development of preferences for sweet tastants. In one of these studies, Levine and co-workers gave rats a choice between a diet high in sucrose and high in starch for 10 days (Levine *et al.*, 2002). As expected, they found that rats preferred the sucrose-rich diet. After this period, the rats were given the starch diet alone for 10 days. At the end of this phase the rats were implanted with a naltrexone- or saline-filled miniosmotic pump (70 µg/h, 1.7 mg/day) for 10 days and once again given the high sucrose and high starch diet. Those rats that were implanted with the pump containing naltrexone ingested about 33% of their energy from the sucrose diet, whereas the rats implanted with the saline-filled pump ate about 77% of their energy from the sucrose diet. Lynch (1986) reported that injection of naloxone suppressed the increase in the development of a preference for a saccharin solution. Mehiel (1996) found that a conditioned preference for sugar was attenuated by opioid receptor blockade. Ramirez (1997) noted that naloxone decreased flavor acceptance conditioned with intragastric maltodextrin infusion.

In contrast to the above studies, Bodnar and Sclafani's laboratories did not find that opioids are involved in the development of a sweet taste preference. These investigators studied whether naltrexone might alter either acquisition and/or expression of a conditioned flavor preference in sham-fed rats given a flavor paired with sucrose or saccharin solutions. Naltrexone decreased intake of the flavor paired with the preferred sucrose solution, but did not affect acquisition or expression of the preference (Yu *et al.*, 1999); an identical pattern of effects was found using fructose as the conditioned stimulus in real-feeding rats (Baker *et al.*, 2004). While naltrexone decreased intake, it also did not affect acquisition or expression of a preference associated with an intragastric infusion of a 16% sucrose solution (Azzara *et al.*, 2000). Yet Bodnar and Sclafani also reported that naltrexone inhibited expression, but not acquisition of a place preference associated with sucrose (Delamater *et al.*, 2000). Given that all of these studies are dependent on conditioning and/or learning, and since opioids affect learning (Canli et al., 1990), it seems feasible that conditioned-taste preferences might respond differently to opioid receptor blockade than unconditioned ingestion of food or fluids.

Levine and colleagues have suggested that a "hedonic deprivation state" might involve endogenous opioids (Levine & Billington, 2004; Lowe & Levine, 2005). When rats were fed an isocaloric amount of a high corn starch diet and a high fat/sucrose diet, gene expression of endogenous opioids resembled that seen after energy deprivation (Welch et al., 1996). Others have also reported that restriction of a preferred diet results in altered opioid gene expression similar to that seen with food deprivation or restriction (Levin & Dunn-Meynell, 2002; Kelley et al., 2003). Thus, restraining the intake of a palatable diet results in a "neural opioid state," that resembles energy restriction, even though energy was not restricted. Colantuoni and co-workers reported that when a high dose of naloxone was administered to rats chronically ingesting a glucose solution, the rats displayed some behaviors similar to those observed after opiate withdrawal (Colantuoni et al., 2002). These authors also found increased mu opioid receptor binding in a variety of brain regions in rats chronically exposed to a glucose solution (Colantuoni et al., 2001).

4.   Effects of opioids on macronutrient intake

As discussed above, many investigations have led to the suggestion that opioids are important regulators of hedonic-related eating. Other studies have shown involvement of opioids in macronutrient intake and feeding associated with energy needs. Using techniques originally developed by Richter, some studies indicate that opioid agonists increase and antagonists decrease intake of high-fat diets more than intake of high-carbohydrate diets. Kelley's laboratory reported that injection of DAMGO, a mu opioid agonist, into the nucleus accumbens (NAC) resulted in a fourfold increase in the amount of a fat diet ingested, while only increasing intake of the carbohydrate intake by 75% (Zhang et al., 1998). When animals were given both diets concurrently, injection of DAMGO into the NAC increased intake of the high-fat diet compared with saline controls. Gosnell and co-workers first suggested that a rat's preference for a high-fat diet might affect whether opioids preferentially increase fat intake (Gosnell et al., 1990a). These investigators divided rats into carbohydrate or fat preferrers according to their baseline preference for such diets when presented at the same time. Morphine increased intake of the high-fat diet to a greater degree in rats that preferred the high-fat to the high-carbohydrate diet. Morphine increased intake of the high-carbohydrate diet to a greater extent in those rats that preferred the high-carbohydrate diet to the high-fat diet. Others have noted that opioid receptor blockade inhibits intake of preferred diets much more effectively than non-preferred diets. For example, peripheral injection of naloxone at a low 0.01 mg/kg dose decreased intake of a preferred diet, whereas a higher 3 mg/kg dose did not change intake of a non-preferred diet (Glass *et al.*, 1996). Welch and co-workers also found that diet preferences affect morphine-induced intake of high-carbohydrate and high-fat diets (Welch *et al.*, 1994). However, these investigators reported that morphine still increased high fat intake to a greater degree than high carbohydrate intake, even when baseline preferences were considered. Glass and co-workers reported that the site of injection can influence the efficacy of naltrexone on preferred and non-preferred diets (Glass *et al.*, 2000). Naltrexone decreased preferred diet intake more effectively than non-preferred diet intake after injection in the central nucleus of the amygdala, but decreased intake independent of preference when injected into the paraventricular nucleus of the hypothalamus (PVN).

5.   Effect of opioid receptor subtypes and injection sites in food intake

5.1   *Receptor subtype agonists and ventricular studies*

Utilization of opioid subreceptor ligands revealed a very complex system involved in opioid-related feeding. Mu or kappa antagonists inhibit feeding elicited by multiple opioid receptor agonists. For example, BFNA, the mu antagonist (Levine *et al.*, 1991a) and NBNI, the kappa antagonist (Levine *et al.*, 1990b) each reduced feeding elicited by mu, delta and kappa agonists. Morphine-induced feeding is also blocked by the selective mu-1 antagonist, naloxonazine (Mann *et al.*, 1988a). Likewise, intake induced by the endogenous opioid, BEND was significantly reduced by general, mu and kappa, but minimally affected by delta antagonism (Silva *et al.*, 2001). The mu antagonist-induced inhibition of BEND-induced feeding was more potent than delta and kappa opioid antagonists. Delta-selective antagonism decreased feeding under spontaneous and delta agonist-induced feeding (Jackson & Sewell, 1985a, 1985b). Yet, delta-1 (DPDPE) and delta-2 (DELT) agonist-induced feeding was differentially blocked by general, delta-1 and delta-2 antagonist pretreatment (Yu *et al.*, 1997). Further, significant increases in water intake could be induced by either delta-1 (DPDPE) or delta-2 (DELT) agonists, but sub-threshold doses of either agonist failed to alter the ED-50 of drinking induced by ANG II (Yu & Bodnar, 1997). In contrast, DYN-induced feeding was potently reduced by kappa antagonism, and reduced only by high doses of general and mu, but not delta opioid antagonists (Silva *et al.*, 2002a). The kappa agonist, butorphanol induced feeding that was reduced by kappa and mu but not delta antagonists (Levine *et al.*, 1994) and became more sensitive after food restriction (Hagan & Moss, 1991). Kappa agonists stimulated both fat (Drenowski *et al.*, 1992) and sucrose (Lynch & Burns, 1990) intake, yet produced a conditioned place aversion for sucrose (Tang & Collins, 1985). Kappa-1 agonist-induced stimulation of sucrose intake was blocked by insulin and/or kappa antagonism (Sipols *et al.*, 2002). Kappa-3 (NalBzOH) agonist-induced feeding was blocked by general, but not kappa-1 antagonism (Koch *et al.*, 1992). Kappa-1 (U50488H) and kappa-3 (NalBzOH), but not delta-1 (DPDPE) agonists mildly enhanced glucoprivic intake (Yu *et al.*, 1997), whereas all three major agonist classes stimulated intakes of sucrose (Ruegg *et al.*, 1997) and hypotonic saline (Gosnell & Majchrzak, 1990; Gosnell *et al.*, 1990b). Finally, OFQ/N and some of its synthetic pseudopeptides stimulated food intake in a naloxone-reversible manner, and altered c-fos immunoreactivity in the NTS, PVN, supraoptic nuclei, central nucleus of the amygdala, lateral septum and lateral habenula nucleus (Pomonis *et al.*, 1996; Stratford *et al.*, 1997; Olszewski *et al.*, 2000; Rizzi *et al.*, 2002).

Selective opioid antagonists differentially modulate normal food intake and body weight following such regulatory challenges as deprivation, glucoprivation and lipoprivation. Whereas the mu-selective opioid antagonist BFNA significantly reduced food and water intake under spontaneous (Millan & Morris, 1988; Ukai & Holtzman, 1988a) and deprived (Arjune *et al.*, 1990; Levine *et al.*, 1991a) conditions, the mu-1 opioid antagonist, naloxonazine significantly decreased deprivation-induced intake (Simone *et al.*, 1985) and intake and weight in both adult and adolescent animals (Mann *et al.*, 1988b). Kappa, but not delta-1 opioid antagonism also decreased deprivation-induced intake (Arjune & Bodnar, 1990; Levine *et al.*, 1990b; Arjune *et al.*, 1991; Jewett *et al.*, 2001). Chronic mu, mu-1, delta-1 and delta-2, but not kappa opioid antagonist treatment decreased weight and intake of a fat source during development of dietary obesity (Cole *et al.*, 1995). However, rats placed on high-carbohydrate or high-fat diets displayed greater weight gain on the latter diet which was affected to a greater extent by chronic mu, delta-2 or kappa-1 antagonist treatment (Cole *et al.*, 1999). Moreover, weight loss and intake reductions were noted in both lean heterozygote and obese homozygote Zucker rats following chronic mu, mu-1, delta-1, delta-2 or kappa-1 opioid antagonism (Cole *et al.*, 1997). Mu and kappa, but not mu-1, delta or delta-1 antagonists reduced glucoprivic feeding (Arjune & Bodnar, 1990; Arjune *et al.*, 1990, 1991; Beczkowska & Bodnar, 1991), whereas all three major antagonist classes reduced lipoprivic feeding (Stein *et al.*, 2000). Other induced forms of feeding were modulated by selective antagonists as well. Thus, feeding elicited by electrical stimulation of the LH was blocked by mu and kappa antagonists as well as by dynorphin antibodies (Schulz *et al.*, 1984; Carr *et al.*, 1987, 1989, 1993; Carr, 1990; Carr & Bak, 1990; Papadouka & Carr, 1994), an effect also shifted by food restriction (Abrahamsen *et al.*, 1995). In contrast, only mu and mu-1 antagonists reduced feeding elicited by tail-pinch stress (Hawkins *et al.*, 1992; Koch & Bodnar, 1993).

Mu opioid antagonism potently reduces water consumption induced by water deprivation, angiotensin II and isoproterenol (Beczkowska *et al.*, 1992; Glass *et al.*, 1994; Ruegg *et al.*, 1994). However, mu, mu-1, delta-1 and delta-2, but not kappa-1 antagonism decreased water deprivation-induced water intake in sham-drinking rats, indicating an orosensory component (Leventhal & Bodnar, 1996). Whereas mu receptor antagonism decreased intake of dilute sodium chloride solutions (Gosnell & Majchrzak, 1990), none of the selective opioid antagonists altered hypotonic or hypertonic saline intake in water-deprived rats (Bodnar *et al.*, 1995a).

5.2   Site-specific effects of opioid agonists upon feeding

Opioid agonists have been shown to increase food intake after injection into many brain sites. Understanding how opioid circuitry is integrated across a distributed network depends upon an inventory of such sites. Thus, increased food intake occurs following direct injection of mu agonists into the VMH and paraventricular (PVN) hypothalamic nuclei, amygdala, ventral tegmental area (VTA), NAC, parabrachial nucleus and nucleus tractus solitarius (NTS) (Bozarth & Wise, 1981; Tepperman *et al.*, 1981; Leibowitz & Hor, 1982; McLean & Hoebel, 1982; Tepperman & Hirst, 1983; Woods & Leibowitz, 1985; Majeed *et al.*, 1986; Mucha & Iversen, 1986; Jenck *et al.*, 1987; Gosnell, 1988; Stanley *et al.*, 1989; Evans & Vaccarino, 1990; Bakshi & Kelley, 1993a, 1993b; Noel & Wise, 1993, 1995; Devine & Wise, 1994; Badiani *et al.*, 1995; Kotz *et al.*, 1997; Wilson *et al.*, 2003), and an identical pattern of intracerebral effects occurs following enkephalin or delta agonist administration (Tepperman & Hirst, 1983; Cador *et al.*, 1986; Gosnell *et al.*, 1986b; Majeed *et al.*, 1986; Jenck *et al.*, 1987; Stanley *et al.*, 1989; Devine & Wise, 1994; Noel & Wise, 1995; Kotz *et al.*, 1997). Dynorphin, but not other kappa agonists, stimulates feeding following administration into the VMH, PVN, VTA and NAC, but not the amygdala (Gosnell *et al.*, 1986b; Majeed *et al.*, 1986; Gosnell, 1988; Hamilton & Bozarth, 1988; Nencini & Stewart, 1990; Noel & Wise, 1993). OFQ/N administered into the PVN or NAC stimulated food intake in a naloxone-reversible manner (Pomonis *et al.*, 1996; Stratford *et al.*, 1997; Polidori *et al.*, 2000). The opioid eating site within the NAC was shown to be in the medial caudal subregion of the NAC shell and the rostral ventral pallidum using c-fos immunohistochemistry (Pecina & Berridge, 2000).

A mapping study indicated that the ventral striatum (ventrolateral striatum, lateral and core) was more capable than the dorsal striatum to support DAMGO-induced feeding, and that such intake induced c-fos in the hypothalamus, VTA, SN and NTS (Zhang & Kelley, 2000). Further, PVN infusions of mu, but not delta or kappa agonists increased water intake in non-deprived rats (Summy-Long et al., 1981; Spencer et al., 1986; Ukai & Holtzman, 1988b).

5.3   Site-specific effects of opioid antagonists upon feeding

Like opioid agonists, opioid antagonists have been shown to affect feeding in a variety of brain regions. Feeding elicited by either mu or delta-1 opioid agonists in the NAC was significantly reduced by NAC pretreatment with mu, delta-1, delta-2 and kappa-1, but not mu-1 opioid antagonists (Ragnauth et al., 2000).

Correspondingly, mu agonist-induced feeding elicited from the VTA was significantly reduced by VTA same site pretreatment with general, mu and kappa-1, but not delta antagonists (Lamonte et al., 2002). Regional opioid–opioid interactions have also been observed in feeding behavior. Interactions between the PVN and the central nucleus of the amygdala revealed a unidirectional effect such that DAMGO-induced feeding elicited from the central nucleus of the amygdala was blocked by naltrexone pretreatment in the PVN, but DAMGO-induced feeding elicited from the PVN failed to be blocked by naltrexone pretreatment in the central nucleus of the amygdala (Giraudo et al., 1998a). A bidirectional opioid–opioid signaling pathway between the NTS and the central nucleus of the amygdala was observed such that DAMGO-induced feeding elicited from the central nucleus of the amygdala was blocked by naltrexone pretreatment in the NTS, and DAMGO-induced feeding elicited from the NTS was blocked by naltrexone pretreatment in the central nucleus of the amygdala (Giraudo et al., 1998b). Another bidirectional opioid–opioid signaling pathway between the PVN and the VTA has been demonstrated using the same agonist–antagonist approach between the two sites for the general opioid antagonist, naltrexone (Quinn et al., 2003). A final bidirectional opioid agonist–antagonist interaction occurs between the NAC and VTA in that feeding elicited by DAMGO in the NAC or VTA is blocked by naltrexone pretreatment in the alternate site (MacDonald et al., 2003) as well as by mu and kappa, but not delta opioid antagonists in the alternate site (Bodnar et al., 2005). These data argue conclusively that regional pathways interact to elicit coordinated feeding responses, and that opioid peptides and receptors are critical conduits in this process.

Selective antagonists administered into specific sites also affect intake driven by exposure to homeostatic challenges and hedonic stimuli. Thus, mu and kappa, but not delta opioid antagonists administered directly into the PVN strongly reduce deprivation-induced feeding, and to a lesser degree glucoprivic and palatable intake (Koch et al., 1995). Selective mu and kappa, but not mu-1 opioid antagonists administered directly into the NAC shell, but not the VTA significantly also decreased feeding elicited by either food deprivation or 2DG glucoprivation, and to a lesser degree palatable intake, whereas VTA delta-2 antagonists selectively decreased all three forms of intake (Bodnar et al., 1995b; Kelley et al., 1996; Ragnauth et al., 1997). Kappa opioid antagonists in the PBN significantly reduced feeding, but not the reinforcing effects elicited by electrical stimulation of the LH (Carr et al., 1991, 1993).

6.   Opioids and feeding: molecular models

6.1   Ingestive behaviors affect opioid peptide and receptor genes

Chronic food restriction respectively increases (midbrain) and decreases (amygdala, PBN, habenula) mu opioid binding, and respectively increases (BNST, ventral pallidum, medial preoptic area, PBN) and decreases (habenula) kappa opioid binding (Tsujii et al., 1986a; Wolinsky et al., 1994, 1996b). Chronic food restriction increases DYN fragments in the dorsomedial hypothalamus, VMH, PVN, NAC, BNST, cortex, striatum, midbrain and LH, while dynorphin and beta-endorphin are respectively decreased in the central amygdala and hypothalamus (Tsujii et al., 1986b; Berman et al., 1994, 1997; Kim et al., 1996). Indeed, the BNST, central nucleus of the amygdala and NAC display increased c-fos immunoreactivity following naltrexone administration in food-restricted rats, suggesting opioid-mediated inhibitory control (Carr et al., 1998) with similar actions observed for kappa and mu-selective antagonism (Carr et al., 1999). Combinations of food restriction and exercise increase supraoptic hypothalamic DYN as well as arcuate hypothalamic BEND (Aravich et al., 1993). Food deprivation lowers mRNA levels for the NOP receptor in the PVN, LH and amygdala, and pro-OFQ/N mRNA levels in the latter structure (Rodi et al., 2002). Streptozotocin-induced diabetes respectively increased and decreased DYN and BEND fragments in hypothalamic nuclei (Locatelli et al., 1986; Berman et al., 1995, 1997; Kim et al., 1999), whereas combined diabetes and food restriction respectively increased and decreased kappa (medial preoptic area) and mu (habenula) binding (Wolinsky et al., 1996a). Exposure to palatable sweet solutions increases hypothalamic DYN (Welch et al., 1996), and enhances naloxone-induced increases in c-fos activity in the amygdala (Pomonis et al., 2000). Exposure to a high-fat diet increased hypothalamic mu opioid receptors (Barnes et al., 2003), but reduced striatal enkephalin gene expression (Kelley et al., 2003).

6.2   Knockout and antisense approaches alter opioid-mediated ingestion

Two principal methods, the knockout and knockdown approaches, have been used to investigate the functional significance of opioid receptor genes in vivo. The knockout technique involves gene deletion, although pleiotropic effects, caused by potential compensatory expression of genes other than the knockout gene, are a possible confounding variable in functional assessment (Wahlestedt, 1994). Whereas operant food, but not ethanol responding was reduced in mice with met-enkephalin or BEND knockouts, the latter group was hyperphagic and obese, but showed normal stimulatory actions to opioid agonists, and normal inhibitory actions to opioid antagonists (Haywood *et al.*, 2002, 2004; Appleyard *et al.*, 2003; Low *et al.*, 2003). In contrast, mice lacking the pre-proenkephalin gene displayed deficits in emotional responses, but no changes in sensitivity to sucrose (Ragnauth *et al.*, 2001), but enkephalin-knockout mice failed to show naloxone-induced spontaneous and food-conditioned hypoactivity (Haywood & Low, 2005).

The knockdown technique involves the temporary elimination of the expression of a gene by administration of antisense oligodeoxynucleotides (AS ODN) (Pasternak & Standifer, 1995). The technique involves the use of short (18–25 bases) stretches of synthetic nucleic acids that are complementary to regions of cellular mRNA from a specific gene, and theoretically hybridize with complementary targeted mRNA to reduce targeted protein synthesis through translational blockade, splicing arrest, and/or RNase-H degradation of mRNA (Myers & Dean, 2000). AS ODN probes both selectively downregulate relevant mRNA and alter the related behavior in combined in vivo and in vitro studies (Standifer *et al.*, 1994, 1995). Selectivity of the AS technique is controlled by employing a missense (MS) ODN probe, differing from the desired AS ODN probe by the sequence reversal of two or more pairs of bases, and then demonstrating inactivity (Myers & Dean, 2000). This technique provides complimentary and converging evidence for the actions of opioid receptor subtype antagonists in identifying the role of specific opioid receptors in different forms of feeding, and has the two powerful advantages of selectivity and specificity over traditional antagonists. Whereas the mu (MOP) gene has four exons, the kappa (KOP), delta (DOP) and orphan (NOP) gene has three exons, and splice variants for these genes have been identified (Pan *et al.*, 1999, 2001). Thus, AS ODN probes, but not antagonists can specify which segment of the relevant gene is essential for the full expression of the functional ingestive behavior, and thereby provide more precise information about its molecular substrate.

This specificity is demonstrated by dissecting feeding responses induced by DAMGO, morphine and its active metabolite, morphine-6-glucuronide (M6G) which is both sensitive to mu and mu-1, but not delta or kappa-1 antagonists (Mann et al., 1988a; Leventhal et al., 1998b). AS ODN, but not MS ODN probes targeted against coding exon 1 and 4, but not coding exon 2 and 3 of the MOP gene significantly reduced feeding induced by DAMGO and morphine, whereas M6G-induced feeding was blocked by AS ODN probes targeted against either coding exons 2 and 3, but not coding exons 1 or 4 of the MOP gene (Leventhal et al., 1997, 1998b), paralleling AS ODN effects in analgesic assays (Rossi et al., 1995, 1997). Correspondingly AS ODN probes directed respectively against the DOP, KOP and NOP genes reduced feeding elicited by the delta-2 opioid agonist, DELT, the kappa-1 opioid agonist, U50488H and OFQ/N (Leventhal et al., 1998a, 1998b). BEND-induced feeding, primarily reduced by mu opioid antagonists, was especially sensitive to AS ODN, but not MS ODN probes directed against either coding exons 1, 3, or 4, but not exon 2 of the MOP opioid receptor gene, but not sensitive to AS ODN probes directed against coding exons 1, 2 or 3 of either the KOP, NOP or DOP opioid receptor genes (Silva et al., 2001), thereby displaying some similar molecular binding profiles with morphine and DAMGO (sensitivity to exon 1 AS probes) and M6G (sensitivity to exon 2 and 3 AS probes). Thus, BEND-induced feeding is mediated by different isoforms of the MOP gene. DYN-induced feeding, primarily reduced by kappa-1 antagonists, was especially sensitive to AS ODN, but not MS ODN probes directed against coding exons 1 and 2, but not 3 of the KOP and NOP opioid receptor genes, but relatively insensitive to AS ODN probes directed against the MOP or DOP opioid receptor genes (Silva et al., 2002a). Thus, the kappa opioid receptor appears to mediate DYN-induced feeding.

The sensitivity, selectivity and reliability of AS ODN probes to delineate opioid agonist-induced feeding allowed their use in examining opioid modulation of other physiological and pharmacological ingestive situations. Body weight and spontaneous food intake are reduced by AS, but not MS ODN probes targeting coding exons 1, 2, 3 and 4 of the MOP gene suggesting that the receptor responsible for these basal actions is completely encoded by this gene (Leventhal et al., 1996). Glucoprivic feeding, sensitive to mu and kappa, but not delta opioid receptor subtype antagonists, is similarly significantly reduced by AS probes directed against coding exons 1 and 2 of the MOP gene and coding exon 2 of the KOP gene, but not by AS probes directed against the DOP gene (Burdick et al., 1998). Lipoprivic feeding, sensitive to mu, kappa and delta opioid receptor subtype antagonists, is similarly significantly reduced by AS probes directed against coding exons 1, 2 and 3 of the MOP gene, coding exon 3 of the KOP gene, coding exons 1 and 2 of the NOP gene, and coding exon 1 of the DOP gene (Stein et al., 2000). The ability of mu and mu-1 antagonists (50–70%) to more potently reduce deprivation-induced food intake relative to kappa (30%) and delta (minimal) antagonists suggests a role for this receptor in this homeostatic challenge (Simone et al., 1985; Arjune & Bodnar, 1990; Arjune et al., 1990, 1991; Levine et al., 1990b, 1991a). A different pattern emerged in the use of opioid AS ODN probes such that AS ODN probes directed against exon 2 of the KOP gene produced pronounced effects, whereas AS ODN probes directed against exons 2, 3 or 4 of the MOP gene, exon 1 of the DOP gene, and exon 1 of the NOP gene produced significant though modest effects (Hadjimarkou et al., 2003). Thus, whereas antisense and antagonist effects upon deprivation-induced intake were consistent, the pattern of effects suggests that the classic mu opioid receptor MOP gene is not fully responsible for mu-mediated effects, and rather might be mediated by recently identified isoforms of the MOR-1 gene (Pan et al., 1999, 2001). To examine this, the opioid antagonist mediation of deprivation-induced feeding was compared in the rat and the mouse with the former showing the expected mu and kappa mediation, and the latter showing mu, delta and kappa mediation. AS ODN probes directed against exons of the KOP, NOP and DOP genes in the mouse produced significant reductions, whereas AS ODN probes directed against coding exons 2, 4, 7, 8 or 13 of the MOP gene and its isoforms continued to produce modest reductions. Therefore, the molecular target of mu antagonist-mediated effects upon deprivation-induced intake has not been identified (Hadjimarkou et al., 2004).

Given that opioid receptors mediate their effects through putative activation of G-proteins to which they are coupled and modulate the inhibition of cAMP (Reicine & Bell, 1993; Roerig, 1998), one can use the AS ODN technology to examine this inter-relationship. Thus, in complete agreement with opiate analgesic studies (Rossi et al., 1995; Standifer et al., 1996), morphine-induced feeding was significantly reduced by an AS probe directed against G_i alpha$_2$ and increased by an AS probe directed against G_s alpha. In contrast, M6G-induced feeding was significantly reduced by AS probes directed against either G_i alpha$_1$, G_i alpha$_3$ or $G_{x/z}$ alpha (Silva et al., 2000). Further, feeding induced by both BEND and DYN were significantly reduced by an AS probe directed against G_i alpha$_1$, indicating some similarity with that of M6G-induced feeding. However, an AS probe directed against G_o alpha also reduced DYN-induced feeding, whereas AS probes directed against G_i alpha$_2$ and G_i alpha$_3$ significantly increased BEND-induced feeding, implicating these biochemical cascades in these opioid-mediated ingestive responses (Silva et al., 2002b). As with opioid AS ODN probes, AS ODN probes directed against G-protein sub-units also modulate homeostatic ingestive responses. Thus, AS probes directed against G_o alpha and G_{oA} alpha significantly reduced meals at the beginning of the dark cycle (e.g., nocturnal feeding) when rats typically ingest most of their daily food ration (Plata-Salaman *et al.*, 1995). In examining deprivation-induced intake, AS probes directed against G_s alpha and G_q alpha produced the greatest reductions, and AS probes directed against $G_{x/z}$ alpha, G_i alpha$_2$, and G_i alpha$_3$ produced more modest effects (Hadjimarkou *et al.*, 2002).

Given the fact that many of the "selective" opioid agonists and antagonists often display mixed affinities across multiple receptor subtypes together with the emergence of potential isoforms of identified opioid receptor genes, these knockout and knockdown approaches will provide far greater specificity in defining the relative roles of these multiple molecular targets in terms of functional significance in feeding.

7.   Opioid-feeding interactions with dopamine and neuropeptides

Dopamine and opioids are both known to be involved in feeding and other rewarding behaviors. Feeding induced by intra-NAC injection of DAMGO is decreased by injection of a dopamine D1 antagonist into the NAC, but not by injection of a D2 antagonist. Neither blockade of the D1 or D2 receptors in the NAC affected delta-2 opioid-induced feeding. Food intake induced by DAMGO injected unilaterally into the VTA was dose-dependently decreased by bilateral injection of naltrexone or the D1 antagonist SCH 23390 into the NAC shell (MacDonald *et al.*, 2004). When DAMGO was injected into the NAC shell, the resulting food intake was decreased by doses of SCH 23390 ranging from 0.05 to 100 nmol/side injected bilaterally into the VTA, but not by equimolar doses of raclopride, a D2 antagonist.

Opioid antagonists have been shown to decrease intake stimulated by orexin, galanin, agouti-related peptide (AGRP) and neuropeptide Y (NPY). Administration of naltrexone into the nucleus of the solitary tract (NTS) decreases intake due to intra-PVN injection of NPY (Kotz *et al.*, 1995). However, there is no significant decrease in feeding when naltrexone and NPY are injected into the PVN. NPY-induced feeding is decreased by ventricular administration of mu and kappa opioid antagonists, but not by delta receptor blockade (Kotz *et al.*, 1993), and a similar pattern of effects is observed for AS ODN probes directed against MOP, DOP and KOP (Israel *et al.*, 2005). Galanin induced feeding was decreased by mu, but not kappa opioid antagonists (Barton *et al.*, 1996). Orexin-induced feeding elicited from the LH was blocked by systemic and ventricular naltrexone treatment as well as naltrexone administered into the NAC, but not the LH (Sweet *et al.*, 2004). Concurrent blockade of mu and kappa opioid receptors reduced AGRP-induced feeding (Brugman *et al.*, 2002). SHU-9119, like AGRP, is a melanocortin receptor antagonist that increases feeding and this response is eliminated by mu opioid receptor blockade. In turn, the melanotropin receptor agonist, MTII blocks feeding induced by BEND, indicating an inter-relationship between these two POMC-derived systems (Grossman *et al.*, 2003). Established inter-relationships between the endogenous opioid system and GABA have been established in the NAC and VTA and are reviewed elsewhere (Bodnar, 2004).

Opioids also appear to be important to meal maintenance by lengthening the meal. Smith has emphasized that meal size is a major determinant of energy intake (Smith, 1996). Naloxone does not reduce initiation of food intake, but seems to hasten the development of satiety (Kirkham & Blundell, 1984). Naltrexone does not affect latency or goal box running speed in animals running a straight alley maze for food; however, it does decrease food intake in the goal box after contact with the food (Kirkham & Blundell, 1986). Rudski found that naloxone did not affect pressing a lever 80 times to acquire the first pellet of food, but did decrease food intake during the maintenance phase, during which time rats pressed a lever three times to obtain food (Rudski *et al.*, 1994). In addition, naloxone has no effect on sham-fed animals early in the session, but only after eating a sizeable amount of food (Kirkham & Cooper, 1988a, 1988b; Leventhal & Bodnar, 1996).

8.   Conclusions

A host of neuroregulators are distributed across a brain network that is involved in ingestive behavior. The manner in which peptides, catecholamines, amino acids, and endocannabinoids regulate feeding is far from understood. The opioids represent one class of peptides that have effects on energy-related feeding as well as feeding induced by reward. This family of peptides might serve as an important target in treatment of disorders of eating behavior including anorexia, bulimia, binge eating disorder and obesity. Modern molecular and behavioral techniques will assist in understanding the manner in which opioids interact with other neuroregulators to control food intake.

References

Abrahamsen, G. C., Berman, Y. & Carr, K. D. (1995). Curve-shift analysis of self-stimulation in food restricted rats: relationship between daily meal, plasma corticosterone and reward sensitization. *Brain Res.* **695**, 186–94.

Akil, H., Watson, S. J., Young, E. *et al.* (1984). Endogenous opioids: biology and function. *Annu. Rev. Neurosci.* **7**, 223–55.

Apfelbaum, M. & Mandenoff, A. (1981). Naltrexone suppresses hyperphagia induced in the rat by a highly palatable diet. *Pharmacol. Biochem. Behav.* **15**, 89–91.

Appleyard, S. M., Haywood, M., Young, J. I. *et al.* (2003). A role for the endogenous opioid beta-endorphin in energy homeostasis. *Endocrinology* **144**, 1753–60.

Aravich, P. F., Rieg, T. S., Lauterio, T. J. & Doerries, L. E. (1993). Beta-endorphin and dynorphin abnormalities in rats subjected to exercise and restricted feeding: relationship to anorexia nervosa? *Brain Res.* **622**, 1–8.

Arbisi, P. A., Billington, C. J. & Levine, A. S. (1999). The effect of naltrexone on taste detection and recognition threshold. *Appetite* **32**, 241–9.

Arjune, D. & Bodnar, R. J. (1990). Suppression of nocturnal, palatable and glucoprivic intake in rats by the kappa opioid antagonist, nor-binaltorphamine. *Brain Res.* **534**, 313–16.

Arjune, D., Standifer, K. M., Pasternak, G. W. & Bodnar, R. J. (1990). Reduction by central beta-funaltrexamine of food intake in rats under freely-feeding, deprivation and glucoprivic conditions. *Brain Res.* **535**, 101–9.

Arjune, D., Bowen, W. D. & Bodnar, R. J. (1991). Ingestive behavior following central [D-Ala2,Leu5,Cys6]-enkephalin (DALCE), a short-acting agonist and long-acting antagonist at the delta opioid receptor. *Pharmacol. Biochem. Behav.* **39**, 429–36.

Azzara, A. V., Bodnar, R. J, Delamater, A. R. & Sclafani, A. (2000). Naltrexone fails to block the acquisition or expression of a flavor preference conditioned by intragastric carbohydrate infusions. *Pharmacol. Biochem. Behav.* **67**, 545–57.

Badiani, A., Leone, P., Noel, M. B. & Stewart, J. (1995). Ventral tegmental area opioid mechanisms and modulation of ingestive behavior. *Brain Res.* **670**, 264–76.

Baker, R. W., Li, Y., Lee, M. G., Sclafani, A. & Bodnar, R. J. (2004). Naltrexone does not prevent acquisition or expression of flavor preferences conditioned by fructose in rats. *Pharmacol. Biochem. Behav.* **78**, 239–46.

Bakshi, V. P. & Kelley, A. E. (1993a). Feeding induced by opioid stimulation of the ventral striatum: role of opioid receptor subtypes. *J. Pharmacol. Exp. Ther.* **265**, 1253–60.

Bakshi, V. P. & Kelley, A. E. (1993b). Striatal regulation of morphine-induced hyperphagia: an anatomical mapping study. *Psychopharmacology* **111**, 207–14.

Barnes, M. J., Lapanowski, K., Conley, A., Rafols, J. A., Jen, K. L. & Dunbar, J. C. (2003). High fat feeding is associated with increased blood pressure, sympathetic nerve activity and hypothalamic mu opioid receptors. *Brain Res. Bull.* **61**, 511–19.

Barton, C., York, D. A. & Bray, G. A. (1996). Opioid receptor subtype control of galanin-induced feeding. *Peptides* **17**, 237–40.

Beczkowska, I. W. & Bodnar, R. J. (1991). Mediation of insulin hyperphagia by specific central opiate receptor antagonists. *Brain Res.* **547**, 315–18.

Beczkowska, I. W., Bowen, W. D. & Bodnar, R. J. (1992). Central opioid receptor subtype antagonists differentially alter sucrose and deprivation-induced water intake in rats. *Brain Res.* **589**, 291–301.

Beczkowska, I. W., Koch, J. E., Bostock, M. E., Leibowitz, S. F. & Bodnar, R. J. (1993). Central opioid receptor subtype antagonists differentially reduce intake of saccharin and maltose dextrin solutions in rats. *Brain Res.* **618**, 261–70.

Berman, Y., Devi, L. & Carr, K. D. (1994). Effects of chronic food restriction on prodynorphin-derived peptides in rat brain regions. *Brain Res.* **664**, 49–53.

Berman, Y., Devi, L. & Carr, K. D. (1995). Effects of streptozotocin-induced diabetes on prodynorphin-derived peptides in rat brain regions. *Brain Res.* **685**, 129–34.

Berman, Y., Devi, L., Spangler, R., Kreek, M. J. & Carr, K. D. (1997). Chronic food restriction and streptozotocin-induced diabetes differentially alter prodynorphin mRNA levels in rat brain regions. *Mol. Brain Res.* **46**, 25–30.

Bertiere, M. C., Mame Sy, T., Baigts, F., Mandenoff, A. & Apfelbaum, M. (1984). Stress and sucrose hyperphagia: role of endogenous opiates. *Pharmacol. Biochem. Behav.* **20**, 675–9.

Bertino, M., Beauchamp, G. K. & Engelman, K. (1991). Naltrexone, an opiate blocker, alters taste perception and nutrient intake in humans. *Am. J. Physiol.* **261**, R59–63.

Bodnar, R. J. (2004). Endogenous opioids and feeding behavior: a thirty-year historical perspective. *Peptides* **25**, 697–725.

Bodnar, R. J., Glass, M. J. & Koch, J. E. (1995a). Analysis of central opioid receptor subtype antagonism of hypotonic and hypertonic saline intake in water-deprived rats. *Brain Res. Bull.* **36**, 293–300.

Bodnar, R. J., Glass, M. J., Ragnauth, A. & Cooper, M. L. (1995b). General, mu and kappa opioid antagonists in the nucleus accumbens alter food intake under deprivation, glucoprivic and palatable conditions. *Brain Res.* **700**, 205–12.

Bodnar, R. J., Lamonte, N., Israel, Y., Kandov, Y., Ackerman, T. F. & Khaimova, E. (2005). Reciprocal opioid-opioid interactions between the ventral tegmental area and nucleus accumbens regions in mediating mu agonist-induced feeding in rats. *Peptides* **26**, 621–9.

Bozarth, M. A. & Wise, R. A. (1981). Intracranial self-administration of morphine into the ventral tegmental area. *Life Sci.* **28**, 551–5.

Brands, B. J., Thornhill, J. A., Hirst, M. & Gowdey, C. W. (1979). Suppression of food intake and body weight by naloxone in rats. *Life Sci.* **24**, 1773–8.

Brown, D. R. & Holtzman, S. J. (1979). Suppression of deprivation induced food and water intake in rats and mice by naloxone. *Pharmacol. Biochem. Behav.* **11**, 567–83.

Brown, D. R. & Holtzman, S. G. (1980). Evidence that opiate receptors mediate suppression of hypertonic saline-induced drinking in the mouse by narcotic antagonists. *Life Sci.* **26**, 1543–50.

Brown, D. R., Blank, M. S. & Holtzman, S. G. (1980). Suppression by naloxone of water intake induced by deprivation and hypertonic saline in intact and hypophysectomized rats. *Life Sci.* **26**, 1535–42.

Brugman, S., Clegg, D. J., Woods, S. C. & Seeley, R. J. (2002). Combined blockade of both mu- and kappa-opioid receptors prevents the acute orexigenic action of agouti-related protein. *Endocrinology* **143**, 4265–70.

Burdick, K., Yu, W.-Z., Ragnauth, A. et al. (1998). Antisense mapping of opioid receptor clones: effects upon 2-deoxy-D-glucose-induced hyperphagia. *Brain Res.* **794**, 359–63.

Cador, M., Kelley, A. E., LeMoal, M. & Stinus, L. (1986). Ventral tegmental area infusion of substance P, neurotensin and enkephalin: differential effects on feeding behavior. *Neuroscience* **18**, 659–69.

Canli, T., Cook, R. G. & Miczek, K. A. (1990). Opiate antagonists enhance the working memory of rats in the radial maze. *Pharmacol. Biochem. Behav.* **36**, 521–5.

Carr, K. D. (1990). Effects of antibodies to dynorphin A and beta-endorphin on lateral hypothalamic self-stimulation in ad libitum fed and food-deprived rats. *Brain Res.* **534**, 8–14.

Carr, K. D. & Bak, T. H. (1990). Rostral and caudal ventricular infusion of antibodies to dynorphin A (1–17) and dynorphin A (1–8): effects on electrically-elicited feeding in the rat. *Brain Res.* **507**, 289–94.

Carr, K. D. & Simon, E. J. (1983). Effects of naloxone and its quatenary analogue on stimulation-induced feeding. *Neuropharmacology* **22**, 127–30.

Carr, K. D., Bak, T. H., Gioannini, T. L. & Simon, E. J. (1987). Antibodies to dynorphin A(1–13) but not beta-endorphin inhibit electrically-elicited feeding in the rat. *Brain Res.* **422**, 384–8.

Carr, K. D., Bak, T. H., Simon, E. J. & Portoghese, P. S. (1989). Effects of the selective K opioid antagonist, nor-binaltorphamine, on electrically-elicited feeding in the rat. *Life Sci.* **45**, 1787–92.

Carr, K. D., Aleman, D. O., Bak, T. H. & Simon, E. J. (1991). Effects of parabrachial opioid antagonism on stimulation-induced feeding. *Brain Res.* **545**, 283–6.

Carr, K. D., Papadouka, V. & Wolinsky, T. D. (1993). Norbinaltorphamine blocks the feeding but not the reinforcing effect of lateral hypothalamic electrical stimulation. *Psychopharmacology* **111**, 345–50.

Carr, K. D., Park, T. H. & Stone, E. A. (1998). Neuroanatomical patterns of Fos-like immunoreactivity induced by naltrexone in food-restricted and ad libitum fed rats. *Brain Res.* **779**, 26–32.

Carr, K. D., Kutchukhidze, N. & Park, T. H. (1999). Differential effects of mu and kappa opioid antagonists on Fos-like immunoreactivity in extended amygdala. *Brain Res.* **822**, 34–42.

Clark, J. A., Liu, L., Price, M., Hersh, B., Edelson, M. & Pasternak, G. W. (1989). Kappa opiate receptor multiplicity: evidence for two U50,488H-sensitive K-1 subtypes and a novel K-3 subtype. *J. Pharmacol. Exp. Ther.* **251**, 461–8.

Colantuoni, C., Schwenker, J., McCarthy, J. et al. (2001). Excessive sugar intake alters binding to dopamine and mu-opioid receptors in the brain. *Neuroreport* **12**, 3549–52.

Colantuoni, C., Rada, P., McCarthy, J. et al. (2002). Evidence that intermittent, excessive sugar intake causes endogenous opioid dependence. *Obes. Res.* **10**, 478–88.

Cole, J. L., Leventhal, L., Pasternak, G. W., Bowen, W. D. & Bodnar, R. J. (1995). Reductions in body weight following chronic central opioid receptor subtype antagonists during development of dietary obesity in rats. *Brain Res.* **678**, 168–76.

Cole, J. L., Berman, N. & Bodnar, R. J. (1997). Evaluation of chronic opioid receptor antagonist effects upon weight and intake measures in lean and obese Zucker rats. *Peptides* **18**, 1201–7.

Cole, J. L., Ross, A. & Bodnar, R. J. (1999). Dietary history affects the potency of chronic opioid receptor subtype antagonist effects upon body weight in rats. *Nutr. Neurosci.* **1**, 405–18.

Cooper, S. J. (1980). Naloxone: effects on food and water consumption in the non-deprived and deprived rat. *Psychopharmacology* **71**, 1–6.

Cooper, S. J. (1981). Behaviorally-specific hyperdipsia in the non-dependent rat following acute morphine treatment. *Neuropharmacology* **20**, 469–72.

Cooper, S. J. & Gilbert, D. B. (1984). Naloxone suppresses fluid consumption in tests of choice between sodium chloride solutions and water in male and female water-deprived rats. *Psychopharmacology* **84**, 362–7.

Cooper, S. J., Barber, D. J. & Barber-McMullen, J. (1985a). Selective attenuation of sweetened milk consumption by opiate receptor antagonists in male and female rats of the Roman strains. *Neuropeptide* **5**, 349–52.

Cooper, S. J., Jackson, A. & Kirkham, T. C. (1985b). Endorphins and food intake: K opioid receptor agonists and hyperphagia. *Pharmacol. Biochem. Behav.* **23**, 889–901.

Cooper, S. J., Jackson, A., Morgan, R. & Carter, R. (1985c). Evidence for opiate receptor involvement in the consumption of a high palatability diet in non-deprived rats. *Neuropeptide* **5**, 345–8.

Cooper, S. J., Moores, W. R., Jackson, A. & Barber, D. J. (1985d). Effects of tifluadom on food consumption compared with chlordiazepoxide and kappa agonists. *Neuropharmacology* **24**, 877–83.

Czech, D. A. & Stein, E. A. (1980). Naloxone suppresses osmoregulatory drinking in rats. *Pharmacol. Biochem. Behav.* **12**, 987–9.

Czech, D. A., Stein, E. A. & Blake, M. J. (1983). Naloxone-induced hypodipsia: a CNS mapping study. *Life Sci.* **33**, 797–803.

Czech, D. A., Blake, M. J. & Stein, E. A. (1984). Drinking behavior is modulated by CNS administration of opioids. *Appetite* **5**, 15–24.

DeCaro, G., Micossi, L. G. & Venturi, F. (1979). Drinking behavior induced by intracerebroventricular enkephalins in rats. *Nature* **277**, 51–3.

Delamater, A. R., Sclafani, A. & Bodnar, R. J. (2000). Pharmacology of sucrose-reinforced place-preference conditioning: effects of naltrexone. *Pharmacol. Biochem. Behav.* **65**, 697–704.

Devine, D. P. & Wise, R. A. (1994). Self-administration of morphine, DAMGO and DPDPE into the ventral tegmental area of rats. *J. Neurosci.* **14**, 1978–84.

Drewnowski, A., Krahn, D. D., Demitrack, M. A., Nairn, K. & Gosnell, B. A. (1992). Taste responses and preferences for sweet high-fat foods: evidence for opioid involvement. *Physiol. Behav.* **51**, 371–9.

Evans, K. R. & Vaccarino, F. J. (1990). Amphetamine- and morphine-induced feeding: evidence for involvement of reward mechanisms. *Neurosci. Biobehav. Rev.* **14**, 9–22.

Fantino, M., Hosotte, J. & Apfelbaum, M. (1986). An opioid antagonist naltrexone, reduces the preference for sucrose in humans. *Am. J. Physiol.* **251**, R91-6.

Frenk, H. & Rogers, G.H. (1979). The suppressant effects of naloxone on food and water intake in the rat. *Behav. Neur. Biol.* **26**, 23-40.

Giraudo, S.Q., Billington, C.J. & Levine, A.S. (1998a). Effects of the opioid antagonist naltrexone on feeding induced by DAMGO in the central nucleus of the amygdala and in the paraventricular nucleus in the rat. *Brain Res.* **782**, 18-23.

Giraudo, S.Q., Kotz, C.M., Billington, C.J. & Levine, A.S. (1998b). Association between the amygdala and the nucleus of the solitary tract in mu opioid induced feeding in the rat. *Brain Res.* **802**, 184-8.

Glass, M.J., Hahn, B., Joseph, A. & Bodnar, R.J. (1994). Central opioid receptor subtype mediation of isoproterenol-induced drinking in rats. *Brain Res.* **657**, 310-14.

Glass, M.J., Grace, M., Cleary, J.P., Billington, C.J. & Levine, A.S. (1996). Potency of naloxone's anorectic effect in rats is dependent on diet preference. *Am. J. Physiol.* **271**, R217-21.

Glass, M.J., Billington, C.J. & Levine, A.S. (2000). Naltrexone administered to central nucleus of amygdala or PVN: neural dissociation of diet and energy. *Am. J. Physiol. Regul. Integr. Comp. Physiol.* **279**, R86-92.

Goldstein, A., Fischli, W., Lowney, L.I., Hunkapiller, M. & Hood, L. (1981). Porcine pituitary dynorphin: complete amino acid sequence of the biologically active heptadecapeptide. *Proc. Natl. Acad. Sci. USA* **74**, 7219-23.

Gosnell, B.A. (1988). Involvement of mu opioid receptors in the amygdala in the control of feeding. *Neuropharmacology* **27**, 319-26.

Gosnell, B.A. & Majchrzak, M.J. (1989). Centrally administered opioid peptides stimulate saccharin intake in nondeprived rats. *Pharmacol. Biochem. Behav.* **33**, 805-10.

Gosnell, B.A. & Majchrzak, M.J. (1990). Effects of a selective mu opioid receptor agonist and naloxone on the intake of sodium chloride solutions. *Psychopharmacology* **100**, 66-71.

Gosnell, B.A., Levine, A.S. & Morley, J.E. (1986a). The stimulation of food intake by selective agonists of mu, kappa and delta opioid receptors. *Life Sci.* **38**, 1081-8.

Gosnell, B.A., Morley, J.E. & Levine, A.S. (1986b). Opioid-induced feeding: localization of sensitive brain sites. *Brain Res.* **369**, 177-84.

Gosnell, B.A., Grace, M. & Levine, A.S. (1987). Effects of beta-chlornaltrexamine on food intake, body weight and opioid-induced feeding. *Life Sci.* **40**, 1459-67.

Gosnell, B.A., Krahn, D.D. & Majchrzak, M.J. (1990a). The effects of morphine on diet selection are dependent upon baseline diet preferences. *Pharm. Biochem. Behav.* **37**, 207-12.

Gosnell, B.A., Majchrzak, M.J. & Krahn, D.D. (1990b). Effects of preferential delta and kappa opioid receptor agonists on the intake of hypotonic saline. *Physiol. Behav.* **47**, 601-3.

Grandison, L. & Guidotti, A. (1977). Stimulation of food intake by muscimol and beta-endorphin. *Neuropharmacology* **16**, 533-6.

Grossman, H. C., Hadjimarkou, M. M., Silva, R. M., Giraudo, S. Q. & Bodnar, R. J. (2003). Interrelationships between mu opioid and melanocortin receptors in mediating food intake in rats. *Brain Res.* **991**, 240–4.

Hadjimarkou, M. M., Silva, R. M., Rossi, G. C., Pasternak, G. W. & Bodnar, R. J. (2002). Feeding induced by food deprivation is differentially reduced by G-protein alpha-subunit antisense probes in rat. *Brain Res.* **955**, 45–54.

Hadjimarkou, M. M., Khaimova, E., Pan, Y.-X., Rossi, G. C., Pasternak, G. W. & Bodnar, R. J. (2003). Feeding induced by food deprivation is differentially reduced by opioid receptor antisense oligodeoxynucleotide probes in rats. *Brain Res.* **987**, 223–32.

Hadjimarkou, M. M., Singh, A., Kandov, Y. *et al.* (2004). Opioid receptor involvement in food deprivation-induced feeding: evaluation of selective antagonist and antisense oligodeoxynucleotides probe effects in mice and rats. *J. Pharmacol. Exp. Ther.* **311**, 1188–202.

Hagan, M. M. & Moss, D. E. (1991). An animal model of bulimia nervosa: opioid sensitivity to fasting episodes. *Pharmacol. Biochem. Behav.* **39**, 421–2.

Hamilton, M. E. & Bozarth, M. A. (1988). Feeding elicited by dynorphin (1–13) microinjections into the ventral tegmental area. *Life Sci.* **43**, 941–6.

Hawkins, M. F., Cubic, B., Baumeister, A. A. & Bartin, C. (1992). Microinjection of opioid antagonists into the substantia nigra reduces stress-induced eating in rats. *Brain Res.* **584**, 261–5.

Haywood, M. D. & Low, M. J. (2005). Naloxone's suppression of spontaneous and food-conditioned locomotor activity is diminished in mice lacking either the dopamine D(2) receptor or enkephalin. *Mol. Brain Res.* **140**, 91–8.

Haywood, M. D., Pintar, J. E. & Low, M. J. (2002). Selective reward deficit in mice lacking beta-endorphin and enkephalin. *J. Neurosci.* **22**, 8251–8.

Haywood, M. D., Hansen, S. T., Pintar, J. E. & Low, M. J. (2004). Operant self-administration of ethanol in C57BL/6 mice lacking beta-endorphin and enkephalin. *Pharmacol. Biochem. Behav.* **79**, 171–81.

Holtzman, S. G. (1974). Behavioral effects of separate and combined administration of naloxone and d-amphetamine. *J. Pharmacol. Exp. Ther.* **189**, 51–60.

Holtzman, S. G. (1975). Effects of narcotic antagonists on fluid intake in the rat. *Life Sci.* **16**, 1465–70.

Hughes, J., Smith, T., Kosterlitz, H. W., Fothergill, L. A., Morgan, B. A. & Morris, H. R. (1975). Identification of two related penta-peptides from the brain with potent opiate agonist activity. *Nature* **258**, 577–9.

Israel, Y., Kandov, Y., Kest, A., Lewis, S. R. & Bodnar, R. J. (2005). Neuropeptide Y-induced feeding: pharmacological characterization using selective opioid antagonists and antisense probes in rats. *Peptides* **26**, 1167–75.

Jackson, A. & Cooper, S. J. (1985). Effects of K opiate agonists on palatable food consumption in non-deprived rats with and without food preloads. *Brain Res. Bull.* **15**, 391–6.

Jackson, A. & Cooper, S. J. (1986). An observational analysis of the effect of the selective kappa opioid agonist, U50488H, on feeding and related behaviors in the rat. *Psychopharmacology* **90**, 217–21.

Jackson, H.C. & Sewell, R.D.E. (1985a). Are delta opioid receptors involved in the regulation of food and water intake? *Neuropharmacology* **24**, 885–8.

Jackson, H.C. & Sewell, R.D.E. (1985b). Hyperphagia induced by 2-deoxy-D-glucose in the presence of the delta-opioid antagonist, ICI174864. *Neuropharmacology* **24**, 815–17.

Jalowiec, J.E., Panksepp, J., Zolovick, A.J., Najam, N. & Herman, B. (1981). Opioid modulation of ingestive behavior. *Pharmacol. Biochem. Behav.* **15**, 477–84.

Jenck, F., Gratton, A. & Wise, R.A. (1986). Opioid receptor subtypes associated with ventral tegmental facilitation and periaqueductal gray inhibition of feeding. *Brain Res.* **423**, 39–44.

Jenck, F., Gratton, A. & Wise, R.A. (1987). Opioid receptor subtypes associated with ventral tegmental area facilitation of lateral hypothalamic brain stimulation reward. *Brain Res.* **423**, 34–8.

Jewett, D.C., Grace, M.K., Jones, R.M. *et al.* (2001). The kappa-opioid antagonist GNTI reduces U50,488-, DAMGO-, and deprivation-induced feeding, but not butorphanol- and neuropeptide Y-induced feeding in rats. *Brain Res.* **909**, 75–80.

Jiang, Q., Takemori, A.E., Sultana, M. *et al.* (1991). Differential antagonism of opioid delta antinociception by [D-Ala2, Leu5, Cys6]-enkephalin (DALCE) and naltrindole 5′-isothiocyanate (5′-NTII): evidence for delta receptor subtypes. *J. Pharmacol. Exp. Ther.* **257**, 1069–75.

Jones, J.E. & Corp, E.S. (2003). Effect of naltrexone on food intake and body weight in Syrian hamsters depends on metabolic status. *Physiol. Behav.* **78**, 67–72.

Kangawa, K., Minamino, N., Chino, N., Sakakibara, S. & Matsuo, H. (1981). The complete amino acid sequence of alpha-neo-endorphin. *Biochem. Biophys. Res. Commun.* **99**, 871–8.

Kelley, A.E., Bless, E.P. & Swanson, C.J. (1996). Investigation of the effects of opiate antagonists infused into the nucleus accumbens on feeding and sucrose drinking in rats. *J. Pharmacol. Exp. Ther.* **278**, 1499–507.

Kelley, A.E., Will, M.J., Steininger, T.L., Zhang, M. & Haber, S.N. (2003). Restricted daily consumption of a highly palatable food (chocolate Ensure(R)) alters striatal enkephalin gene expression. *Eur. J. Neurosci.* **18**, 2592–8.

Kieffer, B.L. (1995). Recent advances in molecular recognition and signal transduction of active peptides: receptors for opioid peptides. *Cell. Mol. Neurobiol.* **15**, 615–35.

Kim, E.-M., Welch, C.C., Grace, M.K., Billington, C.J. & Levine, A.S. (1996). Chronic food restriction and acute food deprivation decrease mRNA levels of opioid peptides in the arcuate nucleus. *Am. J. Physiol.* **270**, R1019–24.

Kim, E.-M., Grace, M.K., Welch, C.C., Billington, C.J. & Levine, A.S. (1999). STZ-induced diabetes decreases and insulin normalizes POMC mRNA in arcuate nucleus and pituitary in rats. *Am. J. Physiol.* **276**, R1320–6.

Kimura, S., Lewis, R.V., Stern, A.S., Rossier, J., Stein, S. & Undenfriend, S. (1980). Probable precursors of (leu) and (met)-enkephalin in adrenal medulla: peptides of 3-5 kilodaltons. *Proc. Natl. Acad. Sci. USA* **77**, 1681–5.

King, B. M., Castellanos, F. X., Kastin, A. J. *et al.* (1979). Naloxone-induced suppression of food intake in normal and hypothalamic obese rats. *Pharmacol. Biochem. Behav.* **11**, 729-32.

Kirkham, T. C. & Blundell, J. E. (1984). Dual action of naloxone on feeding revealed by behavioral analysis: separate effects on initiation and termination of eating. *Appetite* **5**, 45-52.

Kirkham, T. C. & Blundell, J. E. (1986). Effects of naloxone and naltrexone on the development of satiation measured in the runway: comparisons with d-amphetamine and d-fenfluramine. *Pharm. Biochem. Behav.* **25**, 123-8.

Kirkham, T. C. & Cooper, S. J. (1988a). Attenuation of sham feeding by naloxone is stereospecific: evidence for opioid mediation of orosensory reward. *Physiol. Behav.* **43**, 845-7.

Kirkham, T. C. & Cooper, S. J. (1988b). Naloxone attenuation of sham feeding is modified by manipulation of sucrose concentration. *Physiol. Behav.* **44**, 491-4.

Koch, J. E. & Bodnar, R. J. (1993). Involvement of mu-1 and mu-2 opioid receptor subtypes in tail-pinch feeding in rats. *Physiol. Behav.* **53**, 603-5.

Koch, J. E., Pasternak, G. W., Arjune, D. & Bodnar, R. J. (1992). Naloxone benzoylhydrazone, a kappa-3 opioid agonist, stimulates food intake in rats. *Brain Res.* **581**, 311-14.

Koch, J. E., Glass, M. J., Cooper, M. L. & Bodnar, R. J. (1995). Alterations in deprivation, glucoprivic and sucrose intake following general, mu and kappa opioid antagonists in the hypothalamic paraventricular nucleus of rats. *Neuroscience* **66**, 951-7.

Kotz, C. M., Grace, M. K., Billington, C. J. & Levine, A. S. (1993). The effect of nor-binaltorphamine, beta-funaltrexamine and naltrindole on NPY-induced feeding. *Brain Res.* **631**, 325-8.

Kotz, C. M., Grace, M. K., Briggs, J., Levine, A. S. & Billington, C. J. (1995). Effects of opioid antagonists naloxone and naltrexone on neuropeptide Y-induced feeding and brown fat thermogenesis in the rat. Neural site of action. *J. Clin. Invest.* **96**, 163-70.

Kotz, C. M., Billington, C. J. & Levine, A. S. (1997). Opioids in the nucleus of the solitary tract are involved in feeding in the rat. *Am. J. Physiol.* **272**, R1028-32.

Kumar, R., Mitchell, E. & Stolerman, I. P. (1971). Disturbed patterns of behaviour in morphine tolerant and abstinent rats. *Br. J. Pharmacol.* **42**, 473-84.

Lamonte, N., Echo, J. A., Ackerman, T. F., Christian, G. & Bodnar, R. J. (2002). Analysis of opioid receptor subtype antagonist effects upon mu opioid agonist-induced feeding elicited from the ventral tegmental area of rats. *Brain Res.* **929**, 96-100.

Leibowitz, S. F. & Hor, L. (1982). Endorphinergic and alpha-noradrenergic systems in the paraventricular nucleus: effects on eating behavior. *Peptides* **3**, 421-8.

Leventhal, L. & Bodnar, R. J. (1996). Different central opioid receptor subtype antagonists modify maltose dextrin and deprivation-induced water intake in sham feeding and sham drinking rats. *Brain Res.* **741**, 300-8.

256 Richard J. Bodnar and Allen S. Levine

Leventhal, L., Kirkham, T. C., Cole, J. L. & Bodnar, R. J. (1995). Selective actions of central mu and kappa opioid antagonists upon sucrose intake in sham-feeding rats. *Brain Res.* **685**, 205–10.

Leventhal, L., Cole, J. L., Rossi, G. C., Pan, Y. X., Pasternak, G. W. & Bodnar, R. J. (1996). Antisense oligodeoxynucleotides against the MOR-1 clone alter weight and ingestive responses in rats. *Brain Res.* **719**, 78–84.

Leventhal, L., Stevens, L. B., Rossi, G. C., Pasternak, G. W. & Bodnar, R. J. (1997). Antisense mapping of the MOR-1 opioid receptor clone: modulation of hyperphagia induced by DAMGO. *J. Pharmacol. Exp. Ther.* **282**, 1402–7.

Leventhal, L., Mathis, J. P., Rossi, G. C., Pasternak, G. W. & Bodnar, R. J. (1998a). Orphan opioid receptor antisense probes block orphanin FQ-induced hyperphagia. *Eur. J. Pharmacol.* **349**, R1–3.

Leventhal, L., Silva, R. M., Rossi, G. C., Pasternak, G. W. & Bodnar, R. J. (1998b). Morphine-6beta-glucuronide-induced hyperphagia: characterization of opioid action by selective antagonists and antisense mapping in rats. *J. Pharmacol. Exp. Ther.* **287**, 538–44.

Levin, B. E. & Dunn-Meynell, A. A. (2002). Defense of body weight depends on dietary composition and palatability in rats with diet-induced obesity. *Am. J. Physiol. Regul. Integr. Comp. Physiol.* **282**, R46–54.

Levine, A. S. & Billington, C. J. (2004). Opioids as agents of reward-related feeding: a consideration of the evidence. *Physiol. Behav.* **82**, 57–61.

Levine, A. S. & Morley, J. E. (1981). Peptidergic control of insulin-induced feeding. *Peptides* **2**, 261–4.

Levine, A. S. & Morley, J. E. (1983). Butorphenol tartrate induces feeding in rats. *Life Sci.* **32**, 781–5.

Levine, A. S., Morley, J. E., Brown, D. M. & Handwerger, B. S. (1982a). Extreme sensitivity of diabetic mice to naloxone-induced suppression of food intake. *Physiol. Behav.* **28**, 987–9.

Levine, A. S., Murray, S. S., Kneip, J., Grace, M. & Morley, J. E. (1982b). Flavor enhances the antidipsogenic effect of naloxone. *Physiol. Behav.* **28**, 23–5.

Levine, A. S., Morley, J. E., Kneip, J., Grace, M. & Brown, D. M. (1985). Environment modulates naloxone's suppressive effect on feeding in diabetic and non-diabetic rats. *Physiol. Behav.* **34**, 391–3.

Levine, A. S., Grace, M. & Billington, C. J. (1990a). The effect of centrally administered naloxone on deprivation and drug-induced feeding. *Pharmacol. Biochem. Behav.* **36**, 409–12.

Levine, A. S., Grace, M., Billington, C. J. & Portoghese, P. S. (1990b). Nor-binaltorphamine decreases deprivation and opioid-induced feeding. *Brain Res.* **534**, 60–4.

Levine, A. S., Grace, M. & Billington, C. J. (1991a). B-funaltrexamine (B-FNA) decreases deprivation and opioid-induced feeding. *Brain Res.* **562**, 281–4.

Levine, A. S., Grace, M., Billington, C. J. & Zimmerman, D. M. (1991b). Central administration of the opioid antagonist LY255582 decreases short- and long-term food intake in rats. *Brain Res.* **566**, 193–7.

Levine, A. S., Grace, M., Portoghese, P. S. & Billington, C. J. (1994). The effect of selective opioid antagonists on butorphanol-induced feeding. *Brain Res.* **637**, 242–8.

Levine, A. S., Weldon, D. T., Grace, M., Cleary, J. P. & Billington, C. J. (1995). Naloxone blocks that portion of feeding driven by sweet taste in food-restricted rats. *Am. J. Physiol.* **268**, R248–52.

Levine, A. S., Grace, M. K., Cleary, J. P. & Billington, C. J. (2002). Naltrexone infusion inhibits the development of preference for a high-sucrose diet. *Am. J. Physiol. Regul. Integr. Comp. Physiol.* **283**, R1149–54.

Locatelli, V., Petraglia, F., Tirloni, N. & Muller, E. E. (1986). Beta-endorphin concentrations in the hypothalamus, pituitary and plasma of streptozotocin-diabetic rats with and without insulin substitution therapy. *Life Sci.* **38**, 379–86.

Locke, K. W., Brown, D. R. & Holtzman, S. G. (1982). Effects of opiate antagonists and putative mu- and kappa-agonists on milk intake in rat and squirrel monkey. *Pharmacol. Biochem. Behav.* **17**, 1275–9.

Lord, J. A. H., Waterfield, A. A., Hughes, J. & Kosterlitz, H. (1977). Endogenous opioid peptides: multiple agonists and receptors. *Nature* **267**, 495–9.

Low, M. J., Haywood, M. D., Appleyard, S. M. & Rubinstein, M. (2003). State-dependent modulation of feeding behavior by proopiomelanocortin-derived beta-endorphin. *Ann. N. Y. Acad. Sci.* **994**, 192–201.

Lowe, M. R. & Levine, A. S. (2005). Eating motives and the controversy over dieting: eating less than needed versus less than wanted. *Obes. Res.* **13**, 797–806.

Lowy, M. T. & Yim, G. K. W. (1983). Stimulation of food intake following opiate agonists in rats but not hamsters. *Psychopharmacology* **81**, 28–32.

Lowy, M. T., Maickel, R. P. & Yim, G. K. W. (1980). Naloxone reduction of stress-related feeding. *Life Sci.* **26**, 2113–18.

Lynch, W. C. (1986). Opiate blockade inhibits saccharin intake and blocks normal preference acquisition. *Pharmacol. Biochem. Behav.* **24**, 833–6.

Lynch, W. C. & Burns, G. (1990). Opioid effects on intake of sweet solutions depend both on prior drug experience and on prior ingestive experience. *Appetite* **15**, 23–32.

Lynch, W. C. & Libby, L. (1983). Naloxone suppresses intake of highly preferred saccharin solutions in food deprived and sated rats. *Life Sci.* **33**, 1909–14.

MacDonald, A. F., Billington, C. J. & Levine, A. S. (2003). Effects of the opioid antagonist naltrexone on feeding induced by DAMGO in the ventral tegmental area and in the nucleus accumbens shell region in the rat. *Am. J. Physiol.* **285**, R999–1004.

MacDonald, A. F., Billington, C. J. & Levine, A. S. (2004). Alterations in food intake by opioid and dopamine signaling pathways between the ventral tegmental area and the shell of the nucleus accumbens. *Brain Res.* **1018**, 78–85.

Maickel, R. P., Braude, M. C. & Zabik, J. E. (1977). The effects of various narcotic agonists and antagonists on deprivation-induced fluid consumption. *Neuropharmacology* **16**, 863–6.

258   Richard J. Bodnar and Allen S. Levine

Mains, R. E., Eipper, B. A. & Ling, N. (1977). Common precursor to corticotropins and endorphin. *Proc. Natl. Acad. Sci. USA* **197**, 3014–18.

Majeed, N. H., Przewlocka, B., Wedzony, K. & Przewlocki, R. (1986). Stimulation of food intake following opioid microinjection into the nucleus accumbens septi in rats. *Peptides* **7**, 711–16.

Mandenoff, A., Fumeron, F., Apfelbaum, M. & Margules, D. L. (1982). Endogenous opiates and energy balance. *Science* **215**, 1536–7.

Mann, P. E., Arjune, D., Romero, M. T., Pasternak, G. W., Hahn, E. F. & Bodnar, R. J. (1988a). Differential sensitivity of opioid-induced feeding to naloxone and naloxonazine. *Psychopharmacology* **94**, 330–41.

Mann, P. E., Pasternak, G. W., Hahn, E. F., Curreri, G., Lubin, E. & Bodnar, R. J. (1988b). Comparison of chronic naloxone and naloxonazine effects upon food intake and body weight maintainance in rats. *Neuropharmacology* **27**, 349–55.

Margules, D. L., Moisset, B., Lewis, M. J., Shibuya, H. & Pert, C. B. (1978). Beta-endorphin is associated with overeating in genetically-obese mice (ob/ob) and rats (fa/fa). *Science* **202**, 988–91.

Marks-Kaufman, R., Balmagiya, T. & Gross, E. (1984). Modifications in food intake and energy metabolism in rats as a function of chronic naltrexone infusions. *Pharmacol. Biochem. Behav.* **20**, 911–16.

Martin, W. R., Wikler, A., Eades, C. G. & Pescor, F. T. (1963). Tolerance to and physical dependence on morphine in rats. *Psychopharmacology* **4**, 247–60.

Martin, W. R., Eades, C. G., Thompson, J. A., Huppler, R. E. & Gilbert, P. E. (1976). The effects of morphine- and nalorphine-like drugs in the nondependent and morphine-dependent chronic spinal dog. *J. Pharmacol. Exp. Ther.* **197**, 517–32.

Mattia, A., Vanderah, T., Mosberg, H. I. & Porreca, F. (1991). Lack of antinociceptive cross-tolerance between [D-Pen2, D-Pen5]-enkephalin and [D-Ala2]-deltorphan II in mice: evidence for delta receptor subtypes. *J. Pharmacol. Exp. Ther.* **258**, 583–7.

McLaughlin, C. L. & Baile, C. A. (1983). Nalmefene decreases meal size, food and water intake and weight gain in Zucker rats. *Pharmacol. Biochem. Behav.* **19**, 235–40.

McLaughlin, C. L. & Baile, C. A. (1984). Feeding behavior responses of Zucker rats to naloxone. *Physiol. Behav.* **32**, 755–61.

McLean, S. & Hoebel, B. G. (1982). Opiate and norepinephrine-induced feeding from the paraventricular nucleus of the hypothalamus are dissociable. *Life Sci.* **31**, 2379–82.

Mehiel, R. (1996). The effects of naloxone on flavor-calorie preference learning indicate involvement of opioid reward systems. *Psychol. Rec.* **46**, 435–50.

Meunier, J. C., Mollereau, C., Toll, L. et al. (1995). Isolation and structure of the endogenous agonist of the opioid receptor like ORL1 receptor. *Nature* **377**, 532–5.

Millan, M. J. & Morris, B. J. (1988). Long-term blockade of mu-opioid receptors suggests a role in control of ingestive behavior, body weight and core temperature in the rat. *Brain Res.* **450**, 247–58.

Morley, J. E. & Levine, A. S. (1980). Stress-induced eating is mediated through endogenous opiates. *Science* **209**, 1259–61.

Morley, J. E. & Levine, A. S. (1981). Dynorphin (1–13) induces spontaneous feeding in rats. *Life Sci.* **29**, 1901–3.

Morley, J. E. & Levine, A. S. (1983). Involvement of dynorphin and the kappa opioid receptor in feeding. *Peptides* **4**, 797–800.

Morley, J. E., Levine, A. S., Grace, M. & Kneip, J. (1982). An investigation of the role of kappa opiate receptors in the initiation of feeding. *Life Sci.* **31**, 2617–26.

Morley, J. E., Levine, A. S., Kneip, J., Grace, M., Zeugner, H. & Shearman, G. T. (1985). The K opioid receptor and food intake. *Eur. J. Pharmacol.* **112**, 17–25.

Mucha, R. F. & Iversen, S. D. (1986). Increased food intake after opioid microinjections into nucleus accumbens and ventral tegmental area of rat. *Brain Res.* **397**, 214–24.

Myers, K. J. & Dean, N. M. (2000). Sensible use of antisense: how to use oligonucleotides as research tools. *Trends Pharmacol. Sci.* **21**, 19–23.

Nencini, P. & Stewart, J. (1990). Chronic systemic administration of amphetamine increases food intake to morphine, but not to U50488H, microinjected into the ventral tegmental area in rats. *Brain Res.* **527**, 254–8.

Nock, B., Rajpara, A., O'Connor, L. H. & Cicero, T. J. (1988). Autoradiography of [3-H]-U69,593 binding sites in rat brain: evidence for K opioid receptor subtypes. *Eur. J. Pharmacol.* **154**, 27–34.

Noel, M. B. & Wise, R. A. (1993). Ventral tegmental injections of morphine but not U50488H enhance feeding in food-deprived rats. *Brain Res.* **632**, 68–73.

Noel, M. B. & Wise, R. A. (1995). Ventral tegmental injections of a selective mu or delta opioid enhance feeding in food-deprived rats. *Brain Res.* **673**, 304–12.

O'Hare, E., Cleary, J. P., Billington, C. J. & Levine, A. S. (1997). Naloxone administration following operant training of sucrose/water discrimination in the rat. *Psychopharmacology* **129**, 289–94.

Olson, G. A., DeLatte, S. W., Kastin, A. J., McLean, J. H., Phillpott, D. F. & Olson, R. D. (1985). Naloxone and fluid consumption in rats: dose-response relationship for 15 days. *Pharmacol. Biochem. Behav.* **23**, 1065–8.

Olszewski, P. K., Grace, M. K., Billington, C. J. & Levine, A. S. (2000). The effect of [Phe (1)psi(CH(2)-NH)Gly(2)]-nociceptin(1–13)NH(2) on feeding and c-Fos immunoreactivity in selected brain sites. *Brain Res.* **876**, 95–102.

Ostrowski, N. L., Rowland, N., Foley, T. L., Nelson, J. L. & Reid, L. D. (1981). Morphine antagonists and consummatory behaviors. *Pharmacol. Biochem. Behav.* **14**, 549–59.

Pan, Y. X., Xu, J., Bolan, E. *et al.* (1999). Identification and characterization of three new alternatively spliced MOR-1 opioid receptor isoforms. *Mol. Pharmacol.* **56**, 396–403.

Pan, Y. X., Xu, J., Mahurter, L., Bolan, E., Xu, M. & Pasternak, G. W. (2001). Generation of the mu opioid receptor (MOR-1) protein by three new splice variants of the Oprm gene. *Proc. Natl. Acad. Sci. USA* **98**, 14084–9.

Papadouka, V. & Carr, K. D. (1994). The role of multiple opioid receptors in the maintenance of stimulation-induced feeding. *Brain Res.* **639**, 42–8.

Parker, L. A., Maier, S., Rennie, M. & Crebolder, J. (1992). Morphine- and naltrexone-induced modification of palatability: analysis by the taste reactivity test. *Behav. Neurosci.* **106**, 999–1010.

Pasternak, G. W. & Standifer, K. M. (1995). Mapping of opioid receptors using antisense oligodeoxynucleotides: correlating their molecular biology and pharmacology. *Trends Pharmacol. Sci.* **16**, 344–50.

Pasternak, G. W. & Wood, P. L. (1986). Multiple mu opiate receptors. *Life Sci.* **38**, 1889–96.

Pecina, S. & Berridge, K. (2000). Opioid site in nucleus accumbens shell mediates eating and hedonic 'liking' for food: map based on microinjection Fos plumes. *Brain Res.* **863**, 71–86.

Pert, C. B. & Snyder, S. H. (1973). Opiate receptor: demonstration in nervous tissue. *Science* **179**, 1011–14.

Plata-Salaman, C. R., Wilson, C. D., Sonti, G., Borkoski, J. P. & ffrench-Mullen, J. M. H. (1995). Antisense oligodeoxynucleotides to G-protein alpha-subunit subclasses identify a transductional requirement for the modulation of normal feeding dependent on Goa alpha subunit. *Mol. Brain Res.* **33**, 72–8.

Polidori, C., deCaro, G. & Massi, M. (2000). The hyperphagic effect of nociceptin/orphanin FQ in rats. *Peptides* **21**, 1051–62.

Pomonis, J. D., Billington, C. J. & Levine, A. S. (1996). Orphanin FQ, agonist of orphan opioid receptor ORL1, stimulates feeding in rats. *Neuroreport* **8**, 369–71.

Pomonis, J. D., Jewett, D. C., Kotz, C. M., Briggs, J. E., Billington, C. J. & Levine, A. S. (2000). Sucrose consumption increases naloxone-induced c-fos immunoreactivity in limbic forebrain. *Am. J. Physiol.* **278**, R712–19.

Quinn, J. G., O'Hare, E., Levine, A. S. & Kim, E. M. (2003). Evidence for a mu-opioid-opioid connection between the paraventricular nucleus and ventral tegmental area in the rat. *Brain Res.* **991**, 206–11.

Ragnauth, A., Ruegg, H. & Bodnar, R. J. (1997). Evaluation of opioid receptor subtype antagonist effects in the ventral tegmental area upon food intake under deprivation, glucoprivic and palatable conditions. *Brain Res.* **767**, 8–16.

Ragnauth, A., Moroz, M. & Bodnar, R. J. (2000). Multiple opioid receptors mediate feeding elicited by mu and delta opioid receptor subtype agonists in the nucleus accumbens shell in rats. *Brain Res.* **876**, 76–87.

Ragnauth, A., Schuller, A., Morgan, M. *et al.* (2001). Female preproenkephalin-knockout mice display altered emotional responses. *Proc. Natl. Acad. Sci. USA* **98**, 1958–63.

Ramirez, I. (1997). Intragastric carbohydrate exerts both intake-stimulating and intake-suppressing effects. *Behav. Neurosci.* **111**, 612–22.

Recant, L., Voyles, N. R., Luciano, M. & Pert, C. B. (1980). Naltrexone reduced weight gain, alters beta-endorphin and reduces insulin output from pancreatic islets of genetically obese mice. *Peptides* **1**, 309–13.

Reicine, T. & Bell, G. I. (1993). Molecular biology of opioid receptors. *Trends Neurosci.* **16**, 506–10.

Reinscheid, R. K., Nothacker, H. P., Bourson, A. *et al.* (1995). Orphanin FQ: a neuropeptide that activates an opioid-like G protein-coupled receptor. *Science* **270**, 792–4.

Rizzi, A., Salis, M. B., Ciccocioppo, R. *et al.* (2002). Pharmacological characterisation of [(pX)Phe4]nociceptin(1–13)NH2 analogues. 2. In vivo studies. *Naunyn Schmiedebergs Arch. Pharmacol.* **365**, 450–6.

Roberts, J. L., Seeburg, P. H., Shine, J., Herbert, E., Baxter, J. D. & Goodman, H. M. (1979). Corticotropin and β-endorphin: construction of analysis of recombinant DNA complementary to mRNA for the common precursor. *Proc. Natl. Acad. Sci. USA* **76**, 2153–7.

Rodi, D., Polidori, C., Bregola, G., Zucchini, S., Simonato, M. & Massi, M. (2002). Pro-nociceptin/orphanin FQ and NOP receptor mRNA levels in the forebrain of food deprived rats. *Brain Res.* **957**, 354–61.

Roerig, S. C. (1998). Opioid regulation of second messenger systems. *Analgesia* **3**, 231–50.

Rossi, G. C., Standifer, K. M. & Pasternak, G. W. (1995). Differential blockade of morphine and morphine-6B-glucuronide analgesia by antisense oligodeoxynucleotides directed against MOR-1 and G-protein alpha subunits in rats. *Neurosci. Lett.* **198**, 99–102.

Rossi, G. C., Leventhal, L., Pan, Y.-X. *et al.* (1997). Antisense mapping of MOR-1 in rats: distinguishing between morphine and morphine-6beta-glucuronide antinociception. *J. Pharmacol. Exp. Ther.* **281**, 109–14.

Rowland, N. (1982). Comparison of the suppression by naloxone of water intake induced in rats by hyperosmolarity, hypovolemia and angiotensin. *Pharmacol. Biochem. Behav.* **16**, 87–91.

Rowland, N. & Bartness, T. J. (1982). Naloxone suppresses insulin-induced food intake in novel and familiar environments, but does not affect hypoglycemia. *Pharmacol. Biochem. Behav.* **16**, 1001–3.

Rudski, J. M., Schaal, D. W., Thompson, T., Cleary, J., Billington, C. J. & Levine, A. S. (1992). Effects of methadone on free feeding in satiated rats. *Pharmacol. Biochem. Behav.* **43**, 1033–7.

Rudski, J. M., Billington, C. J. & Levine, A. S. (1994). Naloxone's effects on operant responding depend upon level of deprivation. *Pharmacol. Biochem. Behav.* **49**, 377–83.

Rudski, J. M., Thomas, D., Billington, C. J. & Levine, A. S. (1995). Buprenorphine increases intake of freely available and operant-contingent food in satiated rats. *Pharmacol. Biochem. Behav.* **50**, 271–6.

Ruegg, H., Hahn, B., Koch, J. E. & Bodnar, R. J. (1994). Differential modulation of angiotensin II and hypertonic saline-induced drinking by opioid receptor subtype antagonists in rats. *Brain Res.* **635**, 203–10.

Ruegg, H., Yu, W.-Z. & Bodnar, R. J. (1997). Opioid receptor subtype agonist-induced enhancements of sucrose intake are dependent upon sucrose concentration. *Physiol. Behav.* **62**, 121–8.

Sanger, D. J. (1981). Endorphinergic mechanisms in the control of food and water intake. *Appetite* **2**, 193–208.

Sanger, D. J. & McCarthy, P. S. (1980). Differential effects of morphine on food and water intake in food deprived and freely feeding rats. *Psychopharmacology* **72**, 103–6.

Sanger, D. J. & McCarthy, P. S. (1981). Increased food and water intake produced by rats by opiate receptor agonists. *Psychopharmacology* **74**, 217–20.

Schulz, R., Wilhelm, A. & Dirlich, G. (1984). Intracerebral microinjection of different antibodies against the endogenous opioids suggests alpha-neoendorphin participation in control of feeding behavior. *Naunyn Schmiedebergs Arch. Pharmacol.* **326**, 222–6.

Shaw, W. N., Mitch, C. H., Leander, J. D. & Zimmerman, D. M. (1990). Effect of phenylpiperidine opioid antagonists on food consumption and weight gain of the obese Zucker rat. *J. Pharmacol. Exp. Ther.* **253**, 85–9.

Shide, D. J. & Blass, E. M. (1991). Opioid mediation of odor preferences induced by sugar and fat in 6-day-old rats. *Physiol. Behav.* **50**, 961–6.

Shimomura, Y., Oku, J., Glick, Z. & Bray, G. A. (1982). Opiate receptors, food intake and obesity. *Physiol. Behav.* **28**, 441–5.

Silva, R. M., Rossi, G. C., Mathis, J. P., Standifer, K. M., Pasternak, G. W. & Bodnar, R. J. (2000). Morphine and morphine-6beta-glucuronide-induced feeding are differentially reduced by G-protein alpha-subunit antisense probes in rats. *Brain Res.* **876**, 62–75.

Silva, R. M., Hadjimarkou, M. M., Rossi, G. C., Pasternak, G. W. & Bodnar, R. J. (2001). Beta-endorphin-induced feeding: pharmacological characterization using selective opioid antagonists and antisense probes in rats. *J. Pharmacol. Exp. Ther.* **297**, 590–6.

Silva, R. M., Grossman, H. C., Hadjimarkou, M. M., Rossi, G. C., Pasternak, G. W. & Bodnar, R. J. (2002a). Dynorphin A1-17-induced feeding: pharmacological characterization using selective opioid antagonists and antisense probes in rats. *J. Pharmacol. Exp. Ther.* **301**, 513–18.

Silva, R. M., Grossman, H. C., Rossi, G. C., Pasternak, G. W. & Bodnar, R. J. (2002b). Pharmacological characterization of beta-endorphin- and dynorphin A-induced feeding using g-protein alpha subunit antisense probes in rats. *Peptides* **23**, 1101–6.

Simon, E. J., Hiller, J. M. & Edelman, I. (1973). Stereospecific binding of the potent narcotic analgesic (3H)etorphine to rat brain homogenate. *Proc. Natl. Acad. Sci. USA* **70**, 1947–9.

Simone, D. A., Bodnar, R. J., Goldman, E. J. & Pasternak, G. W. (1985). Involvement of opioid receptor subtypes in rat feeding behavior. *Life Sci.* **36**, 829–33.

Sipols, A. J., Bayer, J., Bennett, R. & Figlewicz, D. P. (2002). Intraventricular insulin decreases kappa opioid-mediated sucrose intake in rats. *Peptides* **23**, 2181–7.

Siviy, S. M., Bermudez-Rattoni, F., Rockwood, G. A., Dargie, C. M. & Reid, L. D. (1981). Intracerebral administration of naloxone and drinking in water-deprived rats. *Pharmacol. Biochem. Behav.* **15**, 257–62.

Smith, G. P. (1996). The direct and indirect controls of meal size. *Neurosci. Biobehav. Rev.* **20**, 41–6.

Spencer, R. L., Deupree, D., Hsiao, S. *et al.* (1986). Centrally-administered opioid selective agonists inhibit drinking in the rat. *Pharmacol. Biochem. Behav.* **25**, 77–82.

Standifer, K. M., Chien, C. C., Wahlestedt, C., Brown, G. P. & Pasternak, G. W. (1994). Selective loss of delta opioid analgesia and binding by oligodeoxynucleotides to a delta opioid receptor. *Neuron* **12**, 805–10.

Standifer, K. M., Jenab, S., Su, W. *et al.* (1995). Antisense oligodeoxynucleotides to the cloned receptor, DOR-1: Uptake, stability and regulation of gene expression. *J. Neurochem.* **65**, 1981–7.

Standifer, K. M., Rossi, G. C. & Pasternak, G. W. (1996). Differential blockade of opioid analgesia by antisense oligodeoxynucleotides directed against various G protein alpha subunits. *Mol. Pharmacol.* **50**, 293–8.

Stanley, B. G., Lanthier, D. & Leibowitz, S. F. (1989). Multiple brain sites sensitive to feeding stimulation by opioid agonists: a cannula-mapping study. *Pharmacol. Biochem. Behav.* **31**, 825–32.

Stein, J. A., Znamensky, V., Baumer, F., Rossi, G. C., Pasternak, G. W. & Bodnar, R. J. (2000). Mercaptoacetate induces feeding through central opioid-mediated mechanisms in rats. *Brain Res.* **864**, 240–51.

Stratford, T. R., Holahan, M. R. & Kelley, A. E. (1997). Injections of nociceptin into nucleus accumbens shell or ventromedial hypothalamic nucleus increase food intake. *Neuroreport* **8**, 423–6.

Summy-Long, J. Y., Rosella, L. M. & Keil, L. C. (1981). Effects of centrally administered endogenous opioid peptides on drinking behavior, increased plasma vasopressin concentration and pressor response to hypertonic sodium chloride. *Brain Res.* **221**, 343–57.

Sweet, D. C., Levine, A. S. & Kotz, C. M. (2004). Functional opioid pathways are necessary for hypocretin-1 (orexin-A)-induced feeding. *Peptides* **25**, 307–14.

Tang, A. H. & Collins, R. J. (1985). Behavioral effects of a novel kappa opioid analgesic, U50488, in rats and rhesus monkeys. *Psychopharmacology* **85**, 309–14.

Tepperman, F. S. & Hirst, M. (1983). Effects of intrahypothalamic injection of D-Ala-2,D-Leu-5-enkephalin on feeding and temperature in the rat. *Eur. J. Pharmacol.* **96**, 243–9.

Tepperman, F. S., Hirst, M. & Gowdey, C. W. (1981). Hypothalamic injection of morphine: feeding and temperature responses. *Life Sci.* **28**, 2459–67.

Terenius, L. (1973). Stereospecific interaction between narcotic analgesia and a synaptic plasma membrane fraction of rat cerebral cortex. *Acta Pharmacol. Toxicol.* **32**, 317–20.

Thornhill, J. A., Taylor, B., Marshall, W. & Parent, K. (1982). Central, as well as peripheral naloxone administration suppresses feeding in food-deprived Sprague-Dawley and genetically obese (Zucker) rats. *Physiol. Behav.* **29**, 841–6.

Tsujii, S., Nakai, Y., Fukata, J. *et al.* (1986a). Effects of food deprivation and high fat diet on opioid receptor binding in rat brain. *Neurosci. Lett.* **72**, 169–73.

Tsujii, S., Nakai, Y., Koh, T. *et al.* (1986b). Effects of food deprivation on opioid receptor binding in the brain of lean and fatty Zucker rats. *Brain Res.* **399**, 200–3.

Uhl, G. R., Childers, S. R. & Pasternak, G. W. (1994). An opiate receptor gene family reunion. *Trends Neurosci.* **17**, 89–93.

Ukai, M. & Holtzman, S. G. (1988a). Effects of beta-funaltrexamine on ingestive behaviors in the rat. *Eur. J. Pharmacol.* **153**, 161–5.

Ukai, M. & Holtzman, S. G. (1988b). Effects of intrahypothalamic administration of opioid peptides selective for mu, kappa and delta receptors on different schedules of water intake in rats. *Brain Res.* **459**, 275–81.

Ukai, M., Nakayama, S. & Kameyama, T. (1988). The opioid antagonist, MR2266, specifically decreases saline intake in the mouse. *Neuropharmacology* **27**, 1027–31.

Wahlestedt, C. (1994). Antisense oligodeoxynucleotide strategies in neuropharmacology. *Trends Pharmacol. Sci.* **15**, 42–6.

Walker, J. M., Katz, R. J. & Akil, H. (1980). Behavioral effects of dynorphin (1–13) in the mouse and rat: initial observations. *Peptides* **1**, 341–5.

Welch, C. C., Grace, M. K., Billington, C. J. & Levine, A. S. (1994). Preference and diet type affect macronutrient selection after morphine, NPY, norepinephrine, and deprivation. *Am. J. Physiol.* **266**, R426–33.

Welch, C. C., Kim, E.-M., Grace, M. K., Billington, C. J. & Levine, A. S. (1996). Palatability-induced hyperphagia increases hypothalamic dynorphin peptide and mRNA levels. *Brain Res.* **721**, 126–31.

Wilson, J. D., Nicklous, D. M., Aloyo, V. J. & Simansky, K. J. (2003). An orexigenic role for mu-opioid receptors in the lateral parabrachial nucleus. *Am. J. Physiol.* **285**, R1055–65.

Wolinsky, T. D., Carr, K. D., Hiller, J. M. & Simon, E. J. (1994). Effects of chronic food restriction on mu and kappa opioid binding in rat forebrain: a quantitative autoradiographic study. *Brain Res.* **656**, 274–80.

Wolinsky, T. D., Abrahamsen, G. C. & Carr, K. D. (1996a). Diabetes alters mu and kappa opioid binding in rat brain: comparison with effects of food restriction. *Brain Res.* **738**, 167–71.

Wolinsky, T. D., Carr, K. D., Hiller, J. M. & Simon, E. J. (1996b). Chronic food restriction alters mu and kappa opioid receptor binding in the parabrachial nucleus of the rat: a quantitative autoradiographic study. *Brain Res.* **706**, 333–6.

Wolozin, B. L. & Pasternak, G. W. (1981). Classification of multiple morphine and enkephalin binding sites in the central nervous system. *Proc. Natl. Acad. Sci. USA* **78**, 6181–5.

Woods, J. S. & Leibowitz, S. F. (1985). Hypothalamic sites sensitive to morphine and naloxone: effects on feeding behavior. *Pharmacol. Biochem. Behav.* **23**, 431–8.

Yirmiya, R., Lieblich, I. & Liebeskind, J. C. (1988). Reduced saccharin preference in CXBK (opioid receptor-deficient) mice. *Brain Res.* **438**, 339–42.

Yu, W.-Z. & Bodnar, R. J. (1997). Interactions between Angiotensin II and delta opioid receptor subtype agonists upon water intake in rats. *Peptides* **18**, 241–5.

Yu, W.-Z., Ruegg, H. & Bodnar, R. J. (1997). Delta and kappa opioid receptor subtypes and ingestion: antagonist and glucoprivic effects. *Pharmacol. Biochem. Behav.* **56**, 353–61.

Yu, W.-Z., Sclafani, A., Delamater, A. R. & Bodnar, R. J. (1999). Pharmacology of flavor preference conditioning in sham-feeding rats: effects of naltrexone. *Pharmacol. Biochem. Behav.* **64**, 573–84.

Zadina, J. E., Hackler, L., Ge, L.-J. & Kastin, A. J. (1997). A potent and selective endogenous agonist for the mu-opiate receptor. *Nature* **386**, 499–502.

Zhang, M. & Kelley, A. E. (2000). Enhanced intake of high-fat food following striatal mu-opioid stimulation: microinjection mapping and fos expression. *Neuroscience* **99**, 267–77.

Zhang, M. & Kelley, A. E. (2002). Intake of saccharin, salt, and ethanol solutions is increased by infusion of a mu opioid agonist into the nucleus accumbens. *Psychopharmacology* **159**, 415–23.

Zhang, M., Gosnell, B. A. & Kelley, A. E. (1998). Intake of high-fat food is selectively enhanced by mu opioid receptor stimulation within the nucleus accumbens. *J. Pharmacol. Exp. Ther.* **285**, 908–14.

Zukin, R. S., Eghbalai, M., Olive, D., Unterwald, E. M. & Tempel, A. (1988). Characterization and visualization of rat and guinea pig brain K opioid receptors: evidence for K-1 and K-2 opioid receptors. *Proc. Natl. Acad. Sci. USA* **85**, 4061–5.

9

Ghrelin: an orexigenic signal from the stomach

TAMAS HORVATH

1.   Introduction

The discovery of ghrelin, a 28 amino-acid peptide hormone, has generated a substantial amount of attention for a number of reasons. Initially, ghrelin was heralded as the long sought endogenous ligand for the orphan growth hormone secretagogue receptors (GHS-Rs). Indeed, like growth hormone secretagogues (GHS), ghrelin targeted these receptors to potently increase the release of growth hormone (GH) both in vitro and in vivo. Soon, however, it became evident that ghrelin was implicated in a variety of physiological processes that include cell proliferation, metabolism, cell protection, reproduction, etc. Of these, the effects of ghrelin on food intake and metabolism have had the biggest impact; unlike other peripheral signals associated with energy balance, ghrelin increases appetite and leads to the accumulation of body fat. Indeed, the stimulatory effects of ghrelin on food intake and its apparent opposite relation to the anorectic hormone, leptin, have been proposed as the ying/yang model for hormonal regulation of energy balance. Nevertheless, the more is known about ghrelin, the more it becomes obvious that ghrelin produces its metabolic effects via a multitude of central and peripheral mechanisms that work in parallel to modulate the effects of ghrelin in energy regulation. This chapter will review the literature regarding the effects of ghrelin on energy balance. Energy balance implies the regulation of both food intake and energy expenditure, therefore we will discuss both

Neurobiology and Obesity, ed. Jenni Harvey and Dominic J. Withers. Published by Cambridge University Press. © Cambridge University Press 2008

topics in relation to ghrelin. A description of the possible central routes of ghrelin actions on energy balance within the brain will follow. Finally, we will present additional data suggesting that ghrelin targets various brain circuits besides those in the mediobasal hypothalamus involved in energy homeostasis. The effects of ghrelin on other physiological processes can be found in several excellent recent reviews (van der Lely *et al.*, 2004; Kojima & Kangawa, 2005; Smith *et al.*, 2005).

2.   Ghrelin: the endogenous GHS

Much of the work that culminated in the unveiling of the ghrelin protein began with descriptions of peptides that were cleaved from metenkephalin, and that increased the secretion of growth hormone but were devoid of opioidergic effects (Bowers *et al.*, 1984a, 1984b). Because of this, these compounds were named growth hormone secretagogues (GHS). For years, efforts were focused on designing more effective GHS leading to the production of peptide and nonpeptide compounds including growth hormone releasing peptide-6 (GHRP-6), GHRP-2, hexarelin, L-692,429, and MK-0677 to name a few (Bowers, 1993; Smith *et al.*, 1999; Smith, 2005).

The latter compound was used by Howard *et al.* in studies leading to the cloning and characterization of the G-coupled protein receptor named the growth hormone secretagogue receptor (GHS-R) (McKee *et al.*, 1997; Davenport *et al.*, 2005). To date, two subtypes of this receptor have been identified: GHS-R 1a and GHS-R 1b. Most of the current work on the biology of these receptors has focused on GHS-R 1a because GHS-R 1b is devoid of any known ligand-specific responses (McKee *et al.*, 1997). Interestingly, GHS-R 1a and 1b localization is ubiquitous, but high concentrations of these receptors are found in the pituitary and hypothalamus (McKee *et al.*, 1997; Davenport *et al.*, 2005). The presence of a receptor that bound GHS suggested that organisms produced an endogenous substance with biological properties similar to those of these compounds.

The identification of the GHS-R was soon followed by the first description of ghrelin by Kojima *et al.* (1999). In their studies they identified a protein product of oxyntic cells in the stomach that bound to GHS-R, and increased the secretion of growth hormone in a manner that suggested it was the endogenous GHS. The structure of the 28 amino-acid ghrelin protein was peculiar in that its biological activity depended upon the acylation of the hydroxyl group of the serine-3 residue by n-octanoic acid. Several splice variants of ghrelin have been identified, some of which produce similar effects to those of ghrelin (i.e. Des-Gln14-ghrelin) (Hosoda *et al.*, 2000), some of which have no known effect (non-acylated ghrelin) (van der Lely *et al.*, 2004), and some of which have opposite effects to those of ghrelin (Obestatin) (Zhang *et al.*, 2005). In their seminal paper, Kojima *et al.* also showed that the stomach was the main source of circulating ghrelin, although other organs including the brain produced ghrelin. Within the brain, it appeared that ghrelin was secreted by a subset of neurons in the lateral portion of the hypothalamic arcuate nucleus (Kojima *et al.*, 1999). Further studies have confirmed the presence of ghrelin in the hypothalamus and a detailed neuroanatomical distribution of the central ghrelin system has been described (Cowley *et al.*, 2003). The relative contribution of peripheral versus central ghrelin to the regulation of energy balance remains a topic of discussion.

2.1   Ghrelin and food intake

Evidence for the orexigenic effects of ghrelin was predicted by several reports showing that GHS stimulated food intake independently from their effects on GH secretion (Locke *et al.*, 1995; Torsello *et al.*, 1998, 2000; Lall *et al.*, 2001). The identification of the GHS-R and its localization within hypothalamic sites heavily implicated in the regulation of energy balance provided a second clue to the regulatory role of GHS and of ghrelin (Guan *et al.*, 1997). Finally, studies showing that GHS increased the expression of fos immunoreactivity, an index of increased transcriptional activation, in the same hypothalamic sites where the GHS-R was located, were final indicators that the endogenous GHS was a potent regulator of energy balance (Dickson *et al.*, 1995a,1995b, 1996, 1997, 1999, Dickson & Luckman, 1997).

The effects of ghrelin on food intake were first established in three very influential papers (Tschop *et al.*, 2000; Wren *et al.*, 2000; Nakazato *et al.*, 2001). These papers demonstrated that, unlike other orexigenic peptides such as neuropeptide Y (NPY), peripherally delivered ghrelin acted in the brain to stimulate food intake and adipocity. Wren *et al.* determined that acute ghrelin treatment delivered either peripherally or into the cerebral ventricles (icv) produced a potent increase in food intake that was similar to that obtained with equimolar concentrations of NPY (Wren *et al.*, 2000). Soon after, Nakazato and associates showed similar orexigenic effects of central ghrelin administration, and further, they demonstrated that the hypothalamic arcuate nucleus (ARC), and particularly neurons producing NPY/agouti-related peptide (AGRP), were implicated in the food intake effects of ghrelin (Nakazato *et al.*, 2001). Finally, Tschop and colleagues determined that chronic central ghrelin treatment, in addition to potently stimulating food intake, also decreased the utilization of fat as fuel leading ultimately to an increase in the accumulation of body fat (Tschop *et al.*, 2000). Furthermore, Tschop's and Nakazato's groups demonstrated that ghrelin stimulated food intake in growth hormone-deficient mice, showing that the orexigenic effects of ghrelin are not mediated indirectly by increases in GH secretion (Tschop *et al.*, 2000; Nakazato *et al.*, 2001). Several things are evident from these studies. The first is that ghrelin increases food intake dramatically especially when infused directly into the brain. The second is that even though the effects of chronic peripheral ghrelin on food intake subside, they do not decrease when ghrelin is administered chronically into the brain. Finally, these studies show the hypothalamus is sensitive to ghrelin stimulation, as reflected by increases in Fos immunoreactivity in the ARC following ghrelin treatment. In all, these data demonstrated that ghrelin targets cells within the ARC to increase food intake and produce metabolic changes geared to accumulate body fat.

In agreement with these data, circulating levels of ghrelin fluctuate in response to changes in energy status. In rodents, plasma ghrelin concentrations rise just before the onset of the dark phase of the light/dark cycle, the time of day when these animals consume most of their food (Drazen *et al.*, 2006). Moreover, fasting increases circulating plasma levels of ghrelin in both mice and rats (Tschop *et al.*, 2000; Ariyasu *et al.*, 2001; Toshinai *et al.*, 2001; Wren *et al.*, 2001b). Rats treated with streptozotocin, a drug that destroys pancreatic beta cells and that results in a diabetic state, also have high levels of circulating ghrelin levels that correlate with increased food intake (Ishii *et al.*, 2002; Masaoka *et al.*, 2003; Gelling *et al.*, 2004). In humans, ghrelin concentrations rise prior to scheduled meals, and are usually elevated after fasting periods (Cummings *et al.*, 2001). Interestingly, in both laboratory animals and human subjects, ghrelin levels decrease throughout the course of a meal (Cummings *et al.*, 2001; Tschop *et al.*, 2001; Sugino *et al.*, 2002; Drazen *et al.*, 2006). Therefore it is not surprising that hormones that regulate metabolic function such as gonadal and adrenal steroids, and those that are related to short-term regulation of food intake such as glucagon, also appear to regulate plasma ghrelin levels (Toshinai *et al.*, 2001; Nakagawa *et al.*, 2002; Camina *et al.*, 2003; Matsubara *et al.*, 2004; Otto *et al.*, 2004; Arafat *et al.*, 2005; Proulx *et al.*, 2005).

In addition to circulating ghrelin levels being increased, sensitivity to ghrelin may also rise in states of negative energy balance. Fasting, for example, leads to changes in the expression of GHS-R in the hypothalamus and pituitary of rats and mice (Kim *et al.*, 2003; Nogueiras *et al.*, 2004; Park *et al.*, 2004). Within the hypothalamus, increases in the message for GHS-R have been reported in NPY/AGRP cells, but it is likely that this also occurs in cells within other brain regions where the GHS-R is present (Traebert *et al.*, 2002; Seoane *et al.*, 2003; Nogueiras *et al.*, 2004). Importantly, immunoneutralization of ghrelin, or pharmacological blockade of GHS-R using GHS-R antagonists both result in decreases in food intake and adipocity in normal rats and mice, in streptozotocin-treated rats, and in leptin-deficient (^{Lep}/^{Lep}) mice (Nakazato *et al.*, 2001; Ishii *et al.*, 2002; Asakawa *et al.*, 2003). Similar results are seen in rats that over-express an antisense for the GHS-R in the brain under the activity of the tyrosine hydroxylase promoter (Shuto *et al.*, 2002).

As mentioned above, ghrelin and its analogues also produce increases in adipocity. Ghrelin appears to do this via a variety of mechanisms. One is by altering metabolic function in order to preferentially utilize energy derived from carbohydrates, thus decreasing the use of fat as a fuel (Tschop *et al.*, 2000). A second mechanism is one in which ghrelin preferentially increases the ingestion of calories derived from fat (Asakawa *et al.*, 2003; Shimbara *et al.*, 2004). A third mechanism is one where ghrelin decreases metabolic function by lowering the resting metabolic rate and heat production (St-Pierre *et al.*, 2004). A final mechanism identified thus far is one where ghrelin decreases energy expenditure by decreasing spontaneous locomotor activity (Tang-Christensen *et al.*, 2004). These ghrelin-induced changes are of particular importance, especially if ghrelin and its related compounds are to be considered as pharmacological tools to control metabolic function. These changes may also provide clues as to why ghrelin-treated animals are susceptible to accumulate more fat under a high-fat diet regimen than saline-treated animals, and provide insights for the possible causes that lead to metabolic dysfunction in obese individuals.

The role of ghrelin in the regulation of food intake and energy balance has been questioned because initial studies using mice with genetic deletions of either the ghrelin or the GHS-R gene showed no observable phenotypical differences from their wild-type littermates (Sun *et al.*, 2003, 2004; Wortley *et al.*, 2004). Contrary to what was expected, ghrelin ($^{ghrl/ghrl}$) and GHS-R ($^{ghsr/ghsr}$) deficient mice ate and weighed the same as wild-type mice, showed no differential feeding in response to fasting, and were still susceptible to diet-induced obesity when fed a high-fat diet. Nevertheless, recent studies show that both $^{ghrl/ghrl}$ and $^{ghsr/ghsr}$ mice are resistant to diet-induced obesity if they are placed on the diet regimen at a relatively young age (18 weeks) (Wortley *et al.*, 2005; Zigman *et al.*, 2005). Moreover, these mice showed altered metabolic parameters such as increased energy expenditure (in $^{ghrl/ghrl}$), decreased respiratory quotient (in $^{ghsr/ghsr}$), and better glycemic regulation, indicating that ghrelin may play an important role in the development of obesity and metabolic aberrations associated with this disorder (Wortley *et al.*, 2005; Zigman *et al.*, 2005). These results are echoed in recent studies where diet-induced obese mice lost weight after treatment with a mirror (*Spiegel*) L-oligonucleotide that antagonizes the activity of the active form of ghrelin on the GHS-R (Helmling *et al.*, 2004; Kobelt *et al.*, 2005; Shearman *et al.*, 2005).

2.2   Ghrelin receptors: role in energy balance

The above-described reports suggest that the GHS-R 1a is crucial for ghrelin to have an effect on energy balance. The GHS-R 1a is a G-coupled protein receptor that, upon activation, increases the activity of intracellular calcium and protein kinase C (PKC) by increasing the activity of inositol 1,4,5-triphosphate (IP$_3$)/phospholipase C (PLC) and diacylglycerol (Malagon *et al.*, 2003; Camina, 2006). This is a similar signaling cascade activated by GHS (McKee *et al.*, 1997; Kojima *et al.*, 1999). In any event, ghrelin increases the activity of other intracellular pathways via alternate G-coupled protein complexes. Of these, ghrelin-induced increases in the activity of 5′-AMP-activated protein kinase (AMPK), and the cyclic GMP-related release of nitric oxide (NO) are thought to play a role in the hypothalamic regulation of energy balance (Gaskin *et al.*, 2003; Andersson *et al.*, 2004). However, complete characterization of these signaling pathways in relation to ghrelin activation of GHS-R 1a and GHS-R 1b pathways is needed. In addition, it appears that GHS-Rs have a high level of constitutive activity, and can be activated by other ligands such as cortistatin and adenosine (Deghenghi *et al.*, 2001; Broglio *et al.*, 2002; Holst *et al.*, 2003; Carreira *et al.*, 2004; Holst & Schwartz, 2004). The physiological relevance of these phenomena is not yet understood. Furthermore, several studies have suggested the existence of additional GHS-Rs that have not yet been characterized (Halem *et al.*, 2004, 2005; Camina, 2006).

Early descriptions of the localization of GHS-R showed that high concentrations were detected in various endocrine organs. Of these, the hypothalamus and pituitary stood out as potential mediators for the effects of ghrelin on growth hormone secretion (McKee *et al.*, 1997). *In situ* hybridization studies revealed that the hypothalamic arcuate nucleus (ARC) and the ventromedial hypothalamus (VMH) of rats and primates strongly expressed GHS-R mRNA (Guan *et al.*, 1997; Mitchell *et al.*, 2001). These reports additionally showed that the message for the receptor was also localized in hypothalamic and extrahypothalamic brain regions not directly implicated in the regulation of energy balance. Among these, the preoptic area (POA), suprachiasmatic nucleus (SCN), hippocampus, ventral tegmental area (VTA), substantia nigra (SN) and dorsal raphe nucleus (DRN) showed relatively high concentrations of GHS-R mRNA expression (Guan *et al.*, 1997; Mitchell *et al.*, 2001). A recent and more complete study describing the neuroanatomical localization of the GHS-R transcript has confirmed these earlier data and extended them to mice. In addition, they have demonstrated that the receptor is located in brain stem regions also associated with the regulation of food intake such as the parabrachial nucleus, area postrema, and the nucleus of the solitary tract (Zigman et al., 2006).

The number of GHS-Rs that are available for binding is modulated by ghrelin itself and by other hormones. Ghrelin has been shown to produce GHS-R internalization into vesicles in vitro via endosomal trafficking, where it gets recycled back to the membrane without being degraded (Camina et al., 2004). The duration of the cycle of internalization/recycling of the GHS-R corresponds well with the pulsatile nature of ghrelin release (Camina et al., 2004). In contrast, in vivo ghrelin treatment leads to a rapid increase in the expression of GHS-R mRNA in the ARC of rats, whereas leptin treatment results in decreases in GHS-R mRNA in the same region. These effects are specific to the ARC, and the effects of ghrelin at least are dependent on the presence of growth hormone, given that growth hormone deficient rats do not show a ghrelin-induced increase in GHS-R (Nogueiras et al., 2004). Conversely, growth hormone deficient rats (dw/dw dwarf rats) do have significantly higher GHS-R mRNA expression in the hypothalamus than control rats, and the expression of GHS-R is decreased with growth hormone treatment (Nogueiras et al., 2004). The idea that leptin may also play a role is suggested by the fact that genetically obese Zucker rats and fasted animals also show increased levels of GHS-R mRNA expression in the ARC (Nogueiras et al., 2004).

2.3   Ghrelin and the hypothalamic regulation of energy balance

The localization of high levels of GHS-R transcripts in the ARC, as well as the increases in the expression of transcription factors in the ARC following GHS or ghrelin treatment, quickly highlight the ARC as the most relevant hypothalamic site for the regulation of ghrelin's effects on food intake and adipocity (Horvath et al., 2001). Because the ARC lies outside of the blood–brain barrier, it is placed in a position where it can monitor circulating levels of a variety of hormones, including ghrelin. Not surprisingly, the ARC contains first-order sensory neurons that have receptors for most, if not all, hormones associated with energy balance (Elmquist et al., 1998; Woods et al., 1998, 2000; Spiegelman & Flier, 2001; Horvath & Diano, 2004). Orexigenic peptides like NPY and AGRP, and anorexigenic peptides like a-melanocyte stimulating hormone (a-msh) and the cocaine-amphetamine regulated trancript (CART) are both produced by cells in the ARC. Among these, the GHS-R is reportedly expressed in NPY/AGRP secreting cells, but it is likely to be also present in α-msh/CART secreting cells. Because both of these cells groups are also affected by leptin, and represent the cornerstone for the melanocortin hypothesis of body weight regulation, it has been suggested that ghrelin targets the hypothalamus to oppose the anorectic activity of leptin (Woods et al., 1998; Tritos & Maratos-Flier, 1999; Woods et al., 2000; Cone et al., 2001; Cowley, 2003).

Nevertheless, substantial concentrations of GHS-R are present in other hypothalamic nuclei heavily implicated in energy balance including the VMH, paraventricular nucleus (PVN), dorsomedial hypothalamus (DMH), and suprachiasmatic nucleus (SCN) (Guan et al., 1997; Mitchell et al., 2001; Zigman et al., 2006). In addition, central infusions of ghrelin into the lateral hypothalamus increase food intake and the activity of cells that produce hypocretin/orexin, a hypothalamic peptide implicated in arousal and food intake (Olszewski et al., 2003b; Toshinai et al., 2003; Chen et al., 2005). Infusions of ghrelin into the PVN are also effective in increasing food intake, and modulating neuronal activity in PVN cells at picomolar concentrations (Olszewski et al., 2003a; Chen et al., 2005). While no data are yet available on the effects of direct ghrelin infusions into the DMH, SCN, and VMH on food intake, they are all activated by intracerebroventricular (icv) administration of ghrelin as demonstrated by increases in the expression of Fos in these regions (Nakazato et al., 2001; Halem et al., 2005). In contrast to these data, increases in the expression of Fos following peripheral ghrelin treatment are seldom seen outside of the ARC and other regions outside the blood–brain barrier (see Ruter et al., 2003 for exception).

Ghrelin appears to modulate the activity of hypothalamic cells, and particularly cells in the ARC, by modulating their threshold of activation by inhibitory and excitatory neurotransmitters (Cowley, 2003; Cowley et al., 2003; Pinto et al., 2004). Like estrogen and leptin, ghrelin is capable of reorganizing synaptic inputs onto neurons within the ARC (Pinto et al., 2004). In contrast to estrogen or leptin, however, ghrelin increases the number of excitatory inputs and decreases inhibitory inputs onto NPY/AGRP cells, and decreases the number of excitatory inputs and increases the number of inhibitory inputs onto proopiomelanocortin (POMC, the precursor of α-msh) secreting neurons (Pinto et al., 2004). This synaptic re-arrangement correlates with electrophysiological data (see below) and fits well with the stimulatory effects of ghrelin on food intake (Pinto et al., 2004). This, along with the fact that ghrelin appears to target regions of the brain that retain a high degree of plasticity in adulthood, like the hippocampus, SCN and ventral tegmental area (VTA), suggests that ghrelin produces its effects in the hypothalamus and elsewhere by mechanisms that involve synaptic changes.

2.4   Ghrelin and appetite: is it all hypothalamic?

The relatively dense distribution of the GHS-R in the ARC and other mediobasal hypothalamic nuclei has guided researchers to focus primarily on this region as mediating ghrelin's effects on energy regulation. In any event, the widespread distribution of the GHS-R throughout the CNS indicates that ghrelin may modulate a variety of systems associated with appetite.

The brainstem and food intake

The brainstem has been heavily implicated in the regulation of food intake and energy sensing (Grill & Kaplan 2001, 2002). Like the mediobasal hypothalamus, areas within the brainstem such as the area postrema lie outside the blood–brain barrier. Not surprisingly, the area postrema and the adjacent nucleus of the solitary tract have receptors for various metabolic hormones such as cholecystokinin (CCK), estrogen, leptin and ghrelin (Wade & Schneider, 1992; Grill & Kaplan 2001, 2002; Zigman et al., 2006). Neurons in these regions also respond to changes in glucose and free fatty acid utilization suggesting an important role in nutrient sensing (Ritter, 1986; Ritter et al., 2000). In addition, the brainstem receives afferent signals from the gastrointestinal system through the ascending vagus nerve, and sends efferent signals to the gut via the descending vagus (Swanson & Sawchenko, 1980; Sawchenko & Swanson 1981, 1982). Vagal afferent signals target neurons in the nucleus of the solitary tract and the parabrachial nucleus, and from there they are transmitted to hypothalamic and forebrain structures for further processing (Swanson & Sawchenko, 1980). Studies on animals whose brainstem is surgically isolated from the rest of the brain, have demonstrated that this region is sufficient for normal responses to taste and meal size regulation in response to gastrointestinal cues (Grill & Kaplan, 2001, 2002).

Studies show that icv ghrelin infusions increase the expression of the transcription factor Fos in the area postrema and nucleus of the solitary tract (Lawrence et al., 2002). These studies in addition to others showing that ghrelin infused into the fourth ventricle, or directly into the dorsal vagal complex (DVC; a cluster of nuclei that include the area postrema, nucleus of the solitary tract, and others) increase food intake, suggest that this area is sensitive to ghrelin stimulation (Faulconbridge et al., 2003, 2005). Interestingly, ghrelin-induced food intake responses are attenuated by sub-diaphragmic vagotomy in rodents and humans (Williams et al., 2003; le Roux et al., 2005). These data suggest that vagal signals from the gut to the brain and back play a significant role in the regulation of food intake by ghrelin.

Ghrelin and reward circuits

In addition to the hypothalamus and the brainstem, the GHS-R is localized within the ventral tegmental area (VTA) of the mid brain in relatively high concentrations (Guan *et al.*, 1997; Zigman *et al.*, 2006). The VTA contains primarily dopamine cells that play a key role in the neural system that underlie motivated behaviors. The activity of dopamine cells is correlated with increases in behaviors geared to obtain natural rewards like food or a receptive mate, and with behaviors directed towards obtaining drugs of abuse (Berridge, 1996; Wise, 2002). Double labeling studies have determined that about 40% of dopaminergic neurons in the VTA contain GHS-R 1a mRNA signal (Zigman *et al.*, 2006). Ghrelin infusions into the VTA increase food intake, and they seem to do so independent of opioids (Naleid *et al.*, 2005). Ghrelin, like food restriction, enhances the locomotor responses to cocaine, an indication that ghrelin modulates reward circuits (Wellman *et al.*, 2005). In addition, ghrelin can increase food intake when infused into the nucleus accumbens, a major target for VTA dopaminergic cells, and a structure implicated in the appetitive regulation of food intake (Naleid *et al.*, 2005). Interestingly, ghrelin also increases hoarding and foraging behavior, both measures of appetitive behaviors with high motivational components in rodents (Keen-Rhinehart & Bartness, 2005). In humans, ghrelin infusions not only provoke strong feeding responses but they also increase self-report scores on hunger measures and elicit vivid cravings for preferred foods (Wren *et al.*, 2001a; Cummings *et al.*, 2004; Schmid *et al.*, 2005). It is therefore likely that ghrelin targets the VTA and other reward limbic regions to regulate food seeking and hedonic responses to food.

Ghrelin and circadian rhythmicity

Food intake, and most metabolic functions, show fluctuations across the light/dark cycles and these are regulated primarily by a central circadian pacemaker, which in mammals is located in the hypothalamic SCN (Pando & Sassone-Corsi, 2001). It is therefore intriguing, that the SCN contains dense concentrations of GHS-R (Mitchell *et al.*, 2001; Zigman *et al.*, 2006). While there are no data to date as to the role of these receptors in the regulation of circadian rhythms, GHS-R deficient (but not ghrelin deficient) mice show lower levels of locomotor activity in the early dark phase of the light/dark cycle, suggesting the possibility of altered circadian patterns (Zigman *et al.*, 2005). In addition, scheduled meals can produce ghrelin peaks similar to pre-prandial ghrelin increases in the early dark phase of the light/dark cycle (Sugino *et al.*, 2002a, 2002b; Drazen *et al.*, 2006). It could be speculated that ghrelin acts in the SCN to modulate behavioral rhythms according to the timing of food availability in the environment.

2.5   Brain ghrelin?

A hypothesis that has generated a tremendous amount of interest and controversy is that ghrelin is synthesized directly in neurosecretory cells in the brain (Cowley et al., 2003; Mozid et al., 2003) and these are modified by energetic state (Sato et al., 2005). Indeed, several independent groups have shown that hypothalamic cells secrete ghrelin and communicate with cell groups throughout the hypothalamic nuclei shown to contain ghrelin receptors (Cowley et al., 2003). Some papers suggest that the distribution of ghrelin-producing neurons is restricted to the ventro-lateral portion of the ARC (Kojima et al., 1999; Lu et al., 2002; Guan et al., 2003; Toshinai et al., 2003), whereas others have shown an extensive distribution of ghrelin immunoreactive cells that literally envelops all major hypothalamic centers (Cowley et al., 2003). Projections from ghrelin cells make contact with NPY/AGRP cells in the ARC, hypocretin/orexin cells in the lateral hypothalamic region, and corticotropin-releasing hormone (CRH) neurons in the PVN (Lu et al., 2002; Cowley et al., 2003; Toshinai et al., 2003). The electrical activity of these cell groups is modulated by ghrelin as shown using patch clamp electrophysiological studies where ghrelin stimulates the activity of NPY/AGRP and hypocretin/orexin cells, and decreases the activity of POMC and CRH cells (Cowley, 2003; Riediger et al., 2003; Pinto et al., 2004; Chen et al., 2005). This particular pattern of activity is associated with increased food intake and decreased energy expenditure. A caveat to this hypothesis is that the transcript for ghrelin in the hypothalamus can only be detected by amplifying mRNA signals using polymerase chain reaction (PCR), but not by in situ hybridization probes that work to detect the ghrelin transcript on stomach cells. Moreover, mice with the Lac Z reporter gene inserted into the ghrelin promoter do not show Lac Z enzyme activity in the hypothalamus (Wortley et al., 2004), although they do show Lac Z mRNA (Sun et al., 2003). Much work is needed to clarify these discrepancies, yet the widespread distribution of GHS-R in the central nervous system, coupled with the apparent difficulty of ghrelin to enter the brain still point to a central source of ghrelin (Banks et al., 2002).

2.6   Clinical implications

Obesity is currently a primary target for drug development given the rapid increase in the incidence of this condition and the risk factors associated with it. Since animal studies show that the antagonism of ghrelin leads to weight reduction and control of glucopenea in diet-induced and in genetically obese animals, this indicates that antagonists for ghrelin may provide for potential treatments for obesity, type II diabetes and other metabolic disorders (Wortley et al., 2005; Zigman et al., 2005). In addition, ghrelin-based treatments may be used to increase appetite in patients undergoing wasting disorders such as cancer-induced cachexia, or those receiving chemotherapy (Neary *et al.*, 2004).

As we unravel the complexities of the multimodal actions of ghrelin on brain function, we may find that ghrelin and compounds associated with this hormone may be effective in modulating not only metabolism but also the appetitive and cognitive functions related to the human experience of "cravings," something that is key for the treatment of psychiatric conditions associated with eating disorders like anorexia nervosa and bulimia, and for the treatment of drug abuse.

2.7   Conclusion

The discovery of ghrelin and its well-established role in the regulation of feeding and energy balance has provoked an amount of attention that is almost comparable to that generated by leptin. Ghrelin appears to target different CNS regions to modify energy balance and food intake in a multimodal manner. Among these, only the effects of ghrelin on hypothalamic function are somewhat understood, perhaps because we are only beginning to explain the hypothalamic circuits regulating energy homeostasis. Nevertheless, it is becoming more apparent that other systems interact with the hypothalamus to regulate energy balance, and most of these are also targeted by ghrelin as well as other metabolic signals such as leptin and insulin. Future studies will surely provide a clearer picture of the relative contribution of these regions to energy regulation and their responses to changes in metabolism. Gaining knowledge on these networks will surely advance basic understanding of energy regulation and perhaps generate alternative, more effective treatments for obesity.

References

Andersson, U., Filipsson, K. *et al.* (2004). AMP-activated protein kinase plays a role in the control of food intake. *J. Biol. Chem.* **279**, 12 005–8.

Arafat, M. A., Otto, B. *et al.* (2005). Glucagon inhibits ghrelin secretion in humans. *Eur. J. Endocrinol.* **153**, 397–402.

Ariyasu, H., Takaya, K. *et al.* (2001). Stomach is a major source of circulating ghrelin, and feeding state determines plasma ghrelin-like immunoreactivity levels in humans. *J. Clin. Endocrinol. Metab.* **86**, 4753–8.

Asakawa, A., Inui, A. *et al.* (2003). Antagonism of ghrelin receptor reduces food intake and body weight gain in mice. *Gut* **52**, 947–52.

Banks, W. A., Tschop, M. *et al.* (2002). Extent and direction of ghrelin transport across the blood-brain barrier is determined by its unique primary structure. *J. Pharmacol. Exp. Ther.* **302**, 822-7.

Berridge, K. C. (1996). Food reward: brain substrates of wanting and liking. *Neurosci. Biobehav. Rev.* **20**, 1-25.

Bowers, C. Y. (1993). GH releasing peptides - structure and kinetics. *J. Pediatr. Endocrinol.* **6**, 21-31.

Bowers, C. Y., Momany, F. A. *et al.* (1984a). On the in vitro and in vivo activity of a new synthetic hexapeptide that acts on the pituitary to specifically release growth hormone. *Endocrinology* **114**, 1537-45.

Bowers, C. Y., Reynolds, G. A. *et al.* (1984b). New advances on the regulation of growth hormone (GH) secretion. *Int. J. Neurol.* **18**, 188-205.

Broglio, F., Arvat, E. *et al.* (2002). Endocrine activities of cortistatin-14 and its interaction with GHRH and ghrelin in humans. *J. Clin. Endocrinol. Metab.* **87**, 3783-90.

Camina, J. P. (2006). Cell biology of the ghrelin receptor. *J. Neuroendocrin.* **18**, 65-76.

Camina, J. P., Carreira, M. C. *et al.* (2003). Regulation of ghrelin secretion and action. *Endocrine* **22**, 5-12.

Camina, J. P., Carreira, M. C. *et al.* (2004). Desensitization and endocytosis mechanisms of ghrelin-activated growth hormone secretagogue receptor 1a. *Endocrinology* **145**, 930-40.

Carreira, M. C., Camina, J. P. *et al.* (2004). Agonist-specific coupling of growth hormone secretagogue receptor type 1a to different intracellular signaling systems. Role of adenosine. *Neuroendocrinology* **79**, 13-25.

Chen, X., Ge, Y. L. *et al.* (2005). Effects of ghrelin on hypothalamic glucose responding neurons in rats. *Brain Res.* **1055**, 131-6.

Cone, R. D., Cowley, M. A. *et al.* (2001). The arcuate nucleus as a conduit for diverse signals relevant to energy homeostasis. *Int. J. Obes. Relat. Metab. Disord.* **25** (Suppl. **5**), S63-7.

Cowley, M. A. (2003). Hypothalamic melanocortin neurons integrate signals of energy state. *Eur. J. Pharmacol.* **480**, 3-11.

Cowley, M. A., Smith, R. G. *et al.* (2003). The distribution and mechanism of action of ghrelin in the CNS demonstrates a novel hypothalamic circuit regulating energy homeostasis. *Neuron* **37**, 649-61.

Cummings, D. E., Purnell, J. Q. *et al.* (2001). A preprandial rise in plasma ghrelin levels suggests a role in meal initiation in humans. *Diabetes* **50**, 1714-19.

Cummings, D. E., Frayo, R. S. *et al.* (2004). Plasma ghrelin levels and hunger scores in humans initiating meals voluntarily without time- and food-related cues. *Am. J. Physiol. Endocrinol. Metab.* **287**, E297-304.

Davenport, A. P., Bonner, T. I. *et al.* (2005). International Union of Pharmacology. LVI. Ghrelin receptor nomenclature, distribution, and function. *Pharmacol Rev.* **57**, 541-6.

Deghenghi, R., Papotti, M. *et al.* (2001). Cortistatin, but not somatostatin, binds to growth hormone secretagogue (GHS) receptors of human pituitary gland. *J. Endocrinol. Invest.* **24**, RC1-3.

Dickson, S. L. & Luckman, S. M. (1997). Induction of c-fos messenger ribonucleic acid in neuropeptide Y and growth hormone (GH)-releasing factor neurons in the rat arcuate nucleus following systemic injection of the GH secretagogue, GH-releasing peptide-6. *Endocrinology* **138**, 771-7.

Dickson, S. L., Doutrelant-Viltart, O. *et al.* (1995a). GH-deficient dw/dw rats and lit/lit mice show increased Fos expression in the hypothalamic arcuate nucleus following systemic injection of GH-releasing peptide-6. *J. Endocrinol.* **146**, 519-26.

Dickson, S. L., Leng, G. *et al.* (1995b). Central actions of peptide and non-peptide growth hormone secretagogues in the rat. *Neuroendocrinology* **61**, 36-43.

Dickson, S. L., Doutrelant-Viltart, O. *et al.* (1996). Retrogradely labelled neurosecretory neurones of the rat hypothalamic arcuate nucleus express Fos protein following systemic injection of GH-releasing peptide-6. *J. Endocrinol.* **151**, 323-31.

Dickson, S. L., Viltart, O. *et al.* (1997). Attenuation of the growth hormone secretagogue induction of Fos protein in the rat arcuate nucleus by central somatostatin action. *Neuroendocrinology* **66**, 188-94.

Dickson, S. L., Bailey, A. R. *et al.* (1999). Growth hormone (GH) secretagogues and neuroendocrine regulation of GH secretion. *Growth Horm. IGF Res.* **9** (Suppl. **A**), 89-91.

Drazen, D. L., Vahl, T. P. *et al.* (2006). Effects of a fixed meal pattern on ghrelin secretion: evidence for a learned response independent of nutrient status. *Endocrinology* **147**, 23-30.

Elmquist, J. K., Maratos-Flier, E. *et al.* (1998). Unraveling the central nervous system pathways underlying responses to leptin. *Nat. Neurosci.* **1**, 445-50.

Faulconbridge, L. F., Cummings, D. E. *et al.* (2003). Hyperphagic effects of brainstem ghrelin administration. *Diabetes* **52**, 2260-5.

Faulconbridge, L. F., Grill, H. J. *et al.* (2005). Distinct forebrain and caudal brainstem contributions to the neuropeptide Y mediation of ghrelin hyperphagia. *Diabetes* **54**, 1985-93.

Gaskin, F. S., Farr, S. A. *et al.* (2003). Ghrelin-induced feeding is dependent on nitric oxide. *Peptides* **24**, 913-18.

Gelling, R. W., Overduin, J. *et al.* (2004). Effect of uncontrolled diabetes on plasma ghrelin concentrations and ghrelin-induced feeding. *Endocrinology* **145**, 4575-82.

Grill, H. J. & Kaplan, J. M. (2001). Interoceptive and integrative contributions of forebrain and brainstem to energy balance control. *Int. J. Obes. Relat. Metab. Disord.* **25** (Suppl. **5**), S73-7.

Grill, H. J. & Kaplan, J. M. (2002). The neuroanatomical axis for control of energy balance. *Front Neuroendocrinol.* **23**, 2-40.

Guan, J. L., Wang, Q. P. *et al.* (2003). Synaptic interactions between ghrelin- and neuropeptide Y-containing neurons in the rat arcuate nucleus. *Peptides* **24**, 1921-8.

Guan, X. M., Yu, H. *et al.* (1997). Distribution of mRNA encoding the growth hormone secretagogue receptor in brain and peripheral tissues. *Mol. Brain Res.* **48**, 23-9.

Halem, H. A., Taylor, J. E. et al. (2004). Novel analogs of ghrelin: physiological and clinical implications. *Eur. J. Endocrinol.* **151** (Suppl. 1), S71-5.

Halem, H. A., Taylor, J. E. et al. (2005). A novel growth hormone secretagogue-1a receptor antagonist that blocks ghrelin-induced growth hormone secretion but induces increased body weight gain. *Neuroendocrinology* **81**, 339-49.

Helmling, S., Maasch, C. et al. (2004). Inhibition of ghrelin action in vitro and in vivo by an RNA-Spiegelmer. *Proc. Natl. Acad. Sci. USA* **101**, 13174-9.

Holst, B. & Schwartz, T. W. (2004). Constitutive ghrelin receptor activity as a signaling set-point in appetite regulation. *Trends. Pharmacol. Sci.* **25**, 113-17.

Holst, B., Cygankiewicz, A. et al. (2003). High constitutive signaling of the ghrelin receptor - identification of a potent inverse agonist. *Mol. Endocrinol.* **17**, 2201-10.

Horvath, T. L. & Diano, S. (2004). The floating blueprint of hypothalamic feeding circuits. *Nat. Rev. Neurosci.* **5**, 662-7.

Horvath, T. L., Diano, S. et al. (2001). Minireview: ghrelin and the regulation of energy balance - a hypothalamic perspective. *Endocrinology* **142**, 4163-9.

Hosoda, H., Kojima, M. et al. (2000). Purification and characterization of rat des-Gln14-Ghrelin, a second endogenous ligand for the growth hormone secretagogue receptor. *J. Biol. Chem.* **275**, 21 995-2000.

Ishii, S., Kamegai, J. et al. (2002). Role of ghrelin in streptozotocin-induced diabetic hyperphagia. *Endocrinology* **143**, 4934-7.

Keen-Rhinehart, E. & Bartness, T. J. (2005). Peripheral ghrelin injections stimulate food intake, foraging, and food hoarding in Siberian hamsters. *Am. J. Physiol. Regul. Integr. Comp. Physiol.* **288**, R716-22.

Kim, M. S., Yoon, C. Y. et al. (2003). Changes in ghrelin and ghrelin receptor expression according to feeding status. *Neuroreport* **14**, 1317-20.

Kobelt, P., Helmling, S. et al. (2005). Anti-ghrelin Spiegelmer NOX-B11 inhibits neurostimulatory and orexigenic effects of peripheral ghrelin in rats. *Gut.* **55**, 788-92.

Kojima, M. & Kangawa, K. (2005). Ghrelin: structure and function. *Physiol. Rev.* **85**, 495-522.

Kojima, M., Hosoda, H. et al. (1999). Ghrelin is a growth-hormone-releasing acylated peptide from stomach. *Nature* **402**, 656-60.

Lall, S., Tung, L. Y. et al. (2001). Growth hormone (GH)-independent stimulation of adiposity by GH secretagogues. *Biochem. Biophys. Res. Commun.* **280**, 132-8.

Lawrence, C. B., Snape, A. C. et al. (2002). Acute central ghrelin and GH secretagogues induce feeding and activate brain appetite centers. *Endocrinology* **143**, 155-62.

le Roux, C. W., Neary, N. M. et al. (2005). Ghrelin does not stimulate food intake in patients with surgical procedures involving vagotomy. *J. Clin. Endocrinol. Metab.* **90**, 4521-4.

Locke, W., Kirgis, H. D. et al. (1995). Intracerebroventricular growth-hormone-releasing peptide-6 stimulates eating without affecting plasma growth hormone responses in rats. *Life Sci* **56**, 1347-52.

Lu, S., Guan, J. L. et al. (2002). Immunocytochemical observation of ghrelin-containing neurons in the rat arcuate nucleus. *Neurosci. Lett.* **321**, 157-60.

Malagon, M. M., Luque, R. M. *et al.* (2003). Intracellular signaling mechanisms mediating ghrelin-stimulated growth hormone release in somatotropes. *Endocrinology* **144**, 5372–80.

Masaoka, T., Suzuki, H. *et al.* (2003). Enhanced plasma ghrelin levels in rats with streptozotocin-induced diabetes. *FEBS Lett.* **541**, 64–8.

Matsubara, M., Sakata, I. *et al.* (2004). Estrogen modulates ghrelin expression in the female rat stomach. *Peptides* **25**, 289–97.

McKee, K. K., Palyha, O. C. *et al.* (1997). Molecular analysis of rat pituitary and hypothalamic growth hormone secretagogue receptors. *Mol. Endocrinol.* **11**, 415–23.

Mitchell, V., Bouret, S. *et al.* (2001). Comparative distribution of mRNA encoding the growth hormone secretagogue-receptor (GHS-R) in *Microcebus murinus* (Primate, lemurian) and rat forebrain and pituitary. *J. Comp. Neurol.* **429**, 469–89.

Mozid, A. M., Tringali, G. *et al.* (2003). Ghrelin is released from rat hypothalamic explants and stimulates corticotrophin-releasing hormone and arginine-vasopressin. *Horm. Metab. Res.* **35**, 455–9.

Nakagawa, E., Nagaya, N. *et al.* (2002). Hyperglycaemia suppresses the secretion of ghrelin, a novel growth-hormone-releasing peptide: responses to the intravenous and oral administration of glucose. *Clin. Sci. (Lond)* **103**, 325–8.

Nakazato, M., Murakami, N. *et al.* (2001). A role for ghrelin in the central regulation of feeding. *Nature* **409**, 194–8.

Naleid, A. M., Grace, M. K. *et al.* (2005). Ghrelin induces feeding in the mesolimbic reward pathway between the ventral tegmental area and the nucleus accumbens. *Peptides* **26**, 2274–9.

Neary, N. M., Small, C. J. *et al.* (2004). Ghrelin increases energy intake in cancer patients with impaired appetite: acute, randomized, placebo-controlled trial. *J. Clin. Endocrinol. Metab.* **89**, 2832–6.

Nogueiras, R., Tovar, S. *et al.* (2004). Regulation of growth hormone secretagogue receptor gene expression in the arcuate nuclei of the rat by leptin and ghrelin. *Diabetes* **53**, 2552–8.

Olszewski, P. K., Grace, M. K. *et al.* (2003a). Hypothalamic paraventricular injections of ghrelin: effect on feeding and c-Fos immunoreactivity. *Peptides* **24**, 919–23.

Olszewski, P. K., Li, D. *et al.* (2003b). Neural basis of orexigenic effects of ghrelin acting within lateral hypothalamus. *Peptides* **24**, 597–602.

Otto, B., Tschop, M. *et al.* (2004). Endogenous and exogenous glucocorticoids decrease plasma ghrelin in humans. *Eur. J. Endocrinol.* **151**, 113–17.

Pando, M. P. & Sassone-Corsi, P. (2001). Signaling to the mammalian circadian clocks: in pursuit of the primary mammalian circadian photoreceptor. *Sci. STKE* **2001(107)**, RE16.

Park, S., Sohn, S. *et al.* (2004). Fasting-induced changes in the hypothalamic-pituitary-GH axis in the absence of GH expression: lessons from the spontaneous dwarf rat. *J. Endocrinol.* **180**, 369–78.

Pinto, S., Roseberry, A. G. *et al.* (2004). Rapid rewiring of arcuate nucleus feeding circuits by leptin. *Science* **304**, 110–15.

Proulx, K., Vahl, T. P. et al. (2005). The effect of adrenalectomy on ghrelin secretion and orexigenic action. J. Neuroendocrinol. **17**, 445–51.

Riediger, T., Traebert, M. et al. (2003). Site-specific effects of ghrelin on the neuronal activity in the hypothalamic arcuate nucleus. Neurosci. Lett. **341**, 151–5.

Ritter, S. (1986). *Glucoprivation and the Glucoprivic Control of Food Intake.* Orlando, FL: Academic Press.

Ritter, S., Dinh, T. T. et al. (2000). Localization of hindbrain glucoreceptive sites controlling food intake and blood glucose. Brain Res. **856**, 37–47.

Ruter, J., Kobelt, P. et al. (2003). Intraperitoneal injection of ghrelin induces Fos expression in the paraventricular nucleus of the hypothalamus in rats. Brain Res. **991**, 26–33.

Sato, T., Fukue, Y. et al. (2005). Molecular forms of hypothalamic ghrelin and its regulation by fasting and 2-deoxy-d-glucose administration. Endocrinology **146**, 2510–16.

Sawchenko, P. E. & Swanson, L. W. (1981). Central noradrenergic pathways for the integration of hypothalamic neuroendocrine and autonomic responses. Science **214**, 685–7.

Sawchenko, P. E. & Swanson, L. W. (1982). The organization of noradrenergic pathways from the brainstem to the paraventricular and supraoptic nuclei in the rat. Brain Res. **257**, 275–325.

Schmid, D. A., Held, K. et al. (2005). Ghrelin stimulates appetite, imagination of food, GH, ACTH, and cortisol, but does not affect leptin in normal controls. Neuropsychopharmacology **30**, 1187–92.

Seoane, L. M., Lopez, M. et al. (2003). Agouti-related peptide, neuropeptide Y, and somatostatin-producing neurons are targets for ghrelin actions in the rat hypothalamus. Endocrinology **144**, 544–51.

Shearman, L. P., Wang, S. P. et al. (2005). Ghrelin neutralization by an RNA-Spiegelmer ameliorates obesity in diet-induced obese mice. Endocrinology.

Shimbara, T., Mondal, M. S. et al. (2004). Central administration of ghrelin preferentially enhances fat ingestion. Neurosci. Lett. **369**, 75–9.

Shuto, Y., Shibasaki, T. et al. (2002). Hypothalamic growth hormone secretagogue receptor regulates growth hormone secretion, feeding, and adiposity. J. Clin. Invest. **109**, 1429–36.

Smith, R. G. (2005). Development of growth hormone secretagogues. Endocr. Rev. **26**, 346–60.

Smith, R. G., Palyha, O. C. et al. (1999). Growth hormone releasing substances: types and their receptors. Horm. Res. **51** (Suppl. 3); 1–8.

Smith, R. G., Jiang, H. et al. (2005). Developments in ghrelin biology and potential clinical relevance. Trends Endocrinol. Metab. **16**, 436–42.

Spiegelman, B. M. & Flier, J. S. (2001). Obesity and the regulation of energy balance. Cell **104**, 531–43.

St-Pierre, D. H., Karelis, A. D. et al. (2004). Relationship between ghrelin and energy expenditure in healthy young women. J. Clin. Endocrinol. Metab. **89**, 5993–7.

Sugino, T., Hasegawa, Y. *et al.* (2002a). A transient ghrelin surge occurs just before feeding in a scheduled meal-fed sheep. *Biochem. Biophys. Res. Commun.* **295**, 255–60.

Sugino, T., Yamaura, J. *et al.* (2002b). A transient surge of ghrelin secretion before feeding is modified by different feeding regimens in sheep. *Biochem. Biophys. Res. Commun.* **298**, 785–8.

Sun, Y., Ahmed, S. *et al.* (2003). Deletion of ghrelin impairs neither growth nor appetite. *Mol. Cell. Biol.* **23**, 7973–81.

Sun, Y., Wang, P. *et al.* (2004). Ghrelin stimulation of growth hormone release and appetite is mediated through the growth hormone secretagogue receptor. *Proc. Natl. Acad. Sci. USA* **101**, 4679–84.

Swanson, L. W. & Sawchenko, P. E. (1980). Paraventricular nucleus: a site for the integration of neuroendocrine and autonomic mechanisms. *Neuroendocrinology* **31**, 410–17.

Tang-Christensen, M., Vrang, N. *et al.* (2004). Central administration of ghrelin and agouti-related protein (83–132) increases food intake and decreases spontaneous locomotor activity in rats. *Endocrinology* **145**, 4645–52.

Torsello, A., Luoni, M. *et al.* (1998). Novel hexarelin analogs stimulate feeding in the rat through a mechanism not involving growth hormone release. *Eur. J. Pharmacol.* **360**, 123–9.

Torsello, A., Locatelli, V. *et al.* (2000). Differential orexigenic effects of hexarelin and its analogs in the rat hypothalamus: indication for multiple growth hormone secretagogue receptor subtypes. *Neuroendocrinology* **72**, 327–32.

Toshinai, K., Mondal, M. S. *et al.* (2001). Upregulation of Ghrelin expression in the stomach upon fasting, insulin-induced hypoglycemia, and leptin administration. *Biochem. Biophys. Res. Commun.* **281**, 1220–5.

Toshinai, K., Date, Y. *et al.* (2003). Ghrelin-induced food intake is mediated via the orexin pathway. *Endocrinology* **144**, 1506–12.

Traebert, M., Riediger, T. *et al.* (2002). Ghrelin acts on leptin-responsive neurones in the rat arcuate nucleus. *J. Neuroendocrinol.* **14**, 580–6.

Tritos, N. A. & Maratos-Flier, E. (1999). Two important systems in energy homeostasis: melanocortins and melanin-concentrating hormone. *Neuropeptides* **33**, 339–49.

Tschop, M., Smiley, D. L. *et al.* (2000). Ghrelin induces adiposity in rodents. *Nature* **407**, 908–13.

Tschop, M., Wawarta, R. *et al.* (2001). Post-prandial decrease of circulating human ghrelin levels. *J. Endocrinol. Invest.* **24**, RC19–21.

van der Lely, A. J., Tschop, M. *et al.* (2004). Biological, physiological, pathophysiological, and pharmacological aspects of ghrelin. *Endocr. Rev.* **25**, 426–57.

Wade, G. N. & Schneider, J. E. (1992). Metabolic fuels and reproduction in female mammals. *Neurosci. Biobehav. Rev.* **16**, 235–72.

Wellman, P. J., Davis, K. W. *et al.* (2005). Augmentation of cocaine hyperactivity in rats by systemic ghrelin. *Regul. Pept.* **125**, 151–4.

Williams, D. L., Grill, H. J. *et al.* (2003). Vagotomy dissociates short- and long-term controls of circulating ghrelin. *Endocrinology* **144**, 5184–7.

Wise, R. A. (2002). Brain reward circuitry: insights from unsensed incentives. *Neuron* **36**, 229–40.

Woods, S. C., Seeley, R. J. *et al.* (1998). Signals that regulate food intake and energy homeostasis. *Science* **280**, 1378–83.

Woods, S. C., Schwartz, M. W. *et al.* (2000). Food intake and the regulation of body weight. *Annu. Rev. Psychol.* **51**, 255–77.

Wortley, K. E., Anderson, K. D. *et al.* (2004). Genetic deletion of ghrelin does not decrease food intake but influences metabolic fuel preference. *Proc. Natl. Acad. Sci. USA* **101**, 8227–32.

Wortley, K. E., Del Rincon, J. P. *et al.* (2005). Absence of ghrelin protects against early-onset obesity. *J. Clin. Invest.* **115**, 3573–8.

Wren, A. M., Small, C. J. *et al.* (2000). The novel hypothalamic peptide ghrelin stimulates food intake and growth hormone secretion. *Endocrinology* **141**, 4325–8.

Wren, A. M., Seal, L. J. *et al.* (2001a). Ghrelin enhances appetite and increases food intake in humans. *J. Clin. Endocrinol. Metab.* **86**, 5992.

Wren, A. M., Small, C. J. *et al.* (2001b). Ghrelin causes hyperphagia and obesity in rats. *Diabetes* **50**, 2540–7.

Zhang, J. V., Ren, P. G. *et al.* (2005). Obestatin, a peptide encoded by the ghrelin gene, opposes ghrelin's effects on food intake. *Science* **310**, 996–9.

Zigman, J. M., Nakano, Y. *et al.* (2005). Mice lacking ghrelin receptors resist the development of diet-induced obesity. *J. Clin. Invest.* **115**, 3564–72.

Zigman, J. M., Jones, J. E. *et al.* (2006). Expression of ghrelin receptor mRNA in the rat and the mouse brain. *J. Comp. Neurol.* **494**, 528–48.

10

Central nervous system controls of adipose tissue apoptosis

MARY ANNE DELLA-FERA, MARK W. HAMRICK AND
CLIFTON A. BAILE

1.   Background

Increased adipose tissue mass is a common denominator in both obesity and osteoporosis. Obesity is characterized by increased fat storage in subcutaneous and visceral adipose depots resulting from an imbalance between energy intake and energy expenditure, whereas osteoporosis is associated with increased adipocyte production in bone marrow and is not necessarily associated with increased overall adiposity. In obesity a reduction of adipose tissue mass is accompanied by amelioration of the pathophysiological effects. There are currently no therapies that specifically reduce bone marrow adipocyte populations. However, bone formation decreases with increasing proportion of marrow adipocytes (Verma et al., 2002); thus, it is likely that reversal or prevention of bone marrow adiposity may improve bone quality.

In the USA, the prevalence of overweight among adults increased by 61% from 1991 to 2000; currently, more than half of all adults are considered overweight and approximately 20% are extremely overweight or obese (Flegal et al., 1998). Obesity is not just a cosmetic problem – there is much evidence indicating that higher levels of body fat are associated with an increased risk for the development of numerous adverse health consequences (Visscher & Seidell, 2001). There is also a tremendous economic burden associated with the recent rise in prevalence of obesity. The economic costs of obesity are estimated to be ~7% of total healthcare costs in the USA (Colditz, 1999). In addition, approximately 10% of the total costs

Neurobiology and Obesity, ed. Jenni Harvey and Dominic J. Withers. Published by Cambridge University Press. © Cambridge University Press 2008 of loss of productivity due to sick leave and work disability are attributable to obesity-related diseases (Narbro et al., 1996). However, the remedies provided by the $100 billion/year diet industry have failed in providing long-term mainten-ance of weight loss for obese or overweight people (Wadden, 1993).

Approximately 10 million people in the USA are estimated to have osteoporosis, a disease that results in over 1.5 million bone fractures a year. It is now known that the accumulation of adipocytes in bone marrow is a major factor contributing to age-related bone loss. Women with osteoporosis have higher numbers of marrow adipocytes than women with healthy bone (Meunier et al., 1971; Kajkenova et al., 1997; Justesen et al., 2001), and bone formation rate is inversely correlated with adipocyte number in bone tissue biopsies from both men and women (Verma et al., 2002). Recent in vivo and in vitro studies provide important insights into why marrow adipogenesis is associated with bone loss. First, mesenchymal stem cells within bone marrow can differentiate to form adipocytes or osteoblasts. Condi-tions favoring adipocyte differentiation will therefore have adverse effects on bone formation because precursor cells are directed towards the adipocyte lineage rather than the osteoblast lineage (Jilka, 2002; Akune et al., 2004). Second, adipo-cytes secrete osteoclastogenic cytokines such as IL-6 (Fried et al., 1998), and adi-pocytes can inhibit osteoblast activity in culture (Maurin et al., 2000). Finally, adipocyte development and hypertrophy can compress intraosseous capillaries, which decreases blood supply within bone (Laroche, 2002). Experimental studies have shown that treatments that reduce bone marrow adipocyte number are associated with increased bone formation, thus suggesting a new approach to the treatment of osteoporosis (Nuttall et al., 2004).

Weight loss reduces risk factors for and improves symptoms of obesity-related conditions (National Heart Lung and Blood Institute, 1998). Treatments for obesity have traditionally focused on drugs or behavioral strategies that restrict food intake, although surgical options such as gastric reduction are options for those who are morbidly obese. Surgical adipose tissue removal by liposuction is increasingly being used both as a treatment for obesity and for cosmetic body sculpturing. Recent studies have shown that removal of even a relatively small percentage of adipose tissue can lead to significant improve-ments in levels of vascular inflammatory markers and in insulin resistance (Giugliano et al., 2004; D'Andrea et al., 2005). Other findings indicate that a high percentage of patients maintain postoperative weights at least one year after liposuction (Commons et al., 2001). The cost and increased morbidity and mortality associated with this procedure severely limit its use as a treatment for obesity; however, these studies do suggest that stimulation of the endogenous removal of adipose tissue by apoptosis could be a valuable option for obesity treatment.

2.   Molecular mechanisms of apoptosis

Apoptosis is a physiological form of cell suicide that is executed in a precise manner without generating inflammation. Apoptosis is necessary to eliminate excess cells during development and to remove damaged and potentially dangerous cells (Hengartner, 2000; Kaufmann & Hengartner, 2001; Alberts, 2002). Disorders of apoptosis can result in either runaway cellular proliferation, as occurs in cancer, or excessive loss of cells, which occurs in certain immunodeficiency and neurodegenerative disorders.

Apoptosis is characterized by loss of cellular contact with the surrounding matrix, cytoplasmic contraction, chromatin condensation and DNA fragmentation. Other changes that occur include externalization of the phosphatidylserine component of the phospholipid bilayer and formation of apoptotic bodies that are removed through endocytosis by macrophages and other cells. Although a number of stimuli appear to trigger the process of apoptosis, there are two major signaling pathways: the death receptor pathway and the mitochondrial pathway (Figure 10.1) (Gupta, 2001; Mayer & Oberbauer, 2003). In both pathways a series of molecular and biochemical steps leads to the activation of cysteine proteases, or caspases. This results in subsequent cleavage of a number of

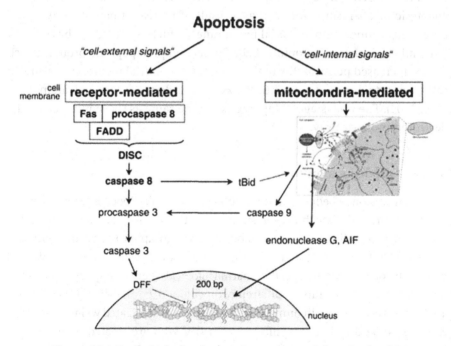

Figure 10.1 Two principal pathways: the receptor and the mitochondria-mediated apoptosis (Mayer & Oberbauer, 2003).

nuclear and cytoplasmic substrates, including those responsible for the maintenance of nuclear integrity, cell cycle progression and DNA repair, resulting in cell death (Hengartner, 2000; Kaufmann & Hengartner, 2001; Alberts, 2002).

The death receptor pathway involves cell membrane receptors that have an extracellular recognition domain and a cytoplasmic sequence, the death domain. Ligands for these receptors belong to the tumor necrosis factor gene family. Binding of a ligand to the extracellular domain leads to formation of an intracellular complex consisting of the death domain, other intracellular molecules and procaspase 8. This aggregation leads to activation of procaspase 8 to caspase 8, which triggers a proteolytic cascade ultimately resulting in formation of enzymes that degrade chromosomal DNA.

The mitochondrial pathway of apoptosis is usually activated by internal stimuli, stress molecules (reactive oxygen species, reactive nitrogen species), chemotherapeutic agents or UV radiation (Mayer & Oberbauer, 2003). Under normal conditions, mitochondria maintain an electrochemical gradient between the inner matrix and the cytoplasm. Mitochondria contain two compartments – the matrix, surrounded by the inner mitochondrial membrane (IMM) and the intermembrane space, surrounded by the outer mitochondrial membrane (OMM).

The intermembrane space contains several apoptosis-inducing factors, including cytochrome c, procaspases and AIF (apoptosis-inducing factor). The apoptotic mechanism is initiated as a result of increased permeability of the outer and/or inner mitochondrial membranes, which is controlled by a variety of members of the anti-apoptotic Bcl-2 family and pro-apoptotic proteins, such as Bax. Increased permeability of the outer mitochondrial membrane results in release of cytochrome c, which triggers the cascade of caspase activation (Page et al., 2004). The final stages of apoptosis are the same as those initiated by the death receptor pathway.

3.   Adipocyte apoptosis

It was once believed that the total number of adipocytes remained constant over one's lifetime; however, studies over the last 10 years have shown that the endogenous elimination of adipocytes through apoptosis occurs normally (Prins & O'Rahilly, 1997), and can also be associated with certain pathological conditions or induced by specific pharmacological agents. Adipocyte apoptosis has been detected in rats with streptozotocin-induced diabetes (Geloen et al., 1989; Loftus et al., 1998), in humans with malignancy-associated weight loss (Prins et al., 1994), and in humans infected with HIV who are treated with protease inhibitors (Dowell et al., 2000; Lagathu et al., 2004, 2005). Recently, several models of inducible adipose tissue apoptosis in rodents have been described (Felmer et al.,

2002; Kolonin *et al.*, 2004; Pajvani *et al.*, 2005; Trujillo *et al.*, 2005). These models have been useful both to study the process of apoptosis in adipose tissue and to demonstrate the beneficial effects of removal of adipocytes in obesity.

Certain natural compounds have also been shown to induce adipocyte apoptosis in vitro, and in some cases, in vivo as well. For example, epigallocatechin gallate (EGCG, a flavonoid in green tea), genistein (an isoflavonoid in soy), esculetin (a coumadin compound), ajoene (from garlic) and conjugated linoleic acid (CLA) all increased apoptosis of 3T3-L1 adipocytes in vitro (Evans *et al.*, 2000; Hargrave *et al.*, 2004; Lin *et al.*, 2005; Yang *et al.*, 2005, 2006; Kim *et al.*, 2006). Both CLA and genistein have also been shown to increase adipose tissue apoptosis in mice in vivo (Tsuboyama-Kasaoka *et al.*, 2000; Hargrave *et al.*, 2002; Kim *et al.*, 2006).

Endogenous factors that may be involved in adipose tissue apoptosis, under either physiological or pathological conditions, have only begun to be explored, and much of this work has involved factors that exert their effects via the CNS, as discussed below. Tumor necrosis factor alpha (TNF*a*), which is produced and secreted by adipocytes, was first shown by Prins *et al.* to induce adipocyte apoptosis in vitro (Prins *et al.*, 1997). Because TNF*a* is produced and secreted by adipocytes, it may act as a paracrine agent to control adipose tissue mass in part through apoptosis, but there is not yet sufficient information to determine whether TNF*a* acts physiologically to regulate apoptosis of adipocytes (Warne, 2003).

4.   Central nervous system control of adipose tissue apoptosis

4.1   *Leptin*

We have shown that the hormone leptin, secreted by adipose tissue, reduces fat mass in rodents not only by increasing lipolysis, but also by stimulating adipocyte apoptosis both in fat depots and in bone marrow (Della-Fera *et al.*, 2001; Gullicksen *et al.*, 2003; Hamrick *et al.*, 2005a). Like TNF*a*, leptin is a cytokine produced and secreted by adipocytes, but our studies have shown that its effect on adipose tissue apoptosis is mediated by the CNS and not locally. As little as 0.1 μg leptin/day administered into the ventromedial nucleus of the hypothalamus (VMH) for four days significantly increased adipose tissue apoptosis in rats (Della-Fera *et al.*, 2005) (Figure 10.2).

4.2   *Melanocortins*

We have recently begun investigating the downstream pathways involved in leptin-induced adipose tissue apoptosis. Because melanocortin receptors appear to mediate a number of leptin's effects, we carried out a study to determine the role of melanocortin receptors in adipose tissue apoptosis

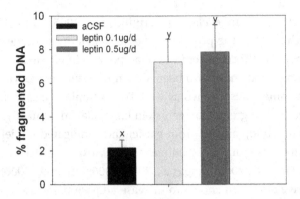

Figure 10.2 Male Sprague–Dawley rats (N = 24) with chronic cannulas directed towards the VMH were injected twice daily with artificial cerebrospinal fluid (aCSF, control), 0.05 μg/injection or 0.25 μg/injection rat recombinant leptin for four consecutive days. Adipose tissue apoptosis (epididymal fat pad) was quantified as the percent of fragmented DNA. Data shown are means ± SEM. x, y: means without a common letter are different, P < 0.01.

(Choi *et al.*, 2003). Rats with cannulas implanted in the lateral cerebral ventricles (LV) were injected icv with either aCSF or the melanocortin receptor blocker SHU9119 (1 nmol) followed one hour later by injection of either aCSF (control), leptin (10 μg) or MTII (0.1 nmol). Treatments were administered for 4 days and food intake and body weight were measured daily. Twenty-four hours after the final injections, the rats were sacrificed and blood and adipose tissues were collected. Both MTII and leptin significantly decreased food intake and body weight. Leptin, but not MTII, significantly decreased serum insulin and leptin concentrations and increased serum free fatty acid concentrations. Both leptin and MTII also decreased epididymal white adipose tissue (eWAT) weight, but only leptin increased adipose tissue apoptosis. Pretreatment of rats with SHU9119 blocked the effects of both MTII and leptin on food intake, body weight and adipose tissue weight and reversed the effects of leptin on serum leptin, insulin and free fatty acid concentrations, but SHU9119 pretreatment had no effect on leptin-induced adipose tissue apoptosis (Figure 10.3). The results of this study indicated that leptin-induced adipose tissue apoptosis is not mediated by downstream melanocortin receptors.

4.3　Cocaine and amphetamine-regulated transcript (CART)

Cocaine and amphetamine-regulated transcript (CART) is one of the most abundantly expressed mRNAs in the rat hypothalamus (Gautvik *et al.*, 1996), and neuroanatomical studies have shown that CART mRNA is expressed

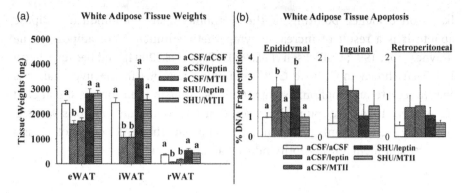

Figure 10.3 (a) White adipose tissue weight of rats pre-injected icv once a day for 4 days with either artificial cerebrospinal fluid (aCSF, 5 μl) or SHU9119 (SHU, 1 nmol/5 μl) followed one hour later with either aCSF (5 μl), leptin (10 μg/5 μl) or MTII (0.1 nmol/5 μl) icv. Food was removed for 1 h between injections. Tissues were collected on day 5 between 24–28 h after the last injections. Epididymal white adipose tissue (eWAT); inguinal WAT (iWAT); retroperitoneal WAT (rWAT). a,b: Means with different letters are significantly different at P < 0.05. Data are means ± SEM (n = 8–10) (Choi et al., 2003a). (b) Fragmented-to-total DNA ratio (%) in fat tissues collected from rats pre-injected icv once a day for 4 days with either artificial cerebrospinal fluid (aCSF, 5 μl) or SHU9119 (SHU, 1 nmol/5 μl) followed one hour later with either aCSF (5 μl), leptin (10 μg/5 μl) or MTII (0.1 nmol/5 μl) icv. Food was removed for 1 h between injections. Fresh tissues, taken on day 5 between 24–28 h after the last injections, were immediately analyzed for DNA. a,b: Means with different letters are significantly different at P < 0.05. Data are means ± SEM (n = 7–10) (Choi et al., 2003).

within hypothalamic areas implicated in the CNS control of feeding behavior and metabolism, including the paraventricular (PVN), arcuate and dorsomedial nuclei (DMN), as well as the lateral hypothalamus (LH) (Koylu et al., 1997, 1998; Dall Vechia et al., 2000). A number of studies indicate that CART peptides act centrally to inhibit feeding (Kristensen et al., 1998; Lambert et al., 1998; Larsen et al., 2000), and CART may be a downstream effector for specific leptin actions in some areas (Elias et al., 1998; Kristensen et al., 1998).

We carried out a study to determine if CART administered icv produced effects similar to leptin on feeding behavior, body weight and adipose tissue. After 4 days of continuous administration, 9.6 μg/d CART decreased food intake and body weight but caused behavioral abnormalities and loss of muscle as well as fat. A dose of 2.4 μg/d CART only reduced food intake. In contrast, rats receiving 15 μg/d leptin had normal behavior, but they ate less and lost weight and body fat, but not muscle.

We had predicted that if CART acted centrally as a downstream mediator of leptin, then it would induce adipose tissue apoptosis. This hypothesis was based on evidence pointing to the possibility that leptin-induced adipose apoptosis is a result of increased sympathetic stimulation of adipose tissue (Haynes et al., 1997; Gullicksen et al., 2003; Page et al., 2004), and because leptin has been shown to activate CART-containing neurons in the hypothalamus that innervate preganglionic sympathetic neurons in the thoracic spinal cord (Elias et al., 1998). We found, however, that adipose tissue apoptosis was significantly increased only by leptin. Thus, it appears that CART does not act as a downstream mediator of leptin-induced adipose tissue apoptosis.

4.4   Ciliary neurotrophic factor

Ciliary neurotrophic factor (CNTF) is a pluripotent neurocytokine expressed by glial cells in peripheral nerves and in the central nervous system (Manthorpe et al., 1993; Ip & Yancopoulos, 1996). However, unlike the prototypical cachectic cytokines, recent studies have shown that CNTF can induce weight loss without exhibiting the typical deleterious characteristics of these cytokines (Xu et al., 1998; Lambert et al., 2001). Ciliary neurotrophic factor has been compared to leptin for its similar effects on food intake, weight loss and energy expenditure. Central administration of CNTF decreases food intake and body weight, and like leptin, after cessation of treatment, there is not an immediate rebound in weight gain (Gloaguen et al., 1997; Kalra et al., 1998; Xu et al., 1998; Lambert et al., 2001; Kokoeva et al., 2005). Because leptin and CNTF have been shown to have similar actions on adipose tissue mass, body weight and food intake, we hypothesized that CNTF administered icv would increase adipose tissue apoptosis. After 4 days of once-daily icv injections (5 μg), both leptin and CNTF significantly increased apoptosis in epididymal and retroperitoneal adipose tissue in rats (Duff et al., 2004).

Although the mechanisms involved in either leptin or CNTF-induced adipose tissue apoptosis are not yet known, both similarities and differences between these two peptides are beginning to suggest a likely CNS pathway. Two important CNS peptides that act as downstream effectors of leptin are α-melanocortin stimulating hormone (αMSH) and neuropeptide Y (NPY) (Inui, 1999). Leptin and CNTF both activate STAT-3 in areas of the hypothalamus involved in feeding behavior and body weight regulation (Sleeman et al., 2000; Lambert et al., 2001). However, CNTF causes weight loss in animal models that are resistant to the effects of leptin, including mice lacking leptin receptors (db/db), mice with diet-induced obesity (DIO) and mice with melanocortin-4 receptor deficiency (Gloaguen et al., 1997; Marsh et al., 1999). It is of interest to note that mice with DIO have enhanced sensitivity to the anorectic effects of melanocortins, suggesting that DIO may involve reduced melanocortin signaling (Hansen et al., 2005). Thus, the effect of CNTF on food intake and body weight appears to be mediated downstream or independently of melanocortin receptors.

In contrast, both leptin and CNTF have been shown to suppress NPY levels and their effects on food intake and body weight can be reversed by concurrent NPY administration (Kotz et al., 1998; Yokosuka et al., 1998; Jang et al., 2000; Lambert et al., 2001). Likewise, the lack of rebound eating after CNTF or leptin treatments are terminated have been suggested to be a result of the decrease in NPY levels, compared with the increase that occurs with food deprivation (Lambert et al., 2001). Because we found that melanocortin receptors are not involved in leptin-induced adipose tissue apoptosis, these findings suggest that NPY is a critical component of the downstream mechanism involved in adipose tissue apoptosis mediated by leptin: both Gong et al. (2003) and Margareto et al. (2000) have shown that inhibition of NPY receptors increases adipose tissue apoptosis in rats; thus, these findings suggest that adipose tissue apoptosis increased by icv injections of leptin or CNTF may be a result of suppression of NPY expression in the hypothalamus.

4.5   Sympathetic nervous system

We have recently found that chronic oral administration of a β2-adrenergic agonist resulted in increased adipose tissue apoptosis in mice (Page et al., 2004). Because leptin has been shown to increase sympathetic nervous system activity (Dunbar et al., 1997; Haynes et al., 1997; Tang-Christensen et al., 1999), while NPY suppresses sympathetic activity (Van Dijk et al., 1994), it is possible that leptin-induced increased β2-adrenergic receptor activation in specific fat depots could trigger adipocyte apoptosis.

There is extensive innervation of white adipose tissue (WAT) by the sympathetic nervous system (SNS) (Bartness & Bamshad, 1998), and adipocytes have been shown to express β-adrenergic receptors, particularly β3 receptors (Collins & Surwit, 2001). Sympathetic denervation of WAT increased fat cell number (Youngstrom & Bartness, 1998), whereas stimulation of β3-adrenergic receptors induced apoptosis through activation of a tyrosine kinase pathway (Ma & Huang, 2002). Indeed, treatment of estrogen-deficient rats with an agonist for the β3-adrenergic receptor significantly decreased bone marrow adiposity in the spine (Kurabayashi et al., 2001).

5.   Role of CNS in bone marrow adipose apoptosis

Preliminary studies suggest that the sympathetic nervous system plays a significant role in the regulation of bone marrow adipocyte populations.

Bone marrow is richly innervated with sympathetic nerve fibers, and neuronal signals appear to play a significant role in the regulation of bone mass. Kellenberger *et al.* showed that β2-agonists increased bone formation (Kellenberger *et al.*, 1998), and β-agonists have been found to decrease bone loss with disuse and muscle atrophy (Zeman *et al.*, 1991; Martin *et al.*, 2005). Moreover, mice lacking the β1- and β2-adrenergic receptors have decreased cortical bone mass (Pierroz, 2004), suggesting that β-adrenergic signaling is necessary for the normal maintenance and accumulation of bone tissue. Signaling through β-adrenergic receptors can also inhibit the expression of adipogenic factors in vivo (Margareto *et al.*, 2001). Other studies, however, suggest that stimulation of β-adrenergic receptors decreases bone formation (Takeda *et al.*, 2002), and mice lacking only β2-adrenergic receptors exhibit a high bone mass phenotype (Elefteriou *et al.*, 2005). Thus, at present, the role of β-adrenergic signaling in regulating bone metabolism is unclear.

We have hypothesized that β-adrenergic signaling in bone marrow, activated centrally via leptin, not only induces bone marrow adipocyte apoptosis but also inhibits bone marrow adipogenesis. Although Ducy *et al.* have shown that leptin-deficient mice (*ob/ob*) and mice with dysfunctional leptin receptors (*db/db*) have increased bone mineralization of the spine (Ducy *et al.*, 2000), others have shown the *ob/ob* mice have lower bone mass and reduced bone density in their femora compared with normal mice (Steppan *et al.*, 2000; Hamrick *et al.*, 2005b) and that *db/db* mice have reduced length, bone mineral density and bone mineral mass of their tibias (Lorentzon *et al.*, 1986). Furthermore, the limb bones of *ob/ob* mice showed increased bone marrow adipogenesis (Hamrick *et al.*, 2005b). Hamrick *et al.* tested the hypothesis that leptin treatment would reduce adipocyte stores in bone marrow and would increase bone formation and bone mass in leptin-deficient *ob/ob* mice (Hamrick *et al.*, 2005b). Leptin (2.5 or 10 μg/d) was administered continuously by subcutaneously implanted osmotic pumps in female *ob/ob* and *OB/?* lean control mice for 14 days. Both doses of leptin significantly decreased the number of marrow adipocytes by more than 20% compared with control-treated *ob/ob* mice. The decrease in adipocyte number with leptin treatment was accompanied by an increase in concentration of the apoptosis marker caspase-3 in bone marrow adipocytes and hematopoietic cells. Both doses also significantly increased the bone-forming endosteal surface by more than 30% compared with control-treated *ob/ob* mice. Leptin treatment increased whole-body bone mineral content by more than 30% in the *ob/ob* mice receiving the highest leptin dose. These results demonstrated that leptin is an osteogenic factor that eliminates bone marrow adipocytes, increases bone formation, and increases bone mineral and density in leptin-deficient animals. More recently, studies have shown that leptin injected directly into the VMH of rats significantly increased endosteal osteoblast surface area, markedly reduced bone marrow adipocyte number by more than 50% and increased bone marrow caspase-3 levels (Hamrick *et al.*, 2005a). Thus, these data indicate that leptin regulates adipocyte apoptosis in bone marrow through a central, hypothalamic signaling pathway (Hamrick *et al.*, 2005a).

6.   Conclusion

Adipose tissue apoptosis is a novel approach that could be useful for treating both obesity and osteoporosis. Activation of adipocyte apoptosis via the CNS has been demonstrated, particularly following leptin treatment, but the neural pathways involved are only beginning to be defined. Although the sympathetic nervous system is the most likely transduction pathway from brain to adipocytes, either in fat pads or in bone marrow, the involvement of an intermediary humoral factor acting directly on adipocytes has not yet been ruled out. It is also possible that adipocyte apoptosis is triggered as a result of alteration of blood supply. Remodeling of tissues is usually accompanied by local changes in angiogenesis, although it can be difficult to determine what is the initiating process. Although there are many technical issues involved in studying adipocyte apoptosis in animals, a better understanding of the biochemical and anatomical pathways involved could lead to development of treatments resulting in the controlled removal of adipocytes in fat depots and bone marrow, and possibly in a site-specific manner.

References

Akune, T., Ohba, S., Kamekura, S. *et al.* (2004). PPARgamma insufficiency enhances osteogenesis through osteoblast formation from bone marrow progenitors. *J. Clin. Invest.* **113**, 846–55.

Alberts, B. (2002). Programmed cell death (apoptosis). In *Molecular Biology of the Cell*, 4th edn, pp. 1010–14. New York: Garland Science.

Bartness, T. J. & Bamshad, M. (1998). Innervation of mammalian white adipose tissue: implications for the regulation of total body fat. *Am. J. Physiol.* **275**, R1399–411.

Choi, Y. H., Li, C., Page, K. *et al.* (2003). Melanocortin receptors mediate leptin effects on feeding and body weight but not adipose apoptosis. *Physiol. Behav.* **79**, 795–801.

Colditz, G. A. (1999). Economic costs of obesity and inactivity. *Med. Sci. Sports Exercise* **31**, S663-7.

Collins, S. & Surwit, R. S. (2001). The beta-adrenergic receptors and the control of adipose tissue metabolism and thermogenesis. *Recent Prog. Horm. Res.* **56**, 309-28.

Commons, G. W., Halperin, B. & Chang, C. C. (2001). Large-volume liposuction: a review of 631 consecutive cases over 12 years. *Plast Reconstr Surg.* **108**, 1753-63; discussion 1764-7.

D'Andrea, F., Grella, R., Rizzo, M. R. *et al.* (2005). Changing the metabolic profile by large-volume liposuction: a clinical study conducted with 123 obese women. *Aesthetic Plast. Surg.* **29**, 472-8.

Dall Vechia, S., Lambert, P. D., Couceyro, P. C., Kuhar, M. J. & Smith, Y. (2000). CART peptide immunoreactivity in the hypothalamus and pituitary in monkeys: analysis of ultrastructural features and synaptic connections in the paraventricular nucleus. *J. Comp. Neurol.* **416**, 291-308.

Della-Fera, M. A., Qian, H. & Baile, C. A. (2001). Adipocyte apoptosis in the regulation of body fat mass by leptin. *Diabetes Obes. Metab.* **3**, 299-310.

Della-Fera, M. A., Choi, Y.-H., Hamrick, M. W., Hartzell, D. L., Pennington, C. & Baile, C. A. (2005). Leptin injected into the ventromedial hypothalamus (VMH) reduces food intake (FI), body weight (BW) and bone marrow adiposity and increases apoptosis of adipose tissue and bone marrow. *FASEB J.* **19**, A1135.

Dowell, P., Flexner, C., Kwiterovich, P. O. & Lane, M. D. (2000). Suppression of preadipocyte differentiation and promotion of adipocyte death by HIV protease inhibitors. *J. Biol. Chem.* **275**, 41 325-32.

Ducy, P., Amling, M., Takeda, S. *et al.* (2000). Leptin inhibits bone formation through a hypothalamic relay: a central control of bone mass. *Cell* **100**, 197-207.

Duff, E., Li, C. L., Hartzell, D. L., Choi, Y. H., Della-Fera, M. A. & Baile, C. A. (2004). Ciliary neurotrophic factor injected icv induces adipose tissue apoptosis in rats. *Apoptosis* **9**, 629-34.

Dunbar, J. C., Hu, Y. & Lu, H. (1997). Intracerebroventricular leptin increases lumbar and renal sympathetic nerve activity and blood pressure in normal rats. *Diabetes* **46**, 2040-3.

Elefteriou, F., Ahn, J. D., Takeda, S. *et al.* (2005). Leptin regulation of bone resorption by the sympathetic nervous system and CART. *Nature* **434**, 514-20.

Elias, C. F., Lee, C., Kelly, J. *et al.* (1998). Leptin activates hypothalamic CART neurons projecting to the spinal cord. *Neuron* **21**, 1375-85.

Evans, M., Geigerman, C., Cook, J., Curtis, L., Kuebler, B. & McIntosh, M. (2000). Conjugated linoleic acid suppresses triglyceride accumulation and induces apoptosis in 3T3-L1 preadipocytes. *Lipids* **35**, 899-910.

Felmer, R., Cui, W. & Clark, A. J. (2002). Inducible ablation of adipocytes in adult transgenic mice expressing the *E. coli* nitroreductase gene. *J. Endocrinol.* **175**, 487-98.

Flegal, K. M., Carroll, M. D., Kuczmarski, R. J. & Johnson, C. L. (1998). Overweight and obesity in the United States: prevalence and trends, 1960-1994. *Int. J. Obes. Rel. Metab. Dis.* **22**, 39-47.

Fried, S. K., Bunkin, D. A. & Greenberg, A. S. (1998). Omental and subcutaneous adipose tissues of obese subjects release interleukin-6: depot difference and regulation by glucocorticoid. *J. Clin. Endocrin. Metab.* **83**, 847–50.

Gautvik, K. M., de Lecea, L., Gautvik, V. T. *et al.* (1996). Overview of the most prevalent hypothalamus-specific mRNAs, as identified by directional tag PCR subtraction. *Proc. Natl. Acad. Sci. USA* **93**, 8733–8.

Geloen, A., Roy, P. E. & Bukowiecki, L. J. (1989). Regression of white adipose tissue in diabetic rats. *Am. J. Physiol.* **257**, E547–53.

Giugliano, G., Nicoletti, G., Grella, E. *et al.* (2004). Effect of liposuction on insulin resistance and vascular inflammatory markers in obese women. *Br. J. Plast. Surg.* **57**, 190–4.

Gloaguen, I., Costa, P., Demartis, A. *et al.* (1997). Ciliary neurotrophic factor corrects obesity and diabetes associated with leptin deficiency and resistance. *Proc. Natl. Acad. Sci. USA* **94**, 6456–61.

Gong, H. X., Guo, X. R., Fei, L., Guo, M., Liu, Q. Q. & Chen, R. H. (2003). Lipolysis and apoptosis of adipocytes induced by neuropeptide Y-Y5 receptor antisense oligodeoxynucleotides in obese rats. *Acta Pharmacol. Sin.* **24**, 569–75.

Gullicksen, P. S., Della-Fera, M. A. & Baile, C. A. (2003). Leptin-induced adipose apoptosis: implications for body weight regulation. *Apoptosis* **8**, 327–35.

Gupta, S. (2001). Molecular steps of death receptor and mitochondrial pathways of apoptosis. *Life Sci.* **69**, 2957–64.

Hamrick, M., Della-Fera, M. A., Hartzell, D. L., Choi, Y.-H. & Baile, C. A. (2005a). Central control of bone marrow adipocyte populations by leptin. *J. Bone Miner. Res.* **20**, S368.

Hamrick, M. W., Della-Fera, M. A., Choi, Y. H., Pennington, C., Hartzell, D. & Baile, C. A. (2005b). Leptin treatment induces loss of bone marrow adipocytes and increases bone formation in leptin-deficient ob/ob mice. *J. Bone Miner. Res.* **20**, 994–1001.

Hansen, M. J., Schioth, H. B. & Morris, M. J. (2005). Feeding responses to a melanocortin agonist and antagonist in obesity induced by a palatable high-fat diet. *Brain Res.* **1039**, 137–45.

Hargrave, K. M., Li, C., Meyer, B. J. *et al.* (2002). Adipose depletion and apoptosis induced by trans-10, cis-12 conjugated linoleic acid in mice. *Obes. Res.* **10**, 1284–90.

Hargrave, K. M., Meyer, B. J., Li, C., Azain, M. J., Baile, C. A. & Miner, J. L. (2004). Influence of dietary conjugated linoleic acid and fat source on body fat and apoptosis in mice. *Obes. Res.* **12**, 1435–44.

Haynes, W. G., Sivitz, W. I., Morgan, D. A., Walsh, S. A. & Mark, A. L. (1997). Sympathetic and cardiorenal actions of leptin. *Hypertension* **30**, 619–23.

Hengartner, M. O. (2000). The biochemistry of apoptosis *Nature* **407**, 770–6.

Inui, A. (1999). Feeding and body-weight regulation by hypothalamic neuropeptides – mediation of the actions of leptin. *Trends Neurosci.* **22**, 62–7.

Ip, N. Y. & Yancopoulos, G. D. (1996). The neurotrophins and CNTF: two families of collaborative neurotrophic factors. *Annu. Rev. Neurosci.* **19**, 491–515.

Jang, M., Mistry, A., Swick, A. G. & Romsos, D. R. (2000). Leptin rapidly inhibits hypothalamic neuropeptide Y secretion and stimulates corticotropin-releasing hormone secretion in adrenalectomized mice. *J. Nutr.* **130**, 2813–20.

Jilka, R. L. (2002). Osteoblast progenitor fate and age-related bone loss. *J. Musculoskelet. Neuronal Interact.* **2**, 581–3.

Justesen, J., Stenderup, K., Ebbesen, E. N., Mosekilde, L., Steiniche, T. & Kassem, M. (2001). Adipocyte tissue volume in bone marrow is increased with aging and in patients with osteoporosis. *Biogerontology* **2**, 165–71.

Kajkenova, O., Lecka-Czernik, B., Gubrij, I. *et al.* (1997). Increased adipogenesis and myelopoiesis in the bone marrow of SAMP6, a murine model of defective osteoblastogenesis and low turnover osteopenia. *J. Bone Miner. Res.* **12**, 1772–9.

Kalra, S. P., Xu, B., Dube, M. G., Moldawer, L. L., Martin, D. & Kalra, P. S. (1998). Leptin and ciliary neurotropic factor (CNTF) inhibit fasting-induced suppression of luteinizing hormone release in rats: role of neuropeptide Y. *Neurosci. Lett.* **240**, 45–9.

Kaufmann, S. C. & Hengartner, M. O. (2001). Programmed cell death: alive and well in the new millennium. *Trends Cell Biol.* **11**, 526–34.

Kellenberger, S., Muller, K., Richener, H. & Bilbe, G. (1998). Formoterol and isoproterenol induce c-fos gene expression in osteoblast-like cells by activating beta2-adrenergic receptors. *Bone* **22**, 471–8.

Kim, H.-K., Nelson-Dooley, C., Della-Fera, M. A. *et al.* (2006). Genistein decreases food intake, body weight and fat pad weight and causes adipose tissue apoptosis in ovariectomized female mice. *J. Nutr.* **136**, 409–14.

Kokoeva, M. V., Yin, H. & Flier, J. S. (2005). Neurogenesis in the hypothalamus of adult mice: potential role in energy balance. *Science* **310**, 679–83.

Kolonin, M. G., Saha, P. K., Chan, L., Pasqualini, R. & Arap, W. (2004). Reversal of obesity by targeted ablation of adipose tissue. *Nat. Med.* **10**, 625–32.

Kotz, C. M., Briggs, J. E., Pomonis, J. D., Grace, M. K., Levine, A. S. & Billington, C. J. (1998). Neural site of leptin influence on neuropeptide Y signaling pathways altering feeding and uncoupling protein. *Am. J. Physiol.* **275**, R478–84.

Koylu, E. O., Couceyro, P. R., Lambert, P. D., Ling, N. C., DeSouza, E. B. & Kuhar, M. J. (1997). Immunohistochemical localization of novel CART peptides in rat hypothalamus, pituitary and adrenal gland. *J. Neuroendocrinol.* **9**, 823–33.

Koylu, E. O., Couceyro, P. R., Lambert, P. D. & Kuhar, M. J. (1998). Cocaine- and amphetamine-regulated transcript peptide immunohistochemical localization in the rat brain. *J. Comp. Neurol.* **391**, 115–32.

Kristensen, P., Judge, M. E., Thim, L. *et al.* (1998). Hypothalamic CART is a new anorectic peptide regulated by leptin. *Nature* **393**, 72–6.

Kurabayashi, T., Tomita, M., Matsushita, H., Honda, A., Takakuwa, K. & Tanaka, K. (2001). Effects of a beta 3 adrenergic receptor agonist on bone and bone marrow adipocytes in the tibia and lumbar spine of the ovariectomized rat. *Calcif Tissue Int.* **68**, 248–54.

Lagathu, C., Bastard, J. P., Auclair, M. *et al.* (2004). Antiretroviral drugs with adverse effects on adipocyte lipid metabolism and survival alter the expression and secretion of proinflammatory cytokines and adiponectin in vitro. *Antivir. Ther.* **9**, 911-20.

Lagathu, C., Kim, M., Maachi, M. *et al.* (2005). HIV antiretroviral treatment alters adipokine expression and insulin sensitivity of adipose tissue in vitro and in vivo. *Biochimie* **87**, 65-71.

Lambert, P. D., Couceyro, P. R., McGirr, K. M., Dall Vechia, S. E., Smith, Y. & Kuhar, M. J. (1998). CART peptides in the central control of feeding and interactions with neuropeptide Y. *Synapse* **29**, 293-8.

Lambert, P. D., Anderson, K. D., Sleeman, M. W. *et al.* (2001). Ciliary neurotrophic factor activates leptin-like pathways and reduces body fat, without cachexia or rebound weight gain, even in leptin-resistant obesity. *Proc. Natl. Acad. Sci. USA* **98**, 4652-7.

Laroche, M. (2002). Intraosseous circulation from physiology to disease. *Joint Bone Spine* **69**, 262-9.

Larsen, P. J., Vrang, N., Petersen, P. C. & Kristensen, P. (2000). Chronic intracerebroventricular administration of recombinant CART(42-89) peptide inhibits and causes weight loss in lean and obese Zucker (fa/fa) rats. *Obes. Res.* **8**, 590-6.

Lin, J., Della-Fera, M. A. & Baile, C. A. (2005). Green tea polyphenol epigallocatechin gallate inhibits adipogenesis and induces apoptosis in 3T3-L1 adipocytes. *Obes. Res.* **13**, 982-90.

Loftus, T. M., Kuhajda, F. P. & Lane, M. D. (1998). Insulin depletion leads to adipose-specific cell death in obese but not lean mice. *Proc. Natl. Acad. Sci. USA* **95**, 14 168-72.

Lorentzon, R., Alehagen, U. & Boquist, L. (1986). Osteopenia in mice with genetic diabetes. *Diabetes Res. Clin. Pract.* **2**, 157-63.

Ma, Y. C. & Huang, X. Y. (2002). Novel signaling pathway through the beta-adrenergic receptor. *Trends Cardiovasc Med.* **12**, 46-9.

Manthorpe, M., Louis, J.C., Hagg, T. & Varon, S. (1993) Ciliary neurotrophic factor. In *Neurotrophic Factors*, ed. Loughlin, S. E. & Fallon, J. H., pp. 443-73. San Diego: Academic Press.

Margareto, J., Aguado, M., Oses-Prieto, J. A. *et al.* (2000). A new NPY-antagonist strongly stimulates apoptosis and lipolysis on white adipocytes in an obesity model. *Life Sci.* **68**, 99-107.

Margareto, J., Larrarte, E., Marti, A. & Martinez, J. A. (2001). Up-regulation of a thermogenesis-related gene (UCP1) and down-regulation of PPARgamma and aP2 genes in adipose tissue: possible features of the antiobesity effects of a beta3-adrenergic agonist. *Biochem. Pharmacol.* **61**, 1471-8.

Marsh, D. J., Hollopeter, G., Huszar, D. *et al.* (1999). Response of melanocortin-4 receptor-deficient mice to anorectic and orexigenic peptides. *Nat Genet.* **21**, 119-22.

Martin, A., de Vittoris, R., David, V. *et al.* (2005). Leptin modulates both resorption and formation while preventing disuse-induced bone loss in tail-suspended female rats. *Endocrinology* **146**, 3652-9.

Maurin, A. C., Chavassieux, P. M., Frappart, L., Delmas, P. D., Serre, C. M. & Meunier, P. J. (2000). Influence of mature adipocytes on osteoblast proliferation in human primary cocultures. *Bone* **26**, 485–9.

Mayer, B. & Oberbauer, R. (2003). Mitochondrial regulation of apoptosis. *News Physiol Sci.* **18**, 89–94.

Meunier, P., Aaron, J., Edouard, C. & Vignon, G. (1971). Osteoporosis and the replacement of cell populations of the marrow by adipose tissue. A quantitative study of 84 iliac bone biopsies. *Clin. Orthop.* **80**, 147–54.

Narbro, K., Jonsson, E., Larsson, B., Waaler, H., Wedel, H. & Sjostrom, L. (1996). Economic consequences of sick-leave and early retirement in obese Swedish women. *Int. J. Obes. Rel. Metab. Dis.* **20**, 895–903.

National Heart Lung and Blood Institute (1998). *Clinical Guidelines of the Identification, Evaluation, and Treatment of Overweight and Obesity in Adults: The Evidence Report.* Bethesda, MD: National Institutes of Health.

Nuttall, M. E. & Gimble, J. M. (2004). Controlling the balance between osteoblastogenesis and adipogenesis and the consequent therapeutic implications. *Curr. Opin. Pharmacol.* **4**, 290–4.

Page, K. A., Hartzell, D. L., Li, C. *et al.* (2004). Beta-adrenergic receptor agonists increase apoptosis of adipose tissue in mice. *Domest. Anim. Endocrinol.* **26**, 23–31.

Pajvani, U. B., Trujillo, M. E., Combs, T. P. *et al.* (2005). Fat apoptosis through targeted activation of caspase 8; a new mouse model of inducible and reversible lipoatrophy. *Nat. Med.* **11**, 797–803.

Pierroz, D. D. (2004). $\beta1\beta2$-adrenergic receptor mice have decreased total body and cortical bone mass despite increased trabecular bone number. *J. Bone Miner. Res.* **19**, 1121.

Prins, J. B. & O'Rahilly, S. (1997). Regulation of adipose cell number in man. *Clin. Sci. (Lond).* **92**, 3–11.

Prins, J. B., Walker, N. I., Winterford, C. M. & Cameron, D. P. (1994). Human adipocyte apoptosis occurs in malignancy. *Biochem. Biophys. Res. Commun.* **205**, 625–30.

Prins, J. B., Niesler, C. U., Winterford, C. M. *et al.* (1997). Tumor necrosis factor-alpha induces apoptosis of human adipose cells. *Diabetes* **46**, 1939–44.

Sleeman, M. W., Anderson, K. D., Lambert, P. D., Yancopoulos, G. D. & Wiegand, S. J. (2000). The ciliary neurotrophic factor and its receptor, CNTFR alpha. *Pharm. Acta. Helv.* **74**, 265–72.

Steppan, C. M., Crawford, D. T., Chidsey-Frink, K. L., Ke, H. & Swick, A. G. (2000). Leptin is a potent stimulator of bone growth in ob/ob mice. *Regul. Pept.* **92**, 73–8.

Takeda, S., Elefteriou, F., Levasseur, R. *et al.* (2002). Leptin regulates bone formation via the sympathetic nervous system. *Cell* **111**, 305–17.

Tang-Christensen, M., Havel, P. J., Jacobs, R. R., Larsen, P. J. & Cameron, J. (1999). Central administration of leptin inhibits food intake and activates the sympathetic nervous system in rhesus macaques. *J. Clin. Endocrinol. Metab.* **84**, 711–17.

Trujillo, M. E., Pajvani, U. B. & Scherer, P. E. (2005). Apoptosis through targeted activation of caspase8 ("ATTAC-mice"): novel mouse models of inducible and reversible tissue ablation. *Cell Cycle* **4**, 1141–5.

Tsuboyama-Kasaoka, N., Takahashi, M., Tanemura, K. *et al.* (2000). Conjugated linoleic acid supplementation reduces adipose tissue by apoptosis and develops lipodystrophy in mice. *Diabetes* **49**, 1534–42.

Van Dijk, G., Bottone, A. E., Strubbe, J. H. & Steffens, A. B. (1994). Hormonal and metabolic effects of paraventricular hypothalamic administration of neuropeptide Y during rest and feeding. *Brain Res.* **660**, 96–103.

Verma, S., Rajaratnam, J. H., Denton, J., Hoyland, J. A. & Byers, R. J. (2002). Adipocytic proportion of bone marrow is inversely related to bone formation in osteoporosis. *J. Clin. Pathol.* **55**, 693–8.

Visscher, T. L. & Seidell, J. C. (2001). The public health impact of obesity. *Annu. Rev. Pub. Health.* **22**, 355–75.

Wadden, T. A. (1993). Treatment of obesity by moderate and severe caloric restriction. Results of clinical research trials. *Ann. Internal Med.* **119**, 688–93.

Warne, J. P. (2003). Tumour necrosis factor alpha: a key regulator of adipose tissue mass. *J. Endocrinol.* **177**, 351–5.

Xu, B., Dube, M. G., Kalra, P. S. *et al.* (1998). Anorectic effects of the cytokine, ciliary neurotropic factor, are mediated by hypothalamic neuropeptide Y: comparison with leptin. *Endocrinology* **139**, 466–73.

Yang, J. Y., Della-Fera, M. A., Nelson-Dooley, C. & Baile, C. A. (2005). Molecular mechanisms of apoptosis induced by ajoene in 3T3-L1 adipocytes. *Obes.* **14**, 388–97.

Yang, J.-Y., Della-Fera, M. A., Hartzell, D. L., Nelson-Dooley, C., Hausman, D. B. & Baile, C. A. (2006). Esculetin induces apoptosis and inhibits adipogenesis in 3T3-L1 cells. *Obes. Res.* **14**, 1691–9.

Yokosuka, M., Xu, B., Pu, S., Kalra, P. S. & Kalra, S. P. (1998). Neural substrates for leptin and neuropeptide Y (NPY) interaction: hypothalamic sites associated with inhibition of NPY-induced food intake. *Physiol. Behav.* **64**, 331–8.

Youngstrom, T. G. & Bartness, T. J. (1998). White adipose tissue sympathetic nervous system denervation increases fat pad mass and fat cell number. *Am. J. Physiol.* **275**, R1488–93.

Zeman, R. J., Hirschman, A., Hirschman, M. L., Guo, G. & Etlinger, J. D. (1991). Clenbuterol, a beta 2-receptor agonist, reduces net bone loss in denervated hindlimbs. *Am. J. Physiol.* **261**, E285–9.

11

Potential therapies to limit obesity

JASON C. G. HALFORD

The chapters within this book have detailed various aspects of the neurobiology of weight control. These include the genetic factors which determined the function of the body's energy regulation and the central mechanisms responsible for maintaining the body's energy balance. Particular focus has been placed on central targets such as the melanocortin and endogenous opioid systems. These systems represent two factors which control food intake: energy balance regulation and pleasure/reward. It is the metabolic demand for energy and the pleasure derived from eating palatable foods which determine when, what and how much we eat. Other chapters have dealt with peripheral generated signals such as ghrelin, leptin and insulin and their role in appetite and energy regulation. Such mechanisms provide episodic meal-by-meal signals of food consumption and the tonic signals of energy storage to the CNS. Organs such as the gut, the pancreas and adipose tissue act as both detectors and effectors in the organism energy regulation system. This diverse peripheral input allows the organism to constantly monitor its current energy status. In turn the CNS does not only adjust the expression of feeding behavior, as the last chapter shows the CNS also exerts control over the storage of energy.

Given the complexity of these systems underpinning energy regulation (episodic and tonic, peripheral and central) it may appear surprising that the state of obesity exists. However, despite the collective action of these many systems it seems many individuals experience great difficulty controlling their own body weight. In fact in many countries, being overweight or obese is

Neurobiology and Obesity, ed. Jenni Harvey and Dominic J. Withers. Published by Cambridge University Press. © Cambridge University Press 2008

now the population norm. The popular scientific explanation for this is that our energy regulatory systems evolved under very differing circumstances. During our development we have never been exposed to the availability of an abundant variety of foods which we experience now. Moreover, the diet which was once consumed did not consist of the hedonic pleasing energy-dense items. Such foods consist of high proportions of refined sugar or fat, and now are a major consistent of the diets of many individuals (Blundell & Halford, 1995).

It appears overall, that the system defends well against under consumption but not over consumption. Authors have referred to this phenomenon as the 'asymmetry' of appetite regulation. It seems in the current obesity promoting (or 'obesogenic') environment the neurobiology of appetite and energy regulation has literally become the neurobiology of obesity. However, through understanding both the functions and the limits of the systems which control energy intake and expenditure we can gain an understanding of where the potential to intervene lies. Thus knowledge of the neurobiology of obesity provides yields targets for obesity treatment (Halford et al., 2003).

For all obesity treatments, even treatments targeting a specific neurobiological mechanism, to achieve a reduction in body mass a negative energy balance has to be attained. With the notable exception of liposuction, all weight loss treatments must either reduce energy intake and/or increase energy expenditure to produce weight loss. Targeting food ingestion has always been the historically favored approach to obesity treatment and the neurobiological approach is no exception. Drugs which reduce intake are still by far the largest class of drugs under development. Such drugs act either centrally or in the periphery on appetite mechanisms to reduce food intake, or act in the gastrointestinal tract to reduce energy absorption (Halford et al., 2004).

Current anti-obesity drugs work exactly by those mechanisms: Sibutramine modulates appetite and Orlistat blocks fat absorption. It is likely that the (provisionally licensed in the USA and approved in the UK) anti-obesity drug Rimonabant also induces weight loss, at least in part by reducing food intake. This does not mean drugs cannot be used to target metabolic processes to promote energy expenditure rather than energy intake. However, no such drugs are currently used to treat obesity and few, if any, of this class of compounds are in clinical trials yet. Peripherally acting drugs such as the β_3-adrenoceptor agonists have been in development for a number of years. Such compounds are thermogenic, increasing metabolic rate and energy expenditure. Interest has focused on the newly characterized thermogenic mitochondrial uncoupling proteins UCP-1, UCP-2 and UCP-3 and a variety of other metabolic targets such as adiponectin-based therapies, Fatty Acid Synthase

(FAS) inhibition, TNF-a inhibition, stearoyl-CoA desaturase (SCD)-1 enzyme inhibition and gene targets such as the human Sir2-like gene sirtunin (SIRT)-1.

1.   Drugs acting centrally on appetite and energy regulation

The CNS receives information generated by the sensory experience of eating, and from the periphery indicating the ingestion, absorption, metabolism and storage of energy. To regulate appetite, a variety of structures within the CNS integrate multiple signals, to assess the biological need for energy, to generate or inhibit conscious experiences of hunger, and subsequently to initiate the appropriate behavioral action. The various anabolic and catabolic circuits with structures such as the hypothalamus have already been detailed elsewhere in this book. This complex neural circuitry containing numerous neuropeptides, both orexogenic (stimulate food intake) and anorexogenic (inhibit food intake) provide a wealth of therapeutic targets. Of particular interest have been the inhibitory and stimulatory neurons that project from the ARC to the PVN and to other hypothalamic nuclei. These "first order" neurons such as the anorexigenic POMC (proopiomelanocortin)-CART (cocaine and amphetamine-regulating transcript) containing neurons and the orexigenic NPY (neuropeptide Y)-AGRP (agouti-related peptide) containing neurons are a key convergence point for peripherally generated episodic and tonic signals (such as leptin, ghrelin, insulin and corticosteroids; Harrold, 2004; Leibowitz & Wortley, 2004; Williams *et al.*, 2004; King, 2005).

1.1   Drugs acting on satiety

Many of the drugs initially used to treat obesity did so, at least in part, by reducing food intake. However, their hypophagic effects may have resulted more from the disruptive effects of these compounds on feeding behavior rather than any appetite enhancing properties they may also have possessed. Drugs such as amphetamine, mazindol, phentermine, phenylpropanolamine (PPA) and diethylpropion have historically been used to treat obesity. However, disruptive side effects such as dizziness, blurred vision, restlessness along with extreme tiredness (caused by lack of sleep), raised blood pressure and heart rate and also its abuse potential have all but stopped the use of amphetamines as clinical compounds. The use of compounds such as mazindol, phentermine and diethylpropion, as well as the ephedrine-like drug phenylpropanolamine (PPA) has also been progressively abandoned. The relative contributions of sympathetic activation, any stimulant properties or any effect on the expression of appetite in their efficacy is difficult to determine in retrospect. However, evidence exists that drugs like amphetamine may have reduced hunger and increased satiety even if they did disrupt the normal pattern of feeding behavior (Halford et al., 2004).

The satiety enhancing effects of serotoninergic enhancing drugs have been well documented in humans. These drugs were possibly the first to be regarded as true satiety enhancing agents (Blundell, 1977). Many laboratory studies in humans using fenfluramine, and later d-fenfluramine, demonstrated the effects of these drugs on hunger, within meal satiation and post-meal satiety (Blundell & Halford, 1998). Their effects on appetite were far more specific than amphetamine and lacked the contaminant behavioral side effects. The use of fenfluramine drugs to treat obesity became widespread and culminated with the prescription release of d-fenfluramine under the trade name Redux in the USA in 1996. However, despite their efficacy, both fenfluramine (which at the time was being used in combination with phentermine) and d-fenfluramine were globally withdrawn within two years due to reports of primary pulmonary hypertension. If the 5-HT system was to be therapeutically targeted again, another means of activating this satiety system was needed (Halford et al., 2005).

The only satiety enhancing drug currently globally licenced to treat obesity is sibutramine. Sibutramine is a noradrenergic and serotoninergic reuptake inhibitor originally developed for the treatment of depression. Sibutramine's first (BTS 54354) and second (BTS 54505) metabolites are potent reuptake inhibitors 5-HT and NA in vivo (Stock, 1997; Heal et al., 1998). Like other ser-otoninergic drugs, sibutramine enhances satiety. In humans, laboratory-based studies have shown sibutramine to reduce both hunger and food intake in the lean. Hansen et al. (1999) demonstrated that a single dose of sibutramine (30 mg) enhanced the satiety response to a fixed breakfast in lean males. With regard to the effect of sibutramine on food intake, a single dose of sibutramine (15 mg) given to lean males also produced a significant decrease in total cal-ories consumed across the day and in self-reported hunger (Chapelot et al., 2000). The effects of sibutramine on food intake and appetite in the obese were first detailed by Rolls et al. (1998). Sibutramine 30 mg reduced total food intake on day 7 (23% from placebo) and sibutramine 10 mg and 30 mg reduced total food intake on day 14 (a 19% and 26% reduction respectively). The hypophagic action of sibutramine appears to persist in the obese during treatment. Barkeling et al. (2003) examined effects of sibutramine on food intake and appetite at the start and end of an open-label trial. Over approximately 10 months the participants had lost 10.9 kg in body weight from baseline on sibutramine. Moreover, the initial effect of sibutramine on appetite predicted the effect of sibutramine on body weight during the subsequent open-label trial. At the end of the trial the effects of sibutramine on appetite were assessed again and the drug still significantly reduced food intake.

The fenfluramines and sibutramine presumably induced satiety by either promoting the release or preventing the reuptake on 5-HT. However, no successful anti-obesity compound to date has targeted the receptors which mediate the transmitter's action on appetite. A variety of studies employing selective 5-HT receptor antagonists, direct agonists, and transgenic animals have confirmed the role of 5-HT_{1B} and 5-HT_{2C} receptors in feeding behavior (Halford et al., 2005). In humans, direct agonism of these 5-HT receptors also potently reduces food intake. Specifically, the drug mCPP ($5\text{-HT}_{1B/2C}$ receptor preferential agonist) has been shown in a number of studies to reduce hunger and enhance satiety, an effect associated with a significant reduction in food intake (Walsh et al., 1994; Cowen et al., 1995; Sargent et al., 1997). A selective 5-HT_{2C} agonist, APD356 from Arena Pharmaceuticals, has successfully progressed into phase 2 clinical trials (Smith et al., 2005a, 2005b), and, recently, phase 3 trials.

In rodents APD356 has been shown to inhibit the development of dietary-induced obesity (Bjenning et al., 2004), an effect associated with an initial phase of hypophagia. According to the company, data from phase 1 trials suggests APD356 is well tolerated and selective to the target receptor in humans (with little affinity to 5-HT_{2A} and 5-HT_{2B} receptors). The drug has completed two phase 2 clinical trials. In the phase 2a study, 352 obese male and female volunteers were given placebo or one of three doses (1 mg, 5 mg or 15 mg) for 28 days (Smith et al., 2005). Weight loss from baseline was 0.318 kg in the placebo, 0.318 kg at 1 mg, 0.408 kg at 5 mg and 1.315 kg at 15 mg (the only significant reduction). The data from the recent 12 week phase 2b study has yet to be presented. However, according to Arena, the highest dose of APD-356 induced a loss in weight of 3.6 kg from baseline over 12 weeks (3.26 kg placebo-subtracted). Given the company chose not to prescribe any diet or lifestyle modification during this 12-week trial, it is difficult to compare these data with other phase 2b studies of other novel anti-obesity agents. Data on the effects of this drug on the expression of human appetite are yet to be published.

As of yet no other CNS satiety enhancing drugs appear to have reached phase 2 clinical trials. Other 5-HT_{2C} agonists are under development and increasing interest is focused on another serotonin receptor 5-HT_6. However, examining the pre-clinical literature and looking at company pipeline information and press releases it seems likely neuropeptide Y5 antagonists and melanocortin 4 receptor agonists will be the next in this class of centrally acting appetite suppressants to emerge. A number of these may already be entering phase 1 and possibly phase 2 trials.

1.2   Drugs acting on appetite through unknown mechanisms

The only anti-obesity drug which has currently completed phase 3 trials is the endocannabinoid CB1 receptor blocker from Sanofi-Aventis, rimonabant (SR141716, Acomplia). This drug has been undergoing concurrent clinical trials for both obesity treatment and smoking cessation. However, the full role of endogenous cannabinoid receptors in the natural operation of appetite has yet to be determined (Kirkham, 2005; Vickers & Kennet, 2005). Rodent and primate data suggest the drug may act by either enhancing satiety, reducing the pleasure derived from consuming palatable foods, and/or reducing the motivation to feed. Therefore, it is the effects of CB1 receptor blockade on the liking and want of food which may be critical to rimonabant actions. In humans, rimonabant has been shown to reduce food intake, hunger and body weight over seven days of treatment in the overweight and obese (Heshmati *et al.*, 2001). However again, the precise effect of rimonabant on human appetite (reducing hedonic value of food, reducing its palatability or enhancing satiety) remains to be fully characterized.

Long before the endogenous endocannabinoid system was characterized, the effects of cannabis on food intake were known. In animals and humans, the administration/use of cannabis and cannabinoid active agents are associated with increased food consumption (Koch, 2001; Williams & Kirkham, 2002; Halford *et al.*, 2004; Kirkham, 2005; Vickers & Kennet, 2005). Moreover, in humans this effect is associated with a prolonged increase in hunger. These hyperphagic properties have lead to the development of cannabinoid-based treatments for cachexia. Dronabinol is used to treat wasting in patients with AIDS and cancer. If activation of this system could be exploited to produce weight gain then it was logical that its blockade may be able to produce weight loss. Rimonabant is a competitive antagonist, not only blocking but reversing the effects of CB1 receptor agonists (Kirkham, 2005; Piomelli, 2005; Vickers & Kennet, 2005). CB1 receptors are found widely in the central nervous system, including the hypothalamus and the nucleus accumbens. CB1 receptors are additionally expressed in gut, liver and adipose tissue, also areas critical to energy regulation.

Rimonabant has undergone four phase 3 clinical trials; RIO (Rimonabant In Obesity) US and RIO Europe were both 2-year studies, RIO-Diabetes and RIO-Lipid were both 1-year studies. Year one data from RIO-Europe was recently published (Van Gaal *et al.*, 2005). During the first year of this trial, those in the placebo control group lost 1.8 kg, whilst those given 20 mg rimonabant lost 6.6 kg. Only some of the changes in fat-related factors could be attributed to weight loss. Data from the RIO-Lipids study were also recently published

(Després *et al.*, 2005). In the 20 mg group placebo subtracted weight loss was 5.4 kg (6.9 kg from baseline). Along with weight loss, rimonabant produced significant improvement in a number of risk factors for obesity-related disease. These data suggest rimonabant 20 mg produces weight loss superior to either sibutramine or orlistat. Whatever the mechanism, the data show that blockade of the endogenous endocannabinoid system can be targeted to produce weight loss. Rimonabant is currently approved in Europe but not the USA.

1.3   Drugs acting centrally which may or may not reduce food intake

Sibutramine was originally developed to treat depression. Its potential weight control indication only became apparent in early clinical trials. It is not uncommon for centrally acting agents, developed to treat various psychiatric or neurological disorders, to be found to have either detrimental or beneficial effects on weight control. For instance early anticonvulsants and some atypical anti-psychotic drugs (e.g. olanzapine) have been shown to produce weight gain (Goudie *et al.*, 2005), whereas other drugs, for instance some of the second generation of anti-convulsants (e.g. topiramate), produce weight loss (Halford, 2004).

Sibutramine is not the only NA reuptake inhibitor shown to produce weight loss in humans. The dopamine and noradrenaline reuptake inhibitor, bupropion (GlaxoSmithKline) also produced weight loss in obese patients (Anderson *et al.*, 2002; Jain *et al.* 2002). Meta-analysis suggests that bupropion placebo subtracted weight loss would be 2.8 kg over 6 to 12 months (Li *et al.*, 2005). The bupropion metabolite radafaxine is under clinical investigation as a potential anti-obesity drug. How either of these two centrally acting drugs reduce body weight, reducing energy intake and/or increasing energy expenditure, remains unclear. However, given that sibutramine enhances satiety and induces thermogenesis, and rodent data suggest that NA receptors are critical to both these effects (Jackson *et al.*, 1997; Hansen *et al.*, 1999), it is possible bupropion and radafaxine could do both.

2.   Drugs acting peripherally

Central appetite and energy regulatory mechanisms are not the only targets for obesity treatment. A variety of peripheral mechanisms provide suitable targets. Perhaps the simplest approach is to block the breakdown of nutrients or the absorption of the products of digestion within the gastro-intestinal tract. Another approach is to enhance satiety signals produced in response to intestinal nutrients. Thirdly, drugs could enhance the metabolism of fat within adipose tissue.

2.1   Blockade of digestion and absorption

Blocking the absorption of nutrients, specifically carbohydrates and fats, from the gut into the body is not a novel idea. Such approaches have employed products which either bind to the nutrients within the gut inhibiting their breakdown or block the action of enzymes on nutrients (i.e. deactivating amylases and/or lipases) so they remain in their unabsorbable forms. Currently no amylase inhibitors appear to be under development as anti-obesity drugs although many are available as weight loss supplements. The only globally licenced gastrointestinal lipase inhibitor is orlistat (Xenical) from Roche. Orlistat works by inhibiting the breakdown of dietary fat. The drug irreversibly blocks the active site of the gastrointestinal lipase. This prevents the hydrolysis of triglycerides into absorbable fatty acids and monoglycerides (Hauptman et al., 1992; Schwizer et al., 1997). Participants given orlistat, consuming a diet containing 30% dietary fats, pass stools which contain approximately a third of this fat (25–30 grams) undigested (at least a 10% reduction in energy absorption) (Zhi et al., 1995; Guerciolini, 1997).

Whilst the drug has no systemic action, the drug may still modulate feeding behavior. The consumption of a high-fat diet in conjunction with orlistat results in aversive gastrointestinal side effects. The avoidance of these effects appears to modulate food choice. In rats, orlistat treatment dose-dependently decreases fat intake but leads to compensatory increases in protein, carbohydrate and total caloric intake (Ackroff & Sclafani, 1996). Similarly, in humans orlistat treatment (72 weeks) has been shown to lead to a significant increase in the consumption of carbohydrate (Ullrich et al., 2003). Those who had lost the least weight (less than 5% from baseline) increased their carbohydrate consumption the most. Other companies have tried to develop similar drugs which do not produce the same side effects. The most advanced of these is cetilistat, also known as ATL-962 (Alizyme Pharmaceuticals) (Kopelman et al., 2004). In a phase 2b trial this lipase inhibitor was shown to produce significant weight loss in the obese. All doses of cetilistat (60, 120 or 240 mg t.i.d.) produced significant weight loss over the 3 months equivalent to that reported to be produced by orlistat. During the trial the average number of adverse events in the treatment groups was not statistically different from placebo (differing from existing data on orlistat). Cetilistat continues to progress through more phase 1 and 2 trials. However, little published data on its efficacy are available.

2.2   Peripheral satiety signaling hormones

The short-term consequences of food ingestion produce a powerful inhibition on further intake. These signals include the release of numerous hormones from various locations in the gut wall and the pancreas. Whilst these hormones control gut function and/or blood sugar levels, they also signal the brain to the presence of nutrients within the gut. This in turn inhibits further eating behavior. Such hormonal signals can potentially be manipulated to reduce meal size and promote post-meal satiety. Currently, there are treatments acting on two gut peptide systems and a pancreatic peptide system, glucagon-like peptide (GLP-1), peptide YY (PYY)$_{3-36}$ and amylin, which have reached the stage of human testing. Data on the effects on appetite and on body weight exist for each of these potential treatments.

Glucagon-like peptide is an incretin (insulin stimulating) hormone, released from L cells in the distal small intestine in response to nutrients (Holst & Gormada, 2004; Bojanowska, 2005). Endogenous GLP-1 levels increase follow-ing food intake, with the largest increase observed in response to the ingestion of carbohydrate (Lavin et al., 1998; Kong et al., 1999) and fat (Frost et al., 2003; Thomsen et al., 2003). Rodent studies indicate that GLP-1 administration into the CNS reduces food intake and GLP-1 receptors are found in the brainstem, particularly in the nucleus of the solitary tract and the area postrema and key hypothalamic nuclei (Turton et al., 1996). There are data suggesting peripheral GLP-1 can also cross the blood–brain barrier and could act directly in other areas of the brain (Kastin et al., 2002). In humans peripheral GLP-1 infusions have been shown to significantly enhance the satiating potential of a fixed caloric load (Flint et al., 1998). Infusions of GLP-1 also produce a reduction in intake at ad libitum meals. These effects are associated with reductions in hunger and enhancements in satiety (Flint et al., 1998; Gutzwiller et al., 1999a). Other studies demonstrate that exogenous infusions of GLP-1 have marked effects on food intake and/or appetite in the overweight and obese (Näslund et al., 1998, 1999; Gutzwiller et al., 1999b; Flint et al., 2001). Meta-analysis of these studies suggests that GLP-1 infusion reduced ad libitum food intake by 727 kJ or 11.7% (13.2% in the lean and 9.3% in the obese) (Verdich et al., 2001). Subcutaneous injections of GLP-1 also induce weight loss in the obese (Näslund et al., 2004). Unfortunately, GLP-1 is normally rapidly inactivated by the enzyme dipeptidyl peptidase IV (DPP IV). Therefore GLP-1 based drugs which are resistant to DPP IV have had to have been developed.

Exendin-4, a naturally occurring GLP-1 agonist, is resistant to DPP IV and possesses a much longer active half-life than GLP-1 itself (Parkes et al., 2001). The peptide has been shown to reduce food intake and body weight gain in rodents (Szayna et al., 2000). Moreover, exendin-4 has been shown to reduce food intake in lean healthy humans (Edwards et al., 2001). In this study, overall daily caloric intake was reduced by 21% following a morning infusion of exendin-4. Exenatide (a.k.a. Byetta for Amylin Pharmaceuticals and Eli Lilly), is a synthetic version of exendin-4 (Nielsen *et al.*, 2004). It has undergone extensive clinical assessment, primarily for the treatment of type 2 diabetes. In these trials moderate weight loss has been observed. Data from a series of 30-week studies in type 2 diabetics, already receiving metformin (M), sulfonylurea (S) or both (M&S), suggests the addition of exenatide to their treatment not only improved their symptomatology but also promoted weight loss (some data is contained in Defronzo *et al.*, 2005 and Kendall *et al.*, 2005). During the subsequent open-label phase, by week 82 all patients had lost about 4.5 kg from baseline, although weight loss of 10.3–12.2 kg during the trial was reported in the 25% most successful patients (Blonde *et al.*, 2005). Its effects in the non-diabetic obese need to be ascertained.

Peptide YY_{3-36} (PYY_{3-36}) is one of the two main endogenous forms of PYY. It is produced from the cleavage of PYY_{1-36} (the other major form of PYY) by dipeptidyl peptidase IV (DPP IV). PYY is a 36 amino acid 'hind gut' peptide released from endocrine cells in response to luminal fat and fatty acids, some forms of fibre and bile acid (Ongaa *et al.*, 2002). In humans, endogenous PYY is released predominantly after rather than during a meal (Ongaa *et al.*, 2002; Batterham *et al.*, 2003) and causes a decrease in gastric emptying (the so-called 'ileal brake'). Endogenous levels of PYY are suppressed by fasting in humans. These data would suggest PYY is a critical nutrient-sensitive satiety signal (Batterham & Bloom, 2003; Renshaw & Batterham, 2005). PYY (including PYY_{3-36}) can cross the blood–brain barrier via a non-saturatable mechanism. However, until recently, CNS PYY was regarded to be a potent stimulator rather than inhibitor of food intake (Hagan, 2002). This remained the consensus until Batterham *et al.* (2002) demonstrated that both peripheral and central doses of the Y2 receptor selective PYY_{3-36} produced a reduction in food intake and weight gain in rodents. These data suggested that PYY_{3-36} inhibited food intake by activating inhibitory Y2 receptors on hypothalamic NPY neurons projecting from the arcuate nucleus into the paraventricular nucleus. Batterham *et al.*'s findings have not been replicated in a number of laboratories (Tschöp *et al.*, 2004), whilst other researchers are able to provide corroborating data (Pittner *et al.*, 2004). Thus, the role of CNS PYY / PYY_{3-36} in appetite regulation still remains controversial, which may have implications for PYY as an anti-obesity treatment (Baggiano *et al.*, 2005).

Batterham *et al.* demonstrated the effect of peripheral PYY_{3-36} infusion on hunger and food intake in lean, healthy volunteers (Batterham *et al.*, 2002). The peptide potently reduced caloric intake and appetite for up to 12 hours. In a second study Batterham *et al.* (2003) demonstrated that an infusion of the peptide produced similar effects in the obese. Over the next 12 hours food intake remained suppressed by 26.3% in the obese. Degen *et al.* (2005) have also demonstrated the effects of PYY$_{3-36}$ on appetite and feeding behavior in lean humans. The highest dose of the exogenous PYY$_{3-36}$ infusion they employed produced suppression in food intake of 32%, at a supra-physiological dose. A number of PYY$_{3-36}$ treatments are undergoing clinical trials; a PYY$_{3-36}$ nasal spray from Nastech Pharmaceuticals and Merck, and AC162352 a synthetic version of human PYY$_{3-36}$ from Amylin Pharmaceuticals. Data on the nasal spray from Nastech Pharmaceuticals have yet to be published. A subcutaneous injection of AC162352 has been shown to decrease the appetite and increase the satiety impact of a set breakfast meal (Lush et al., 2005). In the obese, the breakfast alone also reduced hunger by 12%, but with the addition of 60 μg AC162352 it was reduced by 45%.

Pramlintide (Symlin, AC137) is a human analogue of the 37 amino acid pancreatic beta-cell hormone amylin (developed by Amylin Pharmaceuticals) that is co-secreted with insulin from pancreatic beta-cells in response to nutrient stimuli. Peripheral administration of amylin at near-physiological doses reduces food intake and inhibits body weight gain in rodents. Thus, amylin is hypothesized to be another key satiety factor (Reda et al., 2002; Lutz, 2005). The primary anorexic effects of amylin appear to be mediated by amylin receptors in the area postrema of the brainstem (Lutz et al., 2001). Amylin can also cross the blood–brain barrier and is transported into brain regions such as the hypothalamus. Some authors have suggested that amylin entering the CNS may act like insulin and leptin as a signal of adiposity. This seems plausible as circulating levels of these hormones correlate with body weight (Rushing et al., 2000; Rushing, 2003).

Pramlintide, the amylin analogue, has been developed to manage both common forms of diabetes both of which are characterized by an endogenous amylin deficiency (Weyer et al., 2001; Buse et al., 2002). Trials have also demonstrated pramlintide's potential for the management of body weight (Hollander et al., 2003, 2004). With regard to the expression of appetite, a single subcutaneous injection of pramlintide (120 μg) significantly reduced food intake in the obese and type 2 diabetic patients, an effect associated with enhanced satiety (Chapman et al., 2005). In another study in normal weight male volunteers pramlintide reduced food intake at an ad libitum meal (by 14%) (Weyer et al., 2005), an effect associated with a reduction in pre-meal hunger and an increase in fullness. The reduction in pre-meal hunger ratings correlated with subsequent reduction in caloric intake.

2.3   *Drugs which stimulate energy expenditure*

Although current anti-obesity medications reduce food intake, some also affect energy expenditure. The thermogenic effects of sibutramine are well documented. It has also been suggested that rimonabant also acts directly on fat tissue. For a number of years, companies have been trying to develop treatments which selectively target metabolic processes to increase metabolism and selectively decrease adipose tissue. Drug programs have included beta-3 adrenergic receptor agonists and more recently a variety of other metabolic targets (such as uncoupling proteins) which exist within fat tissue. The only anti-obesity drug acting on expenditure currently known to be undergoing clinical trials is AOD (Advanced Obesity Drug)-9604 from Metabolic Pharmaceuticals.

AOD-9604 is a synthetic peptide based on a peptide derived from the C-terminus of the human growth hormone (Wilding, 2003). Growth Hormone (GH) is a key regulatory hormone that, amongst other actions, stimulates fat metabolism. AOD-9604 has been developed to produce the beneficial effects of GH on fat tissue without its side-effect profile (Wilding, 2003). The drug has been shown to inhibit weight gain in obese rodents (Ng et al., 2000; Heffernan et al., 2001). This effect is thought to be associated with an increase in fat breakdown and a decrease in fat storage. Metabolic Pharmaceuticals recently presented data from their 12-week phase 2b study of its anti-obesity candidate AOD-9604 (Herd et al., 2005). Interestingly, the lowest and the highest doses of AOD-9604 produced the greatest weight loss; only reductions in body weight produced by 1 mg, 20 mg and 30 mg of AOD-9604 were significantly greater than placebo. In 2007, the company terminated development of AOD-9604.

3.   Summary

An understanding of the neurobiology of obesity provides numerous therapeutic targets which could be exploited to treat obesity. Current drugs demonstrate that pharmacotherapy is at least as effective as all other treatments, which the notable exception of baliatric surgery. Sibutramine and orlistat have well-established mechanisms of action and produce a 5–10% loss in body weight from baseline. This corresponds to a placebo-subtracted weight loss of approximately 4.2 kg for sibutramine and 2.7 kg for orlistat (Li et al., 2005). This weight loss produces a significant improvement on a number of obesity-related disease risk factors, and in the case of orlistat has been shown to reduce the incidence of diabetes over the course of a 4-year treatment (Torgerson et al., 2004). In fact, some authors have suggested the improvement in such risk factors is greater than would be expected to be produced by weight loss alone. Despite this, the take-up of existing obesity treatments has been poor with prescription use of both sibutramine and orlistat falling in the Canada and the USA.

The first new anti-obesity drug for 7 years has been approved in Europe. Rimonabant, the endocannabinoid antagonist, appears to reduce food intake by acting on other CNS appetite mechanisms. However, its precise effects on the expression of human appetite require elucidation. Phase 3 data suggest that rimonabant can produce placebo-subtracted weight loss of around 5 kg, which would appear to be a significant improvement on existing treatments. Other CB1 antagonists are now also in clinical trials. A number of other centrally acting appetite suppressing drugs are under development. These include other noradrenergic reuptake inhibitors such as radafaxine, and the selective 5-HT receptor agonists (e.g. APD-356). Melanocortin MC4R receptor agonists and neuropeptide Y5 receptor antagonists may soon be entering clinical trials. MCH1 antagonists and Y2/Y4 receptor agonists have apparently already entered clinical trials. In addition, peripherally acting treatments that target appetite include GLP-1 analogues such as exenatide (Byette), PYY_{3-36} - based treatments and the amylin analogue pramlintide have also produced weight loss. Other peripherally acting drugs undergoing clinical trials include cetilistat.

Acknowledgements

Thanks to Miss Emma Boyland and Miss Lisa D.M. Richards for their help in the preparation of this manuscript. Dr Halford's research has recently been supported by GlaxoSmithKline, Servier, Sanofi-Aventis and Predix Pharmaceuticals.

References

Ackroff, K. & Sclafani, A. (1996). Effects of the lipase inhibitor orlistat on intake and preference for dietary fats in rats. *Am. J. Physiol.* **27**, R48–54.

Anderson, J. W., Greenway, F. L., Fujioka, K., Gadde, K. M., McKenney, J. & O'Neil, P. M. (2002). Buproprion SR enhances weight loss: A 48-week double blind, placebo-controlled trial. *Obes. Res.* **10**, 633–41.

Baggiano, M. M., Chadler, P. C., Oswald, K. D., Rodgers, R. J., Blundell, J. E. & Ishii, Y. (2005). PYY3-36 as an anti-obesity drug target. *Obes. Rev.* **6**, 307–22.

Barkeling, B., Elfhag, K., Rooth, P. & Rössner, S. (2003). Short term effects of sibutramine (Reductil ™) on appetite and eating behaviour and the long term therapeutic outcome. *Int. J. Obes.* **27**, 693–700.

Batterham, R. L. & Bloom, S. R. (2003). The gut hormone peptide YY regulated appetite. *Ann. N.Y. Acad. Sci.* **994**, 162–8.

Batterham, R. L., Cowley, M. A., Small, C. J. et al. (2002). Gut hormone PYY3–36 physiologically inhibits food intake. *Nature* **418**, 650–4.

Batterham, R. L., Cohen, M. A., Ellis, S. M. *et al.* (2003). Inhibition of food intake in obese subjects by Peptide YY3-36. *N. Engl. J. Med.* **349**, 914–18.

Bjenning, C., Whelen, K., Gonzalez, L., Thomsen, W., Saldana, H. & Espitia, S. (2004). Increased sensitivity in female obesity-prone rats; the weight loss effects of APD356, a selective 5-HT2c agonist. *Obes. Res.* **12**, A140.

Blonde, L., Zhang, B., Mac, S., Poon, T., Taylor, K. & Kim, D. (2005). Progressive reductions in body weight with 82 weeks of extenatide treatment in overweight patients with type 2 diabetes. *Obes. Res.* **13**, A102–OR.

Blundell, J. E. (1977). Is there a role for serotonin (5-hydroxytryptamine) in feeding? *Int. J. Obes.* **1**, 15–42.

Blundell, J. E. & Halford, J. C. G. (1995). Pharmacological aspects of obesity treatment: towards the 21st century. *Int. J. Obes.* **19**, 51–5.

Blundell, J. E. & Halford, J. C. G. (1998). Serotonin and appetite regulation: implications for the pharmacological treatment of Obesity. *CNS Drugs* **9**, 473–95.

Bojanowska, E. (2005). Physiology and pathophysiology of glucagon-like peptide 1 (GLP-1): The role of GLP-1 in the pathogenesis of diabetes mellitus, obesity, and stress. *Med. Sci. Monit.* **11**, RA271–8.

Buse, J. B., Weyer, C. & Maggs, D. G. (2002). Amylin replacement with pramlintide in type 1 and type 2 diabetes mellitus: a physiological approach to overcome barriers with insulin therapy. *Clin. Diabetes* **20**, 137–44.

Chapelot, D., Marmonier, C., Thomas, F. & Hanotin, C. (2000). Modalities of the food intake-reducing effect of sibutramine in humans. *Physiol. Behav.* **68**, 299–308.

Chapman, I., Parker, B., Doran, S. *et al.* (2005). Effect of pramlintide on satiety and food intake in obese subjects and subjects with type 2 diabetes. *Diabetologia* **48**, 838–48.

Cowen, P. J., Sargent, P. A., Williams, C., Goodall, E. M. & Olikov, A. B. (1995). *Human Psychopharmacol.* **10**, 385–91.

DeFronzo, R. A., Kim, D. D., Ratner, R. E., Fineman, M. S., Han, J. & Baron, A. D. (2005). Effects of extenatide (exendin-4) on glycemic control over 30 weeks in metformin-treated patients with type 2 diabetes. *Diabetes Care* **28**, 1083–91.

Degen, L., Oesch, S., Casanva, M. *et al.* (2005). Effect of peptide PYY3-36 on food intake in humans. *Gastroenterology.* **129**, 1430–6.

Després, J-P., Golay, A. & Sjöström, L. (2005). Effects of rimonabant on metabolic risk factors in overweight patients with dyslipidemia. *N. Engl. J. Med.* **353**, 2121–34.

Edwards, C. M. B., Stanley, S. A., Davis, R., *et al.* (2001). Exendin-4 reduces fasting and postprandial glucose and decreases energy intake in healthy volunteers. *Am. J. Physiol. Endocr. Metab.* **291**, E155–61.

Flint, A., Raben, A., Astrup, A. & Holst, J. (1998). Glucagon like peptide 1 promotes satiety and suppresses energy intake in humans. *J. Clin. Invest.* **101**, 515–20.

Flint, A., Raben, A.,. Ersböll, A. K., Holst, J. J. & Astrup, A. A. (2001). The effect of physiological levels of glucagon like peptide 1 on appetite, gastric emptying, energy and substrate metabolism in obesity. *Int. J. Obes. Relat. Metab. Disord.* **25**, 781–92.

Frost, G. S., Brynes, A. E., Dhillo, W. S., Bloom, S. R. & McBurney, M. I. (2003). The effects of fibre enrichment of pasta and fat content on gastric emptying, GLP-1, glucose, and insulin responses to a meal. *Eur. J. Clin. Nutr.* **57**, 293–8.

Goudie, A. J., Cooper, G. D. & Halford, J. C. G. (2005). Antipsychotic-induced weight gain. *Diabetes Obes. Metab.* **7**, 478–87.

Guerciolini, R. (1997). Mode of action of orlistat. *Int. J. Obes.* **21**, s12–23.

Gutzwiller, J. P., Goke, B., Drewe, J. et al. (1999a). Glucagon-like peptide-1: a potent regulator of food intake in humans. *Gut* **44**, 81–6.

Gutzwiller, J. P., Drewe, J., Goke, B. et al. (1999b). Glucagon like peptide promotes satiety and reduced food intake in patients with diabetes mellitus. *Am. J. Physiol.* **276**, R1541–5.

Hagan, M. M. (2002). Peptide YY: a key mediator of orexigenic behaviour. *Peptides* **23**, 377–82.

Halford, J. C. G. (2004). Clinical pharmacotherapy for obesity: current drugs and those in advanced development. *Curr. Drug Targets.* **5**, 637–46.

Halford, J. C. G., Cooper, G. D., Dovey, T. M., Ishii, Y., Rodgers, R. J. & Blundell J. E. (2003). Pharmacological approaches to obesity treatment, current medical chemistry. *Central Nervous System Agents*, **3**, 283–310.

Halford, J. C. G., Dovey, T. M. & Cooper, G. D. (2004). Pharmacology of human appetite expression. *Curr. Drug Targets* **5**, 221–40.

Halford, J. C. G., Harrold, J. E., Lawton, C. L. & Blundell, J. E. (2005). Serotonin (5-HT) drugs: effects on appetite expression and use for treatment of obesity. *Curr. Drug Targets* **6**, 201–13.

Hansen, D. L., Toubro, S., Stock, M. J., Macdonald, I. A. & Astrup, A. (1999). The effect of sibutramine on energy expenditure and appetite during chronic treatment without dietary restriction. *Int. J. Obes.* **23**, 10 160–24.

Harrold, J. A. (2004). Hypothalamic control of energy balance. *Curr. Drug Targets* **5**, 207–19.

Hauptman, J. B., Jeunet, F. S. & Hartmann, S. (1992). Initial studies in humans with the novel gastrointestinal lipase inhibitor Ro 18-0647 (tetrahydrolipstatin). *Am. J. Clin. Nutr.* **55**, s309–22.

Heal, D. J., Aspely, A., Prow, M. R., Jackson, H. C., Martin, K. F. & Cheetham, S. C. (1998). Sibutramine: a novel anti-obesity drug. A review of the pharmacological evidence to differentiate from d-amphetamine and d-fenfluramine. *Int. J. Obes. Relat. Metab. Disord.* **22**, s18–28.

Heffernan, M., Summers, R. J., Thorburn, A. et al. (2001). The effects of human GH and its lipolytic fragment (AOD9604) on lipid metabolism following chronic treatment in obese mice and beta(3)-AR knock-out mice. *Endocrinology* **142**, 5182–9.

Herd, C., Wittert, G., Caterson, I., Proietto, J., Srauss, B. & Prins, J. (2005). The effect of AOD9604 on weight loss in obese adults: results of a randomized, double-blind, placebo-controlled, multicenter study. *Obes. Res.* **13** (Suppl.), 106-OR.

Hollander, P., Ratner, R., Fineman, M. et al. (2003). Addition of pramlintide to insulin therapy lowers HbA(1c) in conjunction with weight loss in patients with type 2 diabetes approaching glycaemic targets. *Diabetes Obes. Metab.* **5**, 408–14.

Hollander, P., Maggs, D., Ruggles, J. A. *et al.* (2004). Effect of pramlintide on weight in overweight and obese insulin treated type 2 diabetes patients. *Obes. Res.* **12**, 661–8.

Holst, J. J. & Gromada, J. (2004). Role of incretin hormones in the regulation of insulin secretion in diabetic and nondiabetic humans. *Am. J. Physiol.* **287**, E199–206.

Jackson, H. C., Bearham, M. C., Hutchins, L. J., Mazurkiewicz, S. E., Needham, A. M. & Heal, D. J. (1997). Investigation of the mechanisms underlying the hypophagic effects of the 5-HT and nor-adrenaline reuptake inhibitor sibutramine in the rat. *Br. J. Pharmacol.* **121**, 613–18.

Jain, A. K., Kaplan, R. A., Gadde, K. M. *et al.* (2002). Buproprion SR vs. placebo for weight loss in obese patients with depressive symptoms. *Obes. Res.* **10**, 1049–56.

Kastin, A. J., Akerstrom, V. & Pan, W. (2002). Interaction of glucagon-like petide-1 (GLP-1) with the blood-brain barrier. *J. Mol. Neurosci.* **18**, 7–14.

Kendall, D. M, Riddle, M. C., Rosenstock, J. *et al.* (2005). Effects of extenatide (exendin-4) on glycemic control over 30 weeks in patients with type 2 diabetes treated with metformin and a sulfonylurea. *Diabetes Care* **28**, 1083–91.

King, P. J. (2005). The hypothalamus and obesity. *Curr. Drug Targets* **6**, 225–40.

Kirkham, T. C. (2005). Endocannabinoids in the regulation of appetite and body weight. *Behav. Pharmacol.* **16**, 297–313.

Koch, J. E. (2001). Delta(9)-THC stimulates food intake in Lewis rats – effects on chow, high-fat and sweet high-fat diets. *Pharmacol. Biochem. Behav.* **68**, 539–43.

Kong, M-F., Chapman, I., Goble, A. *et al.* (1999). Effects of oral fructose and glucose on plasma GLP-1 and appetite in normal subjects. *Peptides* **20**, 545–51.

Kopelman, P., Bryson, A. M. & Palmer, R. M. F. (2004). Efficacy and tolerability of ATL-962, a lipase inhibitor in obese patients. *Int. J. Obes.* **28**, AO2–003.

Lavin, J. H., Wittert, G. A., Andrews, J. *et al.* (1998). Interaction of insulin, glucagon-like peptide 1, gastric inhibitory polypeptide, and appetite in response to intraduodenal carbohydrate. *Am. J. Clin. Nutr.* **68**, 591–8.

Leibowitz, S. F. & Wortley, K. E. (2004). Hypothalamic control of energy balance: different peptides, different functions. *Peptides* **25**, 473–504.

Li, Z., Maglione, M., Tu, W. *et al.* (2005). Meta-analysis: pharmacologic treatments of obesity. *Ann. Intern. Med.* **142**, 532–46.

Lush, C., Chen, K., Hompesch, M., Tropin, B., Lacerte, C. & Burns, C. (2005). A phase 1 study to evaluate the safety , tolerability, and pharmacokinetics of rising doses of AC162352 (synthetic human PYY3-36) in lean and obese subjects. *Obes. Rev.* **6** (Suppl. 1), o051.

Lutz, T. A. (2005). Pancreatic amylin as a centrally acting satiating hormone. *Curr. Drug Targets* **6**, 181–9.

Lutz, T. A., Mollet, A., Rushing, P. A. & Riediger, T. (2001). The anorectic effect of a chronic peripheral infusion of amylin is abolished in area postrema/ nucleus of the solitary tract (AP/NTS) lesioned rats. *Int. J. Obes.* **25**, 1005–11.

Näslund, E., Gutniak, M., Skogar, S., Rössner, S. & Hellström, P. M. (1998). Glucagon-like peptide 1 increase the period of postprandial satiety and slows gastric emptying in obese men. *Am. J. Clin. Nutr.* **68**, 525–30.

Näslund, E., Barkeling, B., King, N. *et al.* (1999). Energy intake and appetite are suppressed by glucagon like peptide 1 (GLP-1) in obese men. *Int. J. Obes.* **23**, 304–11.

Näslund, E., King, N., Mansten, S. *et al.* (2004). Prandial subcutaneous injections of glucagon like peptide 1 cause weight loss in obese human subjects. *Br. J. Nutr.* **91**, 439–46.

Ng, F. M., Sun, J., Shama, L., Libinaka, R., Jiang, W. J. & Gianello, R. (2000). Metabolic studies of a synthetic lipolytic domain (A)D9604) of human growth hormone. *Horm. Res.* **53**, 274–8.

Nielsen, L. L., Young, A. A. & Parkes D. G. (2004). Pharmacology of extenatide (synthetic exendin-4): a potential therapeutic for improved glycemic control of type 2 diabetes. *Reg. Peptides* **117**, 766–77.

Ongaa, T., Zabieski, R. & Kato, S. (2002). Multiple regulation of peptide YY in the digestive tract. *Peptide* **23**, 279–90.

Parkes, D., Jodka, C., Smith, P. *et al.* (2001). Pharmacokinetic actions of exendin-4 in the rat: comparison with glucagon like peptide-1. *Drug Dev. Res.* **53**, 260–7.

Piomelli, D. (2005). The endocannabiniod system: a drug discovery perspective. *Curr. Opin. Invest. Drugs* **6**, 272–9.

Pittner, R. A., Moore, C. X., Bhavsar, S. P., Gedulin, B. R. Smith, P. A. & Jodka, C. M. (2004). Effects of PYY[3-36] in rodent models of diabetes and obesity. *Int. J. Obes.* **28**, 963–71.

Reda, T. K., Geliebter, A. & Pi-Sunyer, F. X. (2002). Amylin, food intake and obesity. *Obes. Res.* **10**, 1087–91.

Renshaw, D. & Batterham, R. L. (2005). Peptide YY: a potential therapy for obesity. *Curr. Drug Targets* **6**, 171–8.

Rolls, B. J., Shide, D. J., Thorwart, M. L. & Ulbrecht, J. S. (1998). Sibutramine reduces food intake in non-dieting women with obesity. *Obes. Res.* **6**, 1–11.

Rushing, P. A. (2003). Central amylin signalling and the regulation of energy homeostasis. *Curr. Pharmaceut. Design* **9**, 819–25.

Rushing, P. A., Hagan, M. M., Seeley, R. J., Lutz, T. A. & Woods, S. C. (2000). Amylin: a novel action in the brain to reduced body weight. *Endocrinology* **141**, 850–3.

Sargent, P. A., Sharpley, A. L. & Williams, C. (1997). 5-HT2C activation decreases appetite and body weight in obese subjects. *Psychopharmacology* **133**, 309–12.

Schwizer, A., Asal, K., Kreiss, C., Mettraus, C., Borovicka, J. & Remy, B. (1997). Role of lipase in the regulation of upper gastrointestinal function in humans. *Am. J. Physiol.* **273**, G612–20.

Smith, B. M., Smith, J. M., Tsai, J. H., Schultz, J. A., Gilson, C. A. & Estrada, S. A. (2005b). Discovery and SAR of new benzazapines and potent and selective 5-HT2C receptor agonist for the treatment of obesity. *Bioorg. Med. Chem. Lett.* **12**, 1467–71.

Smith, S., Anderson, J., Frank, A., Fujioka, K., Klein, S. & Perez J. (2005a). The effects of APD356, a selective 5-HT2C agonist, on weight loss in a 4 week study in healthy obese patients. *Obes. Res.* **13**, Abstr. 101-OR.

Stock, M. J. (1997). Sibutramine: a review of the pharmacology of a novel anti-obesity agent. *Int. J. Obes.* **21**, s25–9.

Szayna, M., Doyle, M. E., Betkey, J. A. *et al.* (2000). Exendin-4 decelerates food intake, weight gain, and fat deposition in Zucker rats. *Endocrinology* **141**, 1936–41.

Thomsen, C., Storm, H., Holst, J. J. & Hermansen, K. (2003). Differential effects of saturated and monounsaturated fats on postprandial lipemia and glucagon-like peptide 1 responses in patients with type 2 diabetes. *Am. J. Clin. Nutr.* **77**, 605–11.

Torgerson, J. S., Hauptman, J., Boldrin, M. N. & Sjöström, L. (2004). XENical in the prevention of diabetes in obese subjects (XENDOS) study. A randomised study of orlistat as an adjunct to lifestyle changes for the prevention of type 2 diabetes in obese patients. *Diabetes Care* **27**, 155–61.

Tschöp, M., Castaneda, T. R., Joost, H. G. *et al.* (2004). Does gut hormone PYY3-36 decrease food intake in rodents? *Nature* **430**, 1 following 165.

Turton, M. D., Oshea, D., Gunn, I., Beak, S. A., Edwards, C. M. B. & Meeran, K. (1996). A role for glucagon like peptide 1 in the central regulation of feeding. *Nature* **379**, 69–72.

Ullrich, A., Erdmann, J., Margraf, J. & Schusdziarra, A. (2003). Impact of carbohydrate and fat intake on weight-reducing efficacy of orlistat. *Aliment. Pharmacol. Ther.* **17**, 1007–13.

Van Gaal, L. F., Rissanen, A. M., Scheen, A. J., Ziegler, O. & Rössner, S. (2005). Effects of the cannabinoid-1 receptor blocker rimonabant on weight reduction and cardiovascular risk factors in overweight patients: 1-year experience from the RIO-Europe study. *Lancet* **365**, 1389–97.

Verdich, A., Flint, A, Gutwzwiller, J. P. *et al.* (2001). A meta-analysis of the effects of glucagon-like peptide-1(7-36) amide on ad libitum energy intake in humans. *J. Clin. Endocrinol. Metab.* **86**, 4382–9.

Vickers, S. P. & Kennet G. A. (2005). Cannabinoids and the regulation of ingestive behaviour. *Curr. Drug Targets* **6**, 215–23.

Walsh, A. E., Smith, K. A. & Oldman A. D. (1994). m-Chlorophenylpiperazine decrease food intake in a test meal. *Psychopharmacology* **116**, 120–2.

Weyer, C., Maggs D. G., Young, A. A. & Kolterman, O. G. (2001). Amylin replacement with pramlintide as an adjunct to insulin therapy in type 1 and type 2 diabetes mellitus: a physiological approach towards improved metabolic control. *Curr. Pharmaceut. Design* **7**, 1353–73.

Weyer, C., Chapman, I., Parker B., Doran, S., Feinle-Bisset, C. & Wishart, J. (2005). Pramlintide reduced ad-libitum food intake and meal duration independently of ghrelin, PYY, CKK, and GLP-1: further evidence for a physiological role of amylin agonism in human appetite control. *Obes. Rev.* **6**, Abstr. 0052.

Wilding, J. (2003). AOD-9604 metabolic. *Curr. Opin. Invest. Drugs* **5**, 436–40.

Williams, C. M. & Kirkham T. C. (2002). Reversal of Delta(9)-THC hyperphagia by SR141716 and naloxone but not dexfenfluramine. *Pharmacol. Biochem. Behav.* **71**, 333–40.

Williams, G., Cai, X. J., Elliott, J. C. & Harrold, J. A. (2004). Anabolic neuropeptides. *Physiol. Behav.* **81**, 211–22.

Zhi, J., Melia A. T., Eggers, H., Joly, R. & Patel, I. H. (1995). Review of limited systematic absorption orlistat, a lipase inhibitor, in healthy human volunteers. *J. Clin. Pharmacol.* **35**, 1103–8.

Index

adipocyte apoptosis 287–8,
  288–9
  adrenergic receptors 293,
    294
  bone marrow 294–5
  epigallocatechin gallate
    289
  leptin 289
  melanocortin 290
  NPY 293
  sympathetic nervous
    system 293
  tumor necrosis factor
    alpha 289
adiponectin 58
adipose tissue 2, 286
adiposity signal 84, 88,
  90–1
  basic model 104–5
  body fat mass 89
  insulin 84, 94
  leptin 88, 90–1, 98
  negative feedback 89
  resistance to 105, 106
  termination of
    103–4
agouti-related protein
  (AGRP) 59, 60, 197–9,
    208–9

AMP-activated protein kinase
  (AMPK) 62, 139–40
  therapeutic target 147
amylin 60, 310
anti-obesity drugs 9
  AOD-9604 313
  Cetilistat 309
  Exenatide 12, 310
  Exendin-4 310
  Fenfluramine 305
  Orlistat 9, 303, 309
  peptide $YY_{3–36}$ 11, 310,
    311–12
  Pramlintide 312
  Rimonabant 11, 303,
    307–8
  Sibutramine 9, 303,
    305–6, 308
arcuate nucleus 57,
  59, 91
  access of peripheral
    signals 57, 95
  anabolic 91
  anorexigenic 59
  catabolic 91
  cocaine and
    amphetamine-
    regulated transcript
    (CART) 59, 67–8

circuitry 92–3
  insulin 91, 92, 127
  integrator 59
  leptin 59, 91, 92, 127
  neuropeptide Y (NPY) 59
  NPY/AGRP neurons 91–2
  orexigenic 59
  proopiomelanocortin gene
    (POMC) 59
  POMC/CART neurons 92
  receptors 59
Atkin's diet 110, 111
ATP-sensitive potassium
  channels 62
  insulin 63
  kir 63, 165
  leptin 63
  pancreas 62

body mass index 2
  population variations 2

Cetilistat 309
cholecystokinin 58
ciliary neurotrophic factor
  (CNTF) 28, 292
cocaine and amphetamine-
  regulated transcript
  (CART) 59, 67–8

Printed in the United States
by Baker & Taylor Publisher Services